Mayo Clinic General Surgery

MAYO CLINIC SCIENTIFIC PRESS

Mayo Clinic Atlas of Regional Anesthesia and Ultrasound-Guided Nerve Blockade
Edited by James R. Hebl, MD, and Robert L. Lennon, DO

Mayo Clinic Preventive Medicine and Public Health Board Review
Edited by Prathibha Varkey, MBBS, MPH, MHPE

Mayo Clinic Infectious Diseases Board Review
Edited by Zelalem Temesgen, MD

Just Enough Physiology
By James R. Munis, MD, PhD

Mayo Clinic Cardiology: Concise Textbook, Fourth Edition
Edited by Joseph G. Murphy, MD, and Margaret A. Lloyd, MD

Mayo Clinic Electrophysiology Manual
Edited by Samuel J. Asirvatham, MD

Mayo Clinic Gastrointestinal Imaging Review, Second Edition
By C. Daniel Johnson, MD

Arrhythmias in Women: Diagnosis and Management
Edited by Yong-Mei Cha, MD, Margaret A. Lloyd, MD, and Ulrika M. Birgersdotter-Green, MD

Mayo Clinic Body MRI Case Review
By Christine U. Lee, MD, PhD, and James F. Glockner, MD, PhD

Mayo Clinic Gastroenterology and Hepatology Board Review, Fifth Edition
Edited by Stephen C. Hauser, MD

Mayo Clinic Guide to Cardiac Magnetic Resonance Imaging, Second Edition
Edited by Kiaran P. McGee, PhD, Eric E. Williamson, MD, and Matthew W. Martinez, MD

Mayo Clinic Neurology Board Review, First Edition [2 Volumes]
Edited by Kelly D. Flemming, MD, and Lyell K. Jones Jr, MD

Mayo Clinic Critical Care Case Review
Edited by Rahul Kashyap, MBBS, J. Christopher Farmer, MD, and John C. O'Horo, MD

Mayo Clinic Medical Neurosciences, Sixth Edition
Edited by Eduardo E. Benarroch, MD, Jeremy K. Cutsforth-Gregory, MD, and Kelly D. Flemming, MD

Mayo Clinic Principles of Shoulder Surgery
By Joaquin Sanchez-Sotelo, MD

Mayo Clinic Essential Neurology, Second Edition
By Andrea C. Adams, MD

Mayo Clinic Antimicrobial Handbook: Quick Guide, Third Edition
Edited by John W. Wilson, MD, and Lynn L. Estes, PharmD

Mayo Clinic Critical and Neurocritical Care Board Review
Edited by Eelco F. M. Wijdicks, MD, PhD, James Y. Findlay, MB, ChB, William D. Freeman, MD, and Ayan Sen, MD

Mayo Clinic Internal Medicine Board Review, Twelfth Edition
Edited by Christopher M. Wittich, MD, PharmD, Thomas J. Beckman, MD, Sara L. Bonnes, MD, Nerissa M. Collins, MD, Nina M. Schwenk, MD, Christopher R. Stephenson, MD, and Jason H. Szostek, MD

Mayo Clinic Strategies for Reducing Burnout and Promoting Engagement
By Stephen J. Swensen, MD, and Tait D. Shanafelt, MD

Mayo Clinic General Surgery

Jad M. Abdelsattar, MBBS
Fellow in Gastroenterologic and General Surgery
Mayo Clinic School of Graduate Medical Education
Mayo Clinic College of Medicine and Science

Moustafa M. El Khatib, MB, BCh
Resident in General Surgery
Mayo Clinic School of Graduate Medical Education
Mayo Clinic College of Medicine and Science

T. K. Pandian, MD
Resident in General Surgery
Mayo Clinic School of Graduate Medical Education
Mayo Clinic College of Medicine and Science

Samuel J. Allen
Content Production Specialist
Mayo Clinic Education Innovation Unit
Mayo Clinic College of Medicine and Science

David R. Farley, MD
Consultant, Department of General and
Gastroenterologic Surgery, Mayo Clinic
Professor of Surgery
Mayo Clinic College of Medicine and Science

MAYO CLINIC SCIENTIFIC PRESS   OXFORD UNIVERSITY PRESS

MAYO
CLINIC

The triple-shield Mayo logo and the words MAYO, MAYO CLINIC, and MAYO CLINIC SCIENTIFIC PRESS are marks of Mayo Foundation for Medical Education and Research.

OXFORD
UNIVERSITY PRESS

Oxford University Press is a department of the University of Oxford. It furthers the University's objective of excellence in research, scholarship, and education by publishing worldwide. Oxford is a registered trade mark of Oxford University Press in the UK and certain other countries.

Published in the United States of America by Oxford University Press
198 Madison Avenue, New York, NY 10016, United States of America.

Library of Congress Cataloging-in-Publication Data
Names: Abdelsattar, Jad M., author. | El Khatib, Moustafa M., author. | Pandian, T. K., author. |
Allen, Samuel J., author. | Farley, David R., author. | Mayo Clinic.
Title: Mayo Clinic general surgery / Jad M. Abdelsattar, Moustafa M. El Khatib, T. K. Pandian,
Samuel J. Allen, David R. Farley.
Other titles: Mayo Clinic scientific press (Series)
Description: New York, NY : Oxford University Press, [2020] |
Series: Mayo Clinic scientific press |
Includes bibliographical references and index.
Identifiers: LCCN 2019053140 (print) | LCCN 2019053141 (ebook) |
ISBN 9780190650506 (paperback) | ISBN 9780190650520 (epub)
Subjects: MESH: Surgical Procedures, Operative
Classification: LCC RD31.3 (print) | LCC RD31.3 (ebook) | NLM WO 500 |
DDC 617—dc23
LC record available at https://lccn.loc.gov/2019053140
LC ebook record available at https://lccn.loc.gov/2019053141

9 8 7 6 5 4 3 2 1

Printed by Sheridan Books, Inc., United States of America

Digital Media Accompanying the Book

Individual purchasers of this book are entitled to free personal access to accompanying digital media in the online edition. Please refer to the access token card for instructions on token redemption and access.

These online ancillary materials, where available, are noted with iconography throughout the book.

Video

The corresponding media can be found on *Oxford Medicine Online* at: http://www.oxfordmedicine.com/mayoclinicgeneralsurgery.

If you are interested in access to the complete online edition, please consult with your librarian.

Preface

As far back as elementary school, I can remember saving some of my best homework and tests in hopes that they would help my younger brother do well as he followed me in school. More than 50 years later, I am still seeking ways to provide an educational advantage to less experienced learners who seek knowledge and skill. This book was created to provide succinct and accurate information in a written, imaging, and audiovisual format that allows efficient access to surgical learners—especially those with just a few minutes to spare. Ultimately, I hope that this effort better prepares students, residents, and fellows for their surgical experiences and leads to better understanding with long-term retention.

My coauthors and I thank the following persons for their contributions and assistance with this project:

Eduardo Abbott
Mohamed S. Baloul, MBBS
Jacob Billings
EeeLN H. Buckarma, MD
Francisco J. Cardenas Lara, MD
Rachel Cadelina
Abhishek Chandra, PhD
Eric J. Finnesgard
Nicholas L. Fuqua
Becca L. Gas
Miguel Angel Gomez Ibarra, MD
Linda Haigh
Monali Mohan, MBBS
Nimesh D. Naik, MD
Nicole Philipps
Suzy Strubel
Muhammad Hashim Zeb, MBBS

David R. Farley, MD

Contents

Book Abbreviations

ACA	adenocarcinoma
ACC	adrenocortical carcinoma
ASIS	anterior superior iliac spine
BP	blood pressure
BRCA	*br*east *ca*ncer tumor suppressor gene
CBD	common bile duct
CHD	common hepatic duct
CT	computed tomography
CXR	chest radiograph
DES	diffuse esophageal spasm
EGD	esophagogastroduodenoscopy
EO	external oblique
ERCP	endoscopic retrograde cholangiopancreatography
FAST	focused assessment with sonography for trauma
GB	gallbladder
GERD	gastroesophageal reflux disease
GI	gastrointestinal
GIST	gastrointestinal stromal tumor
HCC	hepatocellular carcinoma
HPT	hyperparathyroidism
HU	Hounsfield unit
IMA	inferior mesenteric artery
IV	intravenous
IVC	inferior vena cava
LN	lymph node
MEN	multiple endocrine neoplasia
MRI	magnetic resonance imaging
PMM	pectoralis minor muscle
PTH	parathyroid hormone
PUD	peptic ulcer disease
RLN	recurrent laryngeal nerve
RUQ	right upper quadrant

SBO	small bowel obstruction
SCC	squamous cell carcinoma
SMA	superior mesenteric artery
UGI	upper gastrointestinal
US	ultrasonography

1

Adrenal Glands

Embryology

The adrenal cortex is derived from mesoderm and the medulla, from neural crest ectoderm.

Anatomy

An adrenal gland weighs approximately 5 g. Arterial supply (Figure 1.1) comes from branches of the aorta and phrenic and renal arteries. Venous drainage (Figure 1.2) of the right adrenal gland is through a short, right adrenal vein that empties into the IVC. The left adrenal vein (often joined by the left inferior phrenic vein) empties into the left renal vein. The right gland is located posterior to the IVC; the left gland is posterior to the splenic vessels and pancreatic body. Both glands are retroperitoneal.

Physiology

The cortex (◘ Video 1.1) secretes corticosteroids (cortisol), aldosterone, and sex hormones. The medulla (◘ Video 1.1) secretes catecholamines (epinephrine, norepinephrine, and dopamine). Urinary and serum studies (◘ Video 1.2) are needed to help differentiate adrenal masses and their function.

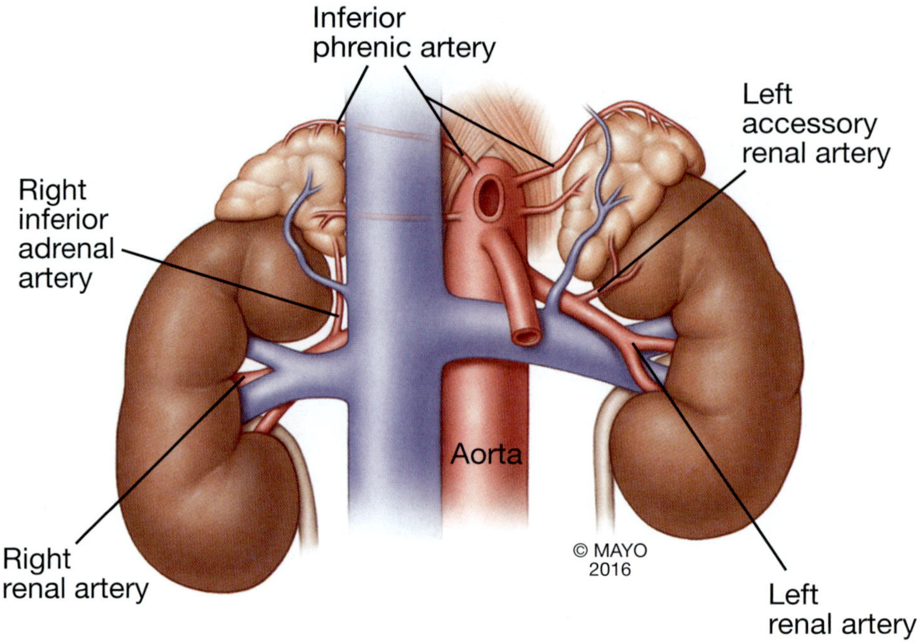

FIGURE 1.1. Arterial Supply to Adrenal Glands.

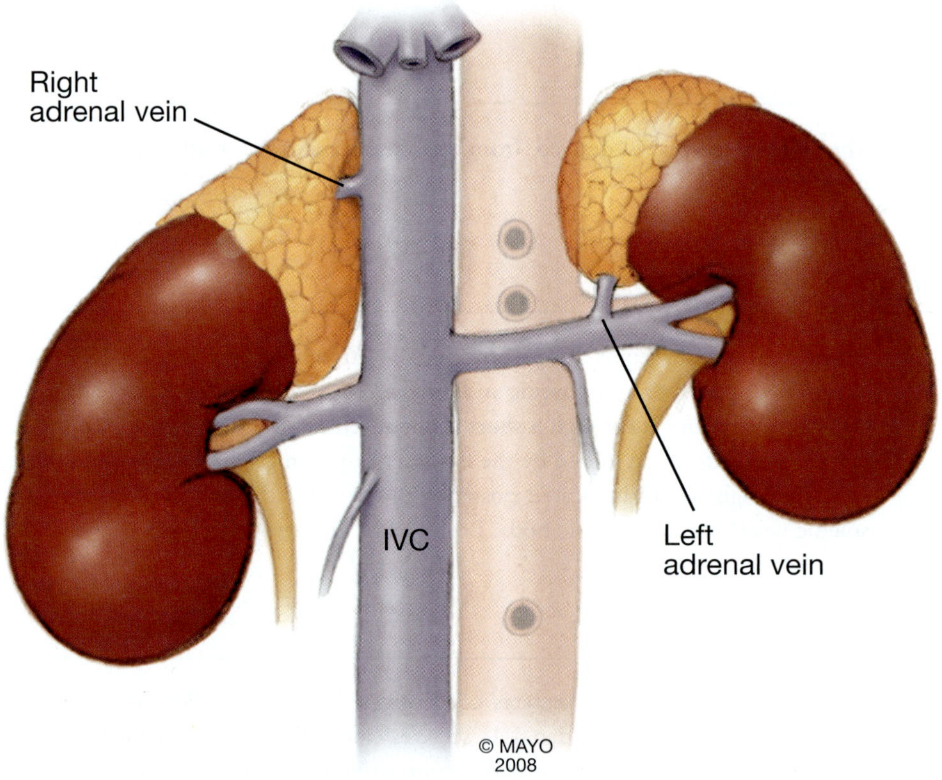

FIGURE 1.2. Venous Drainage of Adrenal Glands. (Modified from McKenzie TJ, Lillegard JB, Young WF Jr, Thompson GB. Aldosteronomas: state of the art. Surg Clin North Am. 2009 Oct; 89[5]:1241–53; used with permission of Mayo Foundation for Medical Education and Research.)

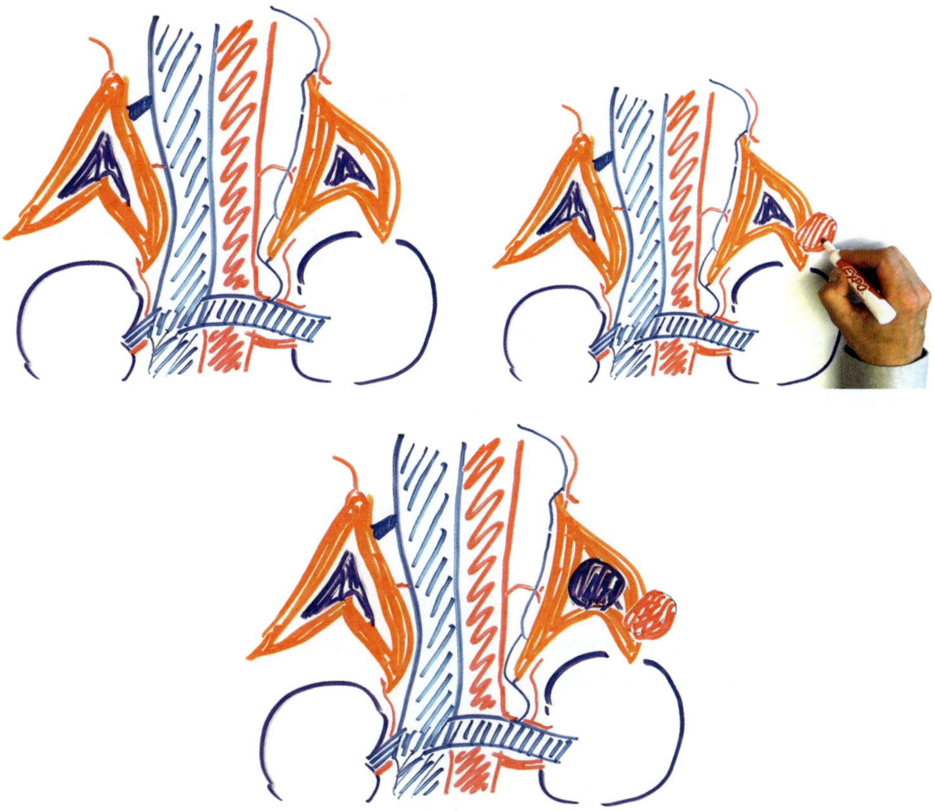

VIDEO 1.1. Adrenal Cortex and Medulla.

Transcript: We have right and left adrenal glands. We have the vena cava and the aorta. These are all retroperitoneal structures; they work in close collaboration. Specifically, take a look at the adrenal glands; they have an outer layer of cortex which tends to be orangish or salmon colored, or tan, golden. On the inside, it's neuroectoderm: it's the medulla. The medulla secretes catecholamines: epinephrine, norepinephrine, and dopamine. The cortex secretes aldosterone, cortisol, and the sex hormones. The cortex is important for regulation of electrolytes, steroids, and a variety of bodily functions. On the inside, the catecholamines are for "fight or flight": response to stress. It's important to know where these tumors come from so that when we identify tumors from the cortex, invariably, if they're functional, they'll deal with or secrete cortisol, aldosterone, or (very rarely) sex hormones. So that allows us to test appropriately for that problem. Whereas, if you have a tumor of the medulla, a so-called pheochromocytoma, as it grows and creates a larger sphere, we know that we should be testing for catecholamines. Cortex and medulla—2 different origins: mesoderm and neuroectoderm. It's important that you know the difference.

Clinical Presentation

Adrenal masses are most commonly asymptomatic; incidentalomas (Video 1.3) are found on imaging studies for other complaints (kidney stones, abdominal pain). A tumor originating from the medulla in adults is a pheochromocytoma (in children, neuroblastoma) (Video 1.4). Cortical neoplasms may cause hypercortisolism (Video 1.5), hyperaldosteronism (Video 1.6), sex hormone excess, or ACC (Video 1.7).

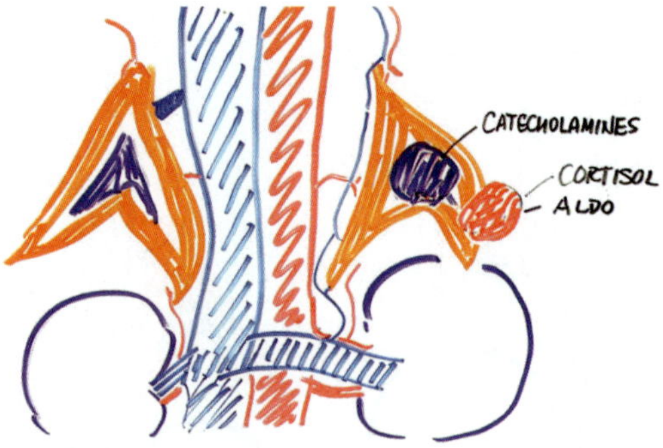

VIDEO 1.2. Urinary and Serum Studies for Adrenal Tumors.
Transcript: We need to make sure that the tumor is not functional. A cortical tumor is either going to secrete cortisol, aldo, or sex hormones—those are so rare I'm not even going to put them on the list. So if we make someone urinate and collect that urine, we can check for cortisol. A simple blood test will check for aldosterone. Those 2 things will show if the tumor is functional; if it is, it should come out. What about the catecholamines in the medulla? We can again have a urinary test to check for epinephrine, norepinephrine, and dopamine or the breakdown products—VMA (vanillylmandelic acid). Those would be vital to knowing the patient has a pheochromocytoma. Most times, lumps and bumps in the adrenal gland are benign—they're nonfunctional; these tests will be negative. If that's the case, smaller tumors, we can watch them. But if any of these tests show a functional tumor—high aldo, high cortisol, or high catecholamines—that lump should be taken out.

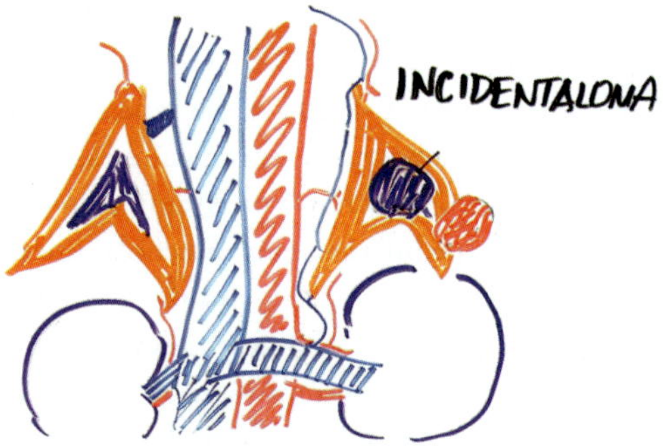

VIDEO 1.3. Incidentalomas.
Transcript: When it comes to the adrenal gland, it's an adrenaloma. It is a tumor that nobody knew was there and was found on an x-ray—a lump inside or on the outside of the adrenal gland that was found maybe for somebody that had kidney stones and they got a CT scan and found an adrenal mass. Maybe it was somebody with a chest x-ray that we could see the adrenal gland and there was a calcified mass. Or maybe somebody had an MRI or a CT or some other structure for abdominal pain and, oops, they found an incidental mass. They happen in about 4% of all CT scans, and they're more common the older you are, such that if the age is greater than 50 or 60, at least 4% of people will have an incidentaloma. For someone that's 10 or 20, there's a less than 1% chance. An incidentaloma is greater than 1 cm in size. It could be in either one or both of the adrenal glands. If it's greater than a centimeter, we should check physiologic studies to see if that lump or bump is functional and secreting hormone.

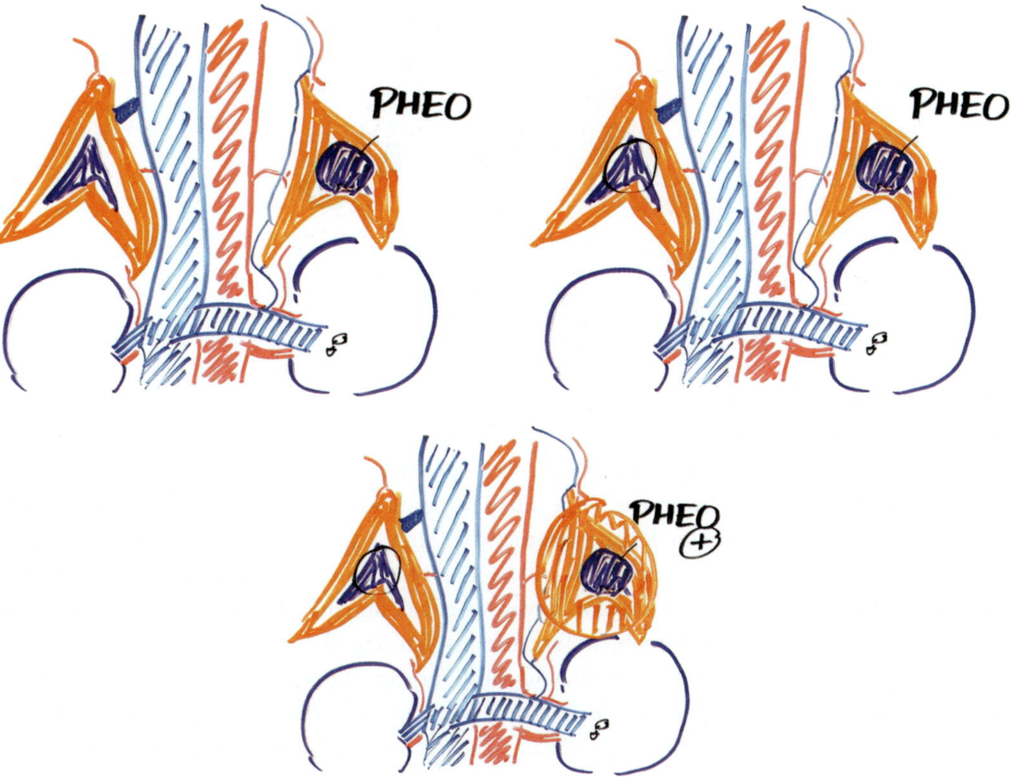

VIDEO 1.4. Pheochromocytoma.

Transcript: Pheochromocytoma is a rare tumor. Maybe 800 of them are identified in the United States every year—half of them being lethal because they secrete catecholamines. Patients can die of excess catecholamines. How so? Myocardial infarction or stroke. Epinephrine, norepinephrine, dopamine generated into the blood stream gets high blood pressure, high heart rates, and people can pass away. About 400 pheos are resected every year in the United States. Again, pheochromocytoma comes from the inside, the medulla, of the adrenal gland. It secretes catecholamines (epinephrine, norepinephrine, dopamine). It's a 10% tumor: 10% of them occur in kids; 10% are familial (typically, MEN2 or von Hippel-Lindau syndrome); 10% are malignant; and 10% are bilateral. It's an unusual tumor and the key thing is, when you find them, test them to make sure that you see they're making hormones. Don't go immediately to the operating room; they need to be blocked with alpha and beta blockade before you operate to take them out.

Last teaching point: A pheochromocytoma, because the cortex is around it, typically over time as it enlarges, the cortex starts to become oval and rounded and no longer has that "witch" shape or comma or some sort of funny little serpentine look. When they become rounded or oval or spherical, and it's an adrenal mass, think pheochromocytoma.

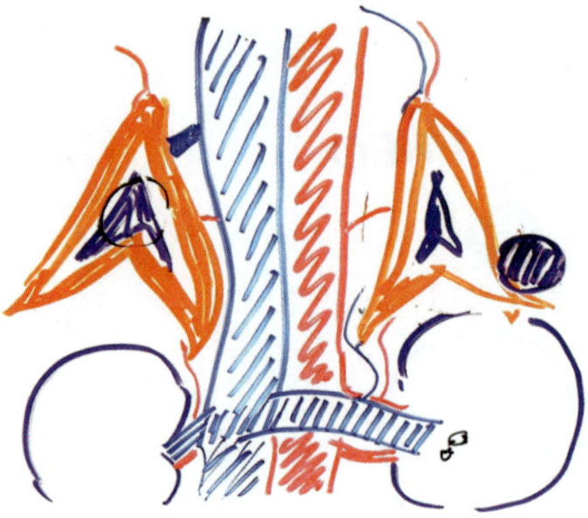

VIDEO 1.5. Hypercortisolism.

Transcript: Hypercortisolism is typically caused by intake of steroids, so it's a medication. I suspect that 99% of all people in the United States with hypercortisolism are taking steroids because of a kidney transplant, because of rheumatoid arthritis, because of some inflammatory condition. So 1% of the people have hypercortisolism related to a body problem. It's rare that they occur in the adrenal gland; they are typically pituitary tumors. But, if there's a lesion in the cortex—it will be kind of a "wart" growing off the side—it will secrete cortisol. That cortisol can easily be eradicated with removal of half the adrenal gland or all of the adrenal gland.

Hypercortisolism can be a deadly problem for patients—causing diabetes, causing weight gain, causing inability to move. Hypercortisolism—how do you check for that? Typically, urinary cortisol levels will let you know that the cortisol is high. Then the question becomes, "Is it because they are taking pills?" "Is it a pituitary problem?" or "Is it an adrenal problem?" There is a variety of tests to check for that.

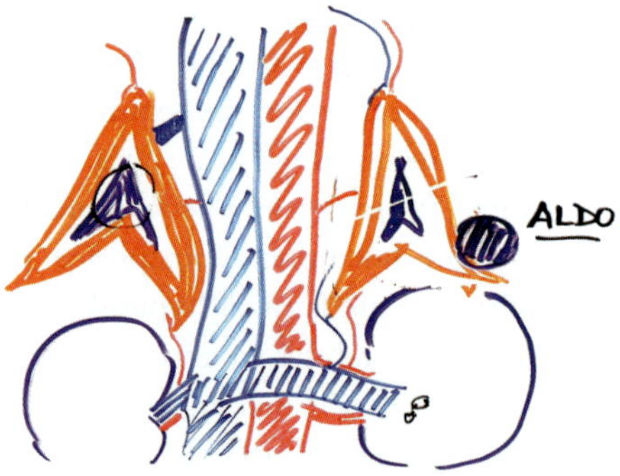

VIDEO 1.6. Hyperaldosteronism.

Transcript: Hyperaldosteronism, so-called Conn's syndrome, is related to a cortical tumor that creates too much aldosterone. Dr Conn was an endocrinologist in the middle 1950s and 60s at the University of Michigan. He did a lot of work on these cortical tumors. Aldosterone eventually holds on to liquid, blood, fluid; secretes potassium; holds on to sodium, and people get hypertension—high blood pressure. By removing half the gland, or all of the gland, and eradicating this aldosteronoma, people are cured—their hypertension drops. If they've had these tumors for a long time (and many have), hypertension may remain. These people are difficult; they'll be on 3, or 4, or 5 blood pressure medicines. If a surgeon takes that lesion out, they'll drop down to 1 or 2, and they're happy about that and they're healthier. Hyperaldosteronism is fairly common; it may be 1% or 2% of all people with high blood pressure have an underlying aldo. Check a CT scan. If there's a "wart" on the cortex, think about an aldo tumor.

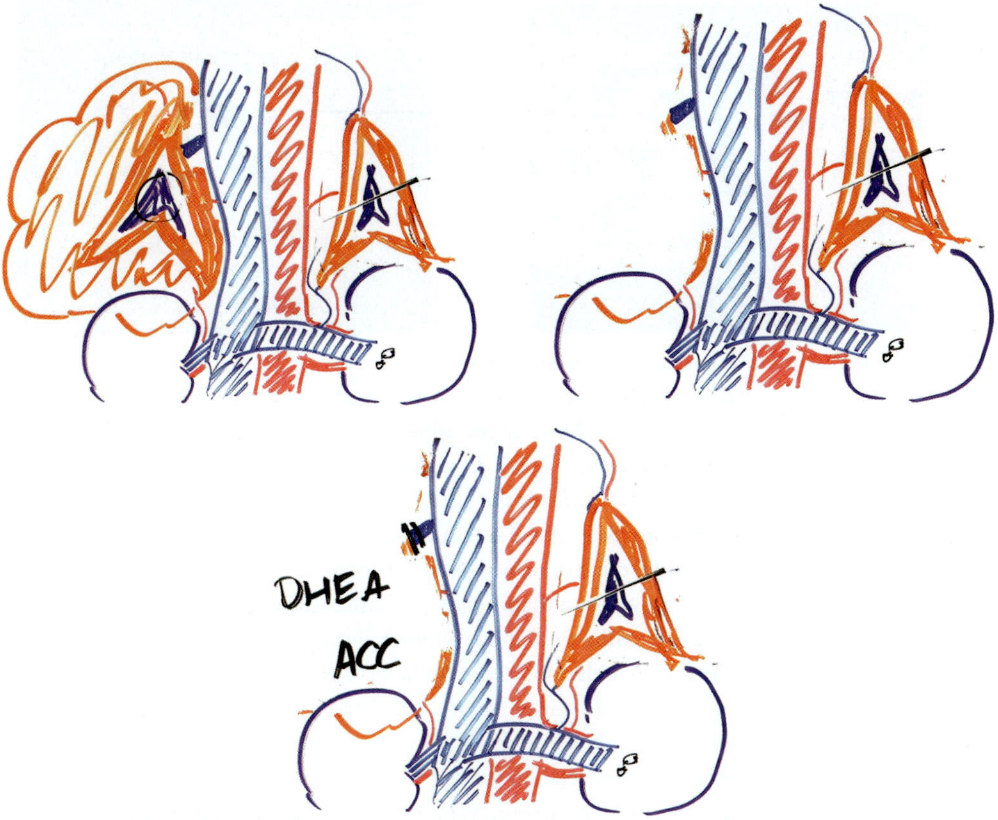

VIDEO 1.7. ACC.

Transcript: Adrenocortical cancer is a lethal problem. It is difficult to eradicate and cure. By the time we see it, it's usually massively large—10, 14, 20 centimeters in size—before there's enough hormone, there's enough malnutrition or cachexia that we see people with these tumors: massive tumors that push the inferior vena cava, the kidney away, the liver away—large tumors. They present subtly initially but later on metastasis to the liver, the lung, the brain, and it's a lethal problem. Having said that, if a tumor is pushing and you eradicate that—you remove the entire tumor—some of these people have long-term survival, and so it's more than adequate and worthwhile to take them out. Oftentimes these tumors will secrete hormone, and these people are miserable because of hypercortisolemia. It's important to eradicate that to make their quality of life better and leave them with nothing there on the side. The other gland will be able to take care of things. How do you find these things early? Careful history and physical examination. Sometimes a dihydroepiandrosterone level (so-called DHEA level) is a marker of adrenocortical cancer. Common things occur commonly; this is a rare tumor, thankfully. A CT scan that shows a huge mass in the retroperitoneum on the left or the right side, we need to think about adrenocortical cancer, and if it's something that we can resect, we should do so ASAP!

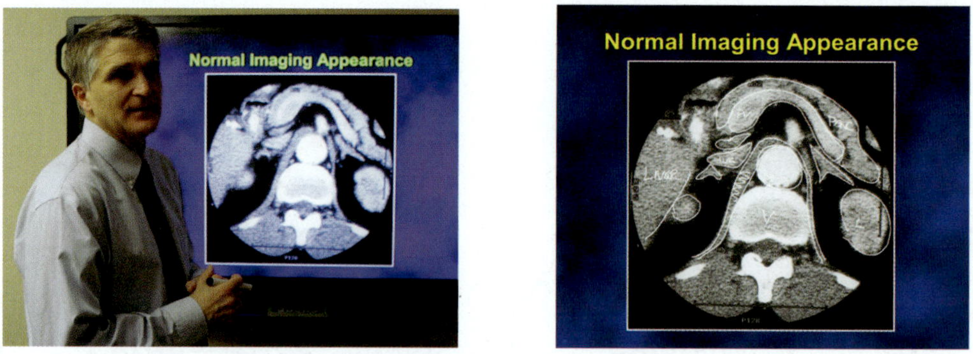

VIDEO 1.8. CT of Abdomen, Focusing on Adrenal Glands.
Transcript: So this is a CT scan of the abdomen, and it's very focused—basically in the retroperitoneum. It's an adrenal CT scan, if you will; people looking for adrenal glands and abnormalities. So hopefully what we can take away here in 90 seconds is, "What do we see?" And as you get more and more expert, think about, "I can see the vertebral body, I can see the aorta" (usually about 2, 2 1/2 centimeters in size). What else do we see? This is going to be liver on the side (the patient's right side). Underneath is going to be the right kidney, and on the left side, the left kidney. Now what's all the rest of this stuff anterior to the aorta and the vertebral body? Well, we've got a diaphragm. Almost everybody's got a diaphragm, and it's in a lot of cuts. It's not terribly large. It's thin, and, quite honestly, it looks like an adrenal gland. It's about the same width as an adrenal gland. What else do we see up here? We see a blood vessel.

This is a contrast-enhanced CT scan, and this is what's called the splenic vein, emptying into what's called the portal vein. So this is the splenic vein, which sits directly posterior to the pancreas. We get a nice cut of the pancreas here; this is all pancreas. So now, if we know our anatomy well, we tell ourselves that the left adrenal gland lies posterior to the splenic vein and the pancreas. And, ta da! Yep, this is our left adrenal gland. I usually think it looks like a little "witch hat," if you will. On the right side, we should be looking for the inferior vena cava. The inferior vena cava is right next to the aorta, and in this cut, it's right here—this is the IVC. Inferior or deep to that is going to be the right adrenal gland, and it too, sometimes looks like a little "witch hat." But it lays posterior. It's not this structure—this is actually a little retrocholedocho lymph node. This is a nice CT scan of 2 normal adrenal glands cut on a CT scan with contrast. The rest of this stuff is fat, and the more fat you have on a CT, the easier it is to see things because it spreads it out. This person is sort of medium build, and the study is a nice one and shows us no abnormalities on this cut with either adrenal gland.

Imaging

Adrenal incidentalomas are masses greater than 1 cm in diameter that are found in 2% to 4% of all CTs (Video 1.8). HU interpretation (Video 1.9) may be diagnostic: adipose tissue density is 20 HUs or less, adrenal cysts have no HU density, and benign adenoma density is less than 10 HUs. Pheochromocytoma, ACC, and metastases are typically greater than 30 HUs.

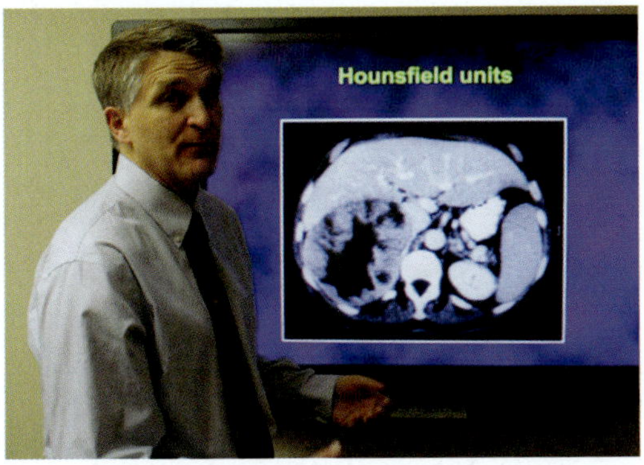

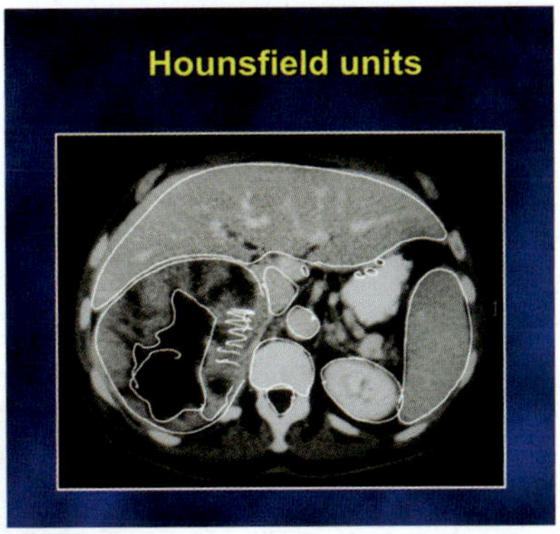

VIDEO 1.9. HU Interpretation on CT.
Transcript: This is an older CT scan—it's not HD, it's not the better quality—but it's an amazing CT scan with a very dangerous problem. We talk about Hounsfield units—Sir Godfrey Hounsfield was a physicist and a computer expert and an Englishman that won the Nobel Prize and was knighted for his work on developing CT scans. The units for density are named after him. Things that are really dense will be white; that means that something like the vertebral bodies might be 200, 300, 400 Hounsfield units. The scale goes up to 1,000 for some titanium or metallic abnormality. Something that is less dense—air—will be −1,000. We don't have much air on this screen; we've got a couple of bubbles of air in the stomach, the intestine, but not much else. That will be −1,000. In the middle will be water. You can always find that because within the spinal cord there is cerebrospinal fluid—that's water. Everything else in the human body is mostly about −10 (which is fat) or +70 (which is blood or dense muscle or organs). This is a nice CT scan of a normal looking kidney. This structure here is—yep—that's the spleen. We've got a liver—nice generous liver here—that looks pretty reasonable. We've got an aorta with contrast in it, and the vena cava is pushed up and out of the way. Why is it pushed up and out of the way? Because we've got a mass that's heterogeneous: it's got hypodense regions here (which is necrotic and it's fluid), and it's got hyperdense regions, which means it's got blood flow. Unfortunately for this young patient, this is a right-sided adrenocortical cancer. These are very difficult to treat and cure. CT scan—what do we take away from it? Hounsfield units: +1,000, metal or dense bone; −1,000, air; water is zero; most bodily tissues—fat is going to be less than zero, −10, −20, −30; and then most organs are going to be 30, 40, or 50. This is a mass—heterogeneous—lots of different densities. It's a mass that's growing so fast that the inside is dying, but the outside is going to lead to the demise of this patient.

Operation

Adrenalectomy is indicated for masses that are enlarging, larger than 4 to 6 cm, or functional (secreting hormone); the operation is fixated on safe transection of adrenal blood vessels. For laparoscopic adrenalectomy (Videos 1.10 and 1.11), 3 or 4 incisions are made at anterior, flank, or posterior access points to gain entry into the retroperitoneum. Open adrenalectomy is reserved for large tumors (>10 cm) and ACC. A laparoscopic right adrenalectomy is shown in Video 1.12.

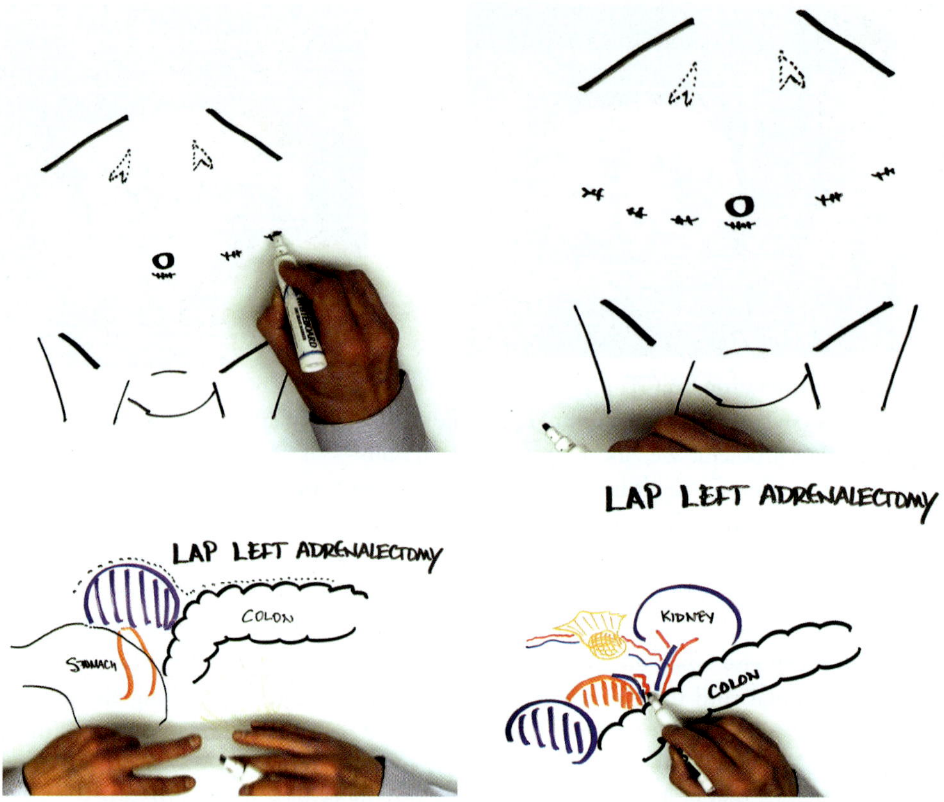

VIDEO 1.10. Laparoscopic (LAP) Left Adrenalectomy.

Transcript: Laparoscopic adrenalectomy is a complex procedure that sneaks behind all these tissues to find these little adrenal glands. On the abdomen, surgeons do it a lot of different ways. Some folks make an incision of the umbilicus—a little 2-cm incision—and then have several others that might be utilized to get out the left adrenal gland. On the right adrenal gland, the liver is in the way and often takes a total of 4 little incisions: 1 near the belly button and 3 others. It can also be done from the back side; a laparoscopic adrenalectomy that truthfully is just in the retroperitoneum, but small incisions give us access to the adrenal glands. Let's take a look at what it looks like inside. We gain access into the abdomen, and what your surgeon and you will see is the colon on the lateral aspect; oftentimes the patient is in the decubitus position (on their side). What the surgeon will do is take the cautery or some sort of gadget and incise that peritoneal attachment and allow this colon to fall back, sneak behind the spleen, and allow the tissue to fall this way, which will expose the underlying kidney and our adrenal gland, which sits right next to the back side of the pancreas. We rarely get to see the pancreas until we flip it over on the back side.

Let me show you what that looks like. With the colon and the spleen rotated medially, the pancreas and the tail rotate medially, exposing the splenic vein and the splenic artery from time to time. Most people have fatty tissue covering this, so you can't always see it as well as it's drawn here, with the kidney and associated adrenal gland. The key to adrenal surgery is finding the veins: the left adrenal vein empties into the left renal vein; there's a phrenic vein. The arteries typically are tiny—coming from the kidney, the diaphragm, or even a couple little branches from the aorta. It's the veins that are crucial. A laparoscopic left adrenalectomy is in a high-rent district. You and your surgeon will have to be careful and find those blood vessels—especially the left adrenal vein.

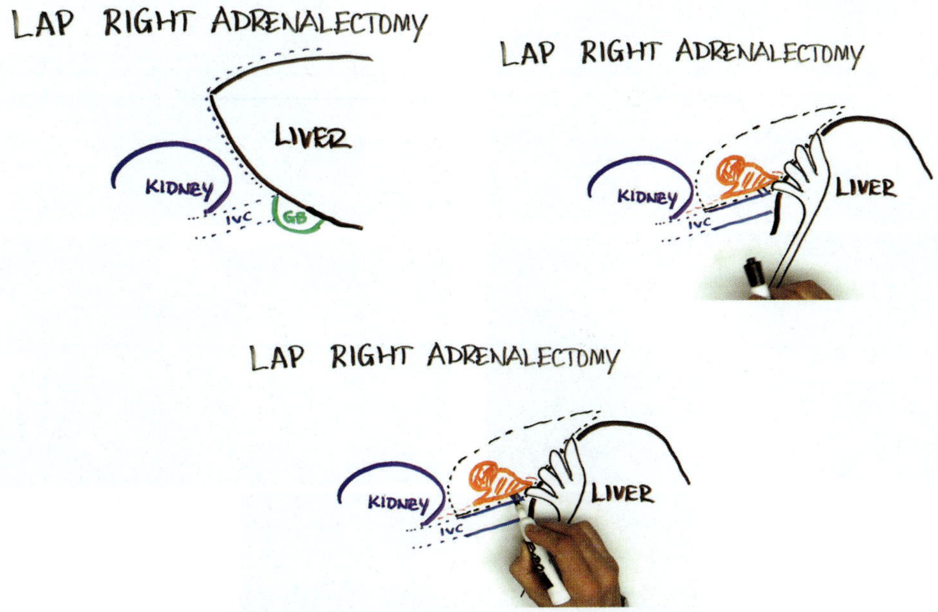

VIDEO 1.11. Laparoscopic (LAP) Right Adrenalectomy.
Transcript: For a laparoscopic right adrenalectomy, the laparoscope near the umbilicus slides in and we can see the liver—sometimes you can see the gallbladder, but if the patient is rotated in the lateral decubitus position the gallbladder will be out of the way. We'll get a sense of a bump of the kidney, there may be fatty tissue here, but we'll definitely see the liver. What the surgeon will try to do is to incise the peritoneal attachments of that liver and allow that liver to rotate medially and fall this way. What that will do is eventually help us expose the IVC that's in the retroperitoneal plane. Let me show you what that kind of looks like with the liver out of the way. Laparoscopically, with the peritoneum incised, the liver can fall, or be rotated, medially. Sometimes a little grasper or ability to retract that liver up will allow us to see the inferior vena cava, sometimes the top of the kidney, and then our adrenal gland. It never looks this clean because there's fatty tissue in the way. Nonetheless, the key for you and your surgeon is to find the small, short right adrenal vein. It's very short, so it means the adrenal gland is close to the inferior vena cava. A couple of clips on that dividing it, and then it's relatively easy to take that adrenal gland out because there's very few arteries going into it, and they're small.

Complications

Complications are relatively uncommon with laparoscopic adrenalectomy, but trauma to surrounding organs (right: liver, kidney, diaphragm; left: pancreas, colon, kidney, diaphragm) can occur. Injury to blood vessels (right: IVC and renal vein; left: splenic and renal veins) is rare but dangerous.

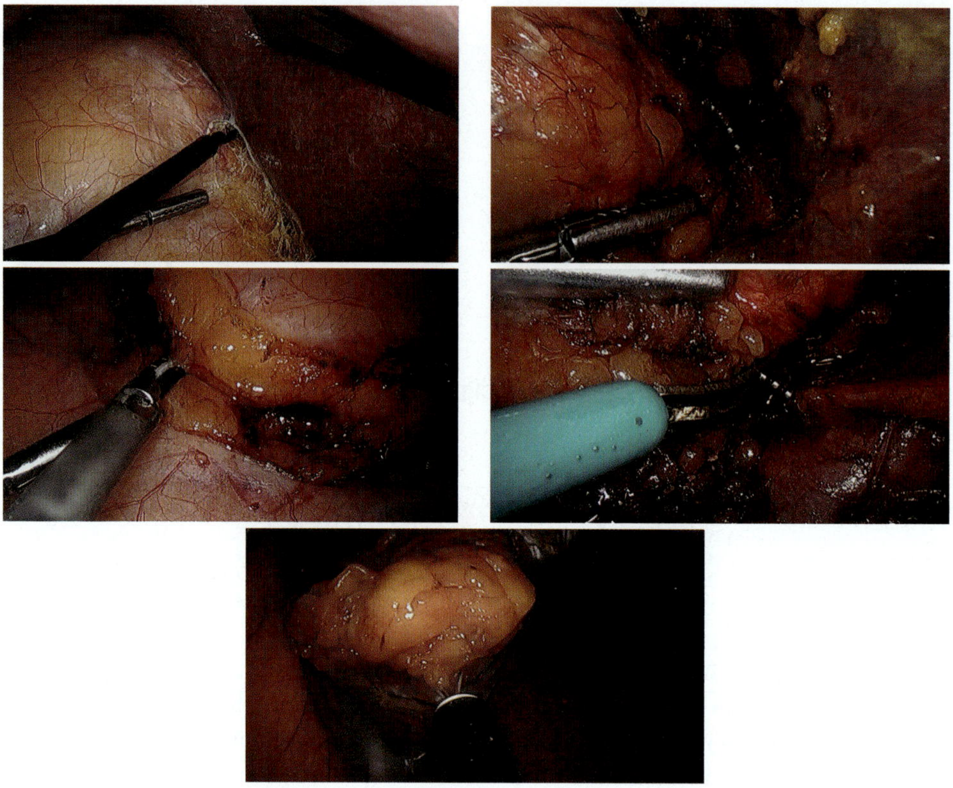

VIDEO 1.12. Laparoscopic Right Adrenalectomy: Intraoperative.

Transcript: This video shows a right-sided laparoscopic adrenalectomy. The liver is to the right, being lifted up by a retracting gadget, so we're kind of from the belly button looking up toward the right shoulder. We see this liver edge and we see something underneath it; there's fatty tissue and kind of an orangish discoloration. These are peritoneal attachments of the liver that hold it in place. That J hook is a cautery—it's a hot stick—and easily goes through fatty tissue or fibrous tissue without any problems. The key thing is the surgeon here has this on tension, so the tissues retract nicely. The adrenal gland lies to the left of the screen within that fat. You can see some reddish and maybe some yellow and tan things. When we do a right-sided adrenalectomy—as opposed to the left side—we think about the vena cava, which runs posterior to the liver. The caudate lobe is back there; there's a variety of structures that are dangerous in this small little space.

The key thing is finding the little blood vessels. Using a clip applier, that basically deploys a clip that can ligate or occlude a vessel and then either with scissors or cautery or a variety of thermal instruments, we can transsect the blood supply to the adrenal gland. We're using a laparoscopic camera—you can see from time to time it shakes and moves a little bit. These are human beings tackling this effort. The adrenal gland is to the left; you don't see it very well because it's well protected in the fatty tissue. Several little vessels—arterial vessels, from the phrenic, from the renal artery, from the aorta—go into the adrenal gland, and on the right side, just the main right hepatic adrenal vein. We've got a mass now: liver to the right, adrenal above, and we're incising the peritoneum using electrocautery.

Again, we're on the lookout for blood vessels—the arterial vessels from the phrenic, from the kidney, from the aorta and typically just 1 blood vessel in the right adrenal gland. We're to the patient's right of that adrenal gland, the diaphragm is up on the top of the screen, liver to the right. And in the

VIDEO 1.12. Continued

retroperitoneum, especially for folks that are a little chubbier, there's more fatty tissue. Several hands working here: one hand is grasping, one hand has a cautery tool. This is a thermal dissecting tool; it's called a harmonic scalpel. It does pretty doggone well at cutting through fatty and fibrous tissue and sealing off blood vessels. You've got to be careful though, within the jaws, and make sure we don't hurt anything we're not trying to injure.

Here, the harmonic scalpel takes a little bitty arterial vessel and easily cuts through it—makes it quick. We've now got the blood vessel draining from the adrenal gland—the right adrenal vein going into the vena cava, which lies on the back side of that liver. It's dangerous here—it's tented up. A rip in the vena cava can be a dangerous problem—a deadly problem! It's important that the team of surgeons carefully places clips, occludes vessels, and then cuts between them. As you see this very difficult right adrenal vein transection, you can realize there's not much space here. Everything is magnified; those 4 clips are being placed in a space less than a centimeter. It's going to be hard to cut between them. Adrenal surgery sometimes is very, very dangerous, and it gets us nervous. But if we can cut through this right adrenal vein and let it release from the vena cava, we no longer have troubles.

This is one of the harder adrenal vein transections I've seen because the space was so narrow, and it was difficult to place the clips far enough apart that you can cut between them. We can see the surgeon is finally getting through there, and we get a sense that now the gland is far more mobile, and we can safely take the gland out without hurting the vena cava to the right. It's a tough video to look at because there's so much fatty tissue. The vena cava is to the right, liver to the right, working in the right upper quadrant, up behind the liver. We finally get that thing unhooked and put a little plastic bag inside. All that fatty tissue makes it tough to put in there, but eventually we can pull it out through a small little incision and the patient can go home that day or the following day.

Adrenal Glands Challenge Questions

1.1. What arteries supply blood to the adrenal glands?
1.2. Describe the difference in venous drainage of right and left adrenal glands.
1.3. What is the best test to confirm Cushing syndrome?
1.4. What tests are needed for a 60-year-old person with a 2-cm incidentaloma?
1.5. How large is the typical ACC when first identified?
1.6. Why are pheochromocytomas referred to as the "10% tumor"?
1.7. Which patients need corticosteroid replacement after adrenalectomy?
1.8. Can humans live without adrenal glands?
1.9. What functioning tissue must all Federal Aviation Administration–regulated commercial pilots have in their bodies?
1.10. What is the difference between Cushing syndrome and Cushing disease?
1.11. What is the most common type of congenital adrenal hyperplasia?

Answers to Adrenal Glands Challenge Questions

1.1. Small branches of the aorta and renal and phrenic arteries.
1.2. Right, 1 short vein to the IVC. Left, 2 longer veins drain into the left renal vein.
1.3. Overnight dexamethasone suppression test.
1.4. Serum potassium and aldosterone, urinary cortisol, and catecholamine levels.
1.5. Ten to 14 cm in diameter.
1.6. Ten percent are found in children, 10% are bilateral, 10% are familial, and 10% are malignant.
1.7. Those with preoperative hypercortisolism.
1.8. Not well. Cortisone and mineralocorticoids are required daily medications.
1.9. Adrenal and parathyroid.
1.10. Cushing syndrome: hypercortisolism from a pituitary adenoma. Cushing disease: hypercortisolism (exogenous steroids are the number 1 cause).
1.11. A 21-hydroxylase deficiency.

2

Appendix

Embryology

The appendix is an antimesenteric cecal outpouching (midgut) that forms in the fifth month of gestation.

Anatomy

The appendix is a hollow, blind-ending tube approximately 11 cm in length and less than 6 mm in diameter. The base of the appendix is attached to the cecum 2 cm from the ileocecal valve. The appendiceal tip may vary in location and is sometimes retrocecal (Figure 2.1A). The appendicular artery arises from the ileocecal artery.

Pathophysiology

Obstruction of the appendiceal lumen with a fecalith, or less commonly foreign bodies, worms, and lymphadenopathy, may result in swelling of the appendix (Figures 2.1B and 2.2). Venous congestion then causes an increase in pressure that leads to arterial occlusion and resultant ischemia and necrosis.

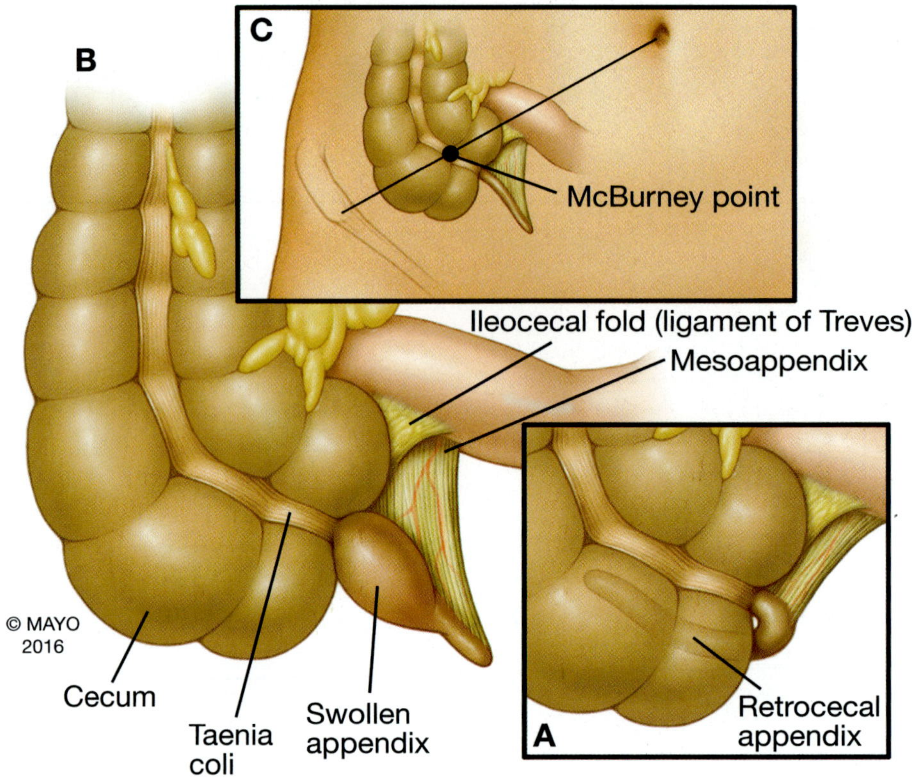

FIGURE 2.1. Anatomy of the Appendix.
A, Retrocecal location. B, Swelling. C, McBurney point.

Clinical Presentation

Patients present with periumbilical abdominal pain that localizes to the right lower quadrant within 24 hours and may be associated with low-grade fever, nausea, vomiting, and anorexia. Tenderness at McBurney point (Figure 2.1C) is typical. Other physical examination findings include rebound tenderness and psoas and Rovsing signs (Video 2.1). Appendiceal neoplasms can be carcinoid tumors (Video 2.2), mucoceles, or, rarely, ACAs.

Imaging

Acute appendicitis is a clinical diagnosis, but CT (axial, Video 2.3A; coronal, Video 2.3B) or US (Video 2.4) is often used to confirm the diagnosis.

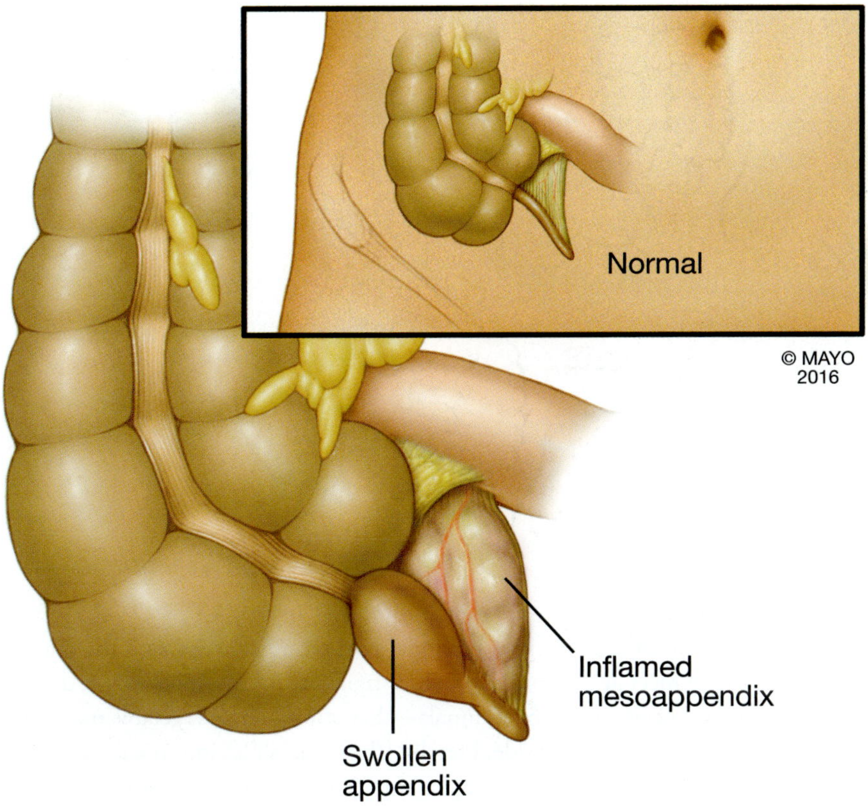

FIGURE 2.2. Normal View (Inset) and Swollen Appendix.

Operation

The majority of patients with signs and symptoms of acute appendicitis should receive prompt surgical intervention (laparoscopic, Video 2.5A; open, Video 2.5B). Patients presenting with a mass in the right lower quadrant that is an abscess should have drainage and later undergo an interval appendectomy (Video 2.6). A laparoscopic appendectomy is shown in Video 2.7.

Complications

Laparoscopic or open appendectomy can be associated with ileus, superficial or deep wound infections, GI leak, bleeding or hematoma, wound dehiscence, or hernia.

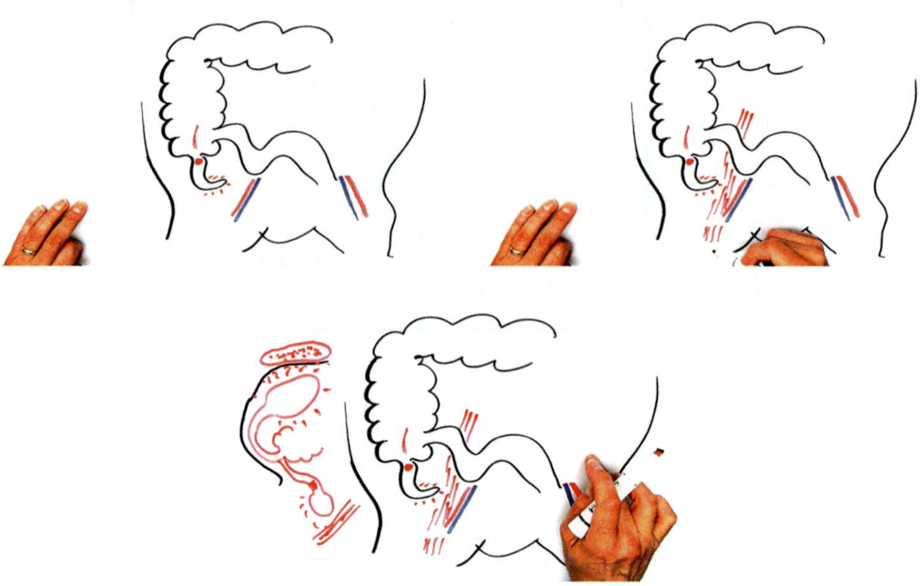

VIDEO 2.1. Psoas and Rovsing Signs.

Transcript: The appendix is located at the very proximal portion of what is called the cecum; as the taenia coli come together, they meet at the base and this vestigial organ, the appendix. It does not really do anything for us in humans; in cows and other animals—they store a lot of vegetable matter there and it is broken down, but for us, it is a pain in the side, literally. The ileum slides into the ileoceceal valve and the appendix is off the base of the cecum. If a fecalith or some sort of material plugs the lumen, the mucus that is secreted out of there gets plugged up and this appendix starts to get swollen and inflamed, and this is what is called appendicitis.

The signs of appendicitis are legendary: it could be a variety of things—from nothing to horrible pain in the right lower quadrant at what is called McBurney's point, sort of the halfway point from the hip bone to the belly button. Two signs to know about: 1) The psoas sign relates to the underlying ileopsoas muscle that sits underneath the iliac vessels and helps us flex the thigh. You could imagine that if you asked someone to flex their hip and this appendix was sitting next to that muscle it would be exquisitely tender. So if you have somebody that flexes their hip, they will have problems with pain. Any time this appendix gets inflamed and touches the peritoneum, the peritoneum is exquisitely sensitive, and this will have discomfort. If a muscle (here that would be rectus or the transversalis above) or if this appendix is posterior and is inflamed because of a stone, any muscle lying near it would be painful. So the psoas sign is flexion of the hip. 2) There are times people have so much inflammation of the appendix that you can push on the opposite side, the left lower quadrant, and because this peritoneum—this lining—is so sensitive (like a trampoline, you touch here and it hurts over there), that is a positive sign for likely inflammation where the appendix is touching the peritoneum, and that is called the Rovsing sign. Push on the left lower quadrant pain in the right, up in the top, Rovsing sign; make the hip flex that is so-called psoas sign: appendicitis.

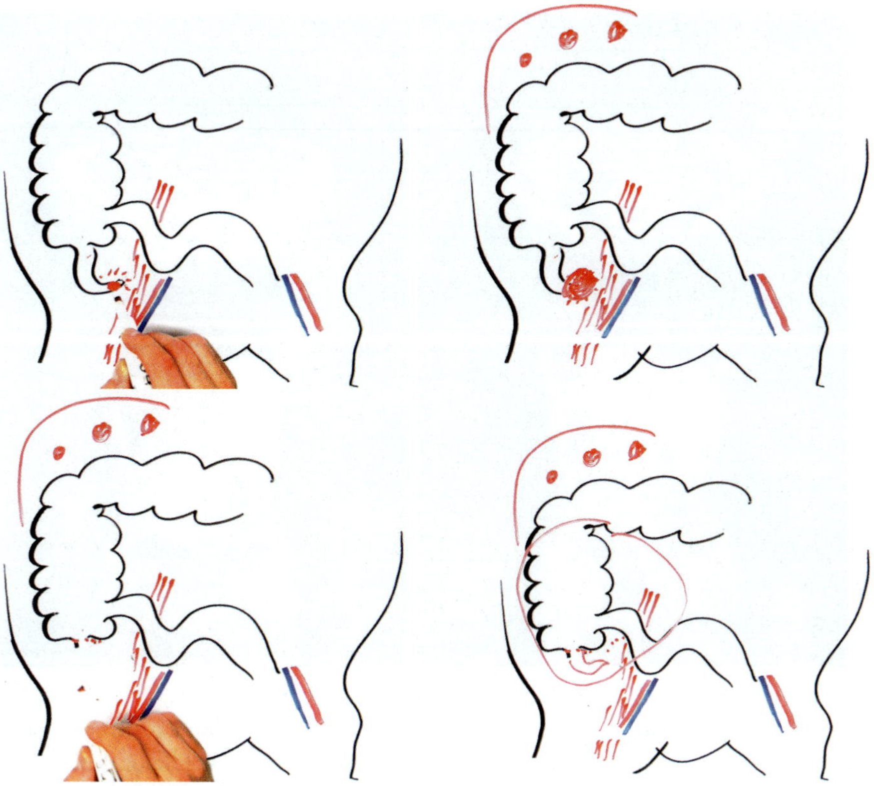

VIDEO 2.2. Carcinoid Tumors.

Transcript: Not everything that causes appendicitis is a fecalith. Sometimes you can grow a mass in the appendix. The most common lump in the appendix is likely what is called a carcinoid tumor. The appendix is common place for these little buggers to grow. They're typically not malignant until they get much larger in size and then they cause problems. But, carcinoid tumors can secrete a variety of hormones—serotonin, histamine, prostaglandins, kallikrein—a variety of different things that may cause flushing or diarrhea. And if these little buggers grow big enough, then tumors—carcinoid tumors—can get into the liver and have metastasis and secrete more hormone. When the hormone level becomes high enough, it gets into the bloodstream and it affects the valves of the heart, and people can have congestive heart failure from a little bitty problem that started out in the appendix. The treatment for carcinoid tumors (ideally when they are small) is to always just remove the appendix. If indeed the tumor is larger (greater than 2 cm) or there is concern for metastasis or lymph node involvement, then likely what is called a right hemicolectomy, including this appendix, can be a cancerous and deadly problem. Fortuitously, it is relatively uncommon; but when you think about appendicitis, or appendiceal problems, carcinoid needs to be high on the list.

A

B

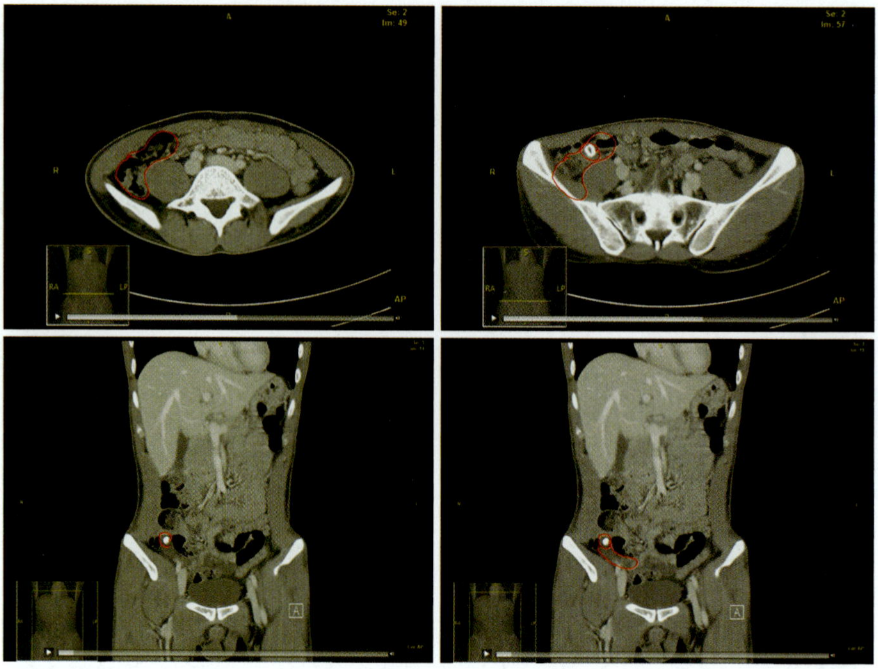

VIDEO 2.3. CT for Diagnosis of Appendicitis. A, Axial view. B, Coronal view.

Transcript A: Most patients with appendicitis develop right lower quadrant pain, fever, and an elevated white blood cell count. They don't always have an ultrasound or a CT scan, but some people do. Sometimes it is very helpful and useful. Let's take a look at this young person with a CT scan that was obtained for right lower quadrant pain. As we cycle through the CT scan, we get down near the cecum and the psoas muscle. We are looking for the appendix. What things should we be looking for? Number 1, we need to look for that cecum and go cut by cut. We are just creeping along, and the cecum is readily identifiable. It is large and it is boggy and it has stool—this is cecum. As we move more caudal, or toward the toes, it ends; at the end of the cecum will be the appendix. So let's see if we can find that appendix, again, just going cut by cut. We can see where the cecum is and it is still sort of there, but now something new.

This is what is called a fecalith. It is calcium, basically. It is sitting inside the appendix, and it commonly happens and obstructs the appendix. So that is the location of the appendix. As we cut down further (let me see if I can't erase this for us), keep our eyes on that fecalith. As we go towards the toes, caudally, it is still there. It is a pretty good size fecalith. Now there is not much left, other than a boggy sort of appendix. This is the ileum sneaking into the cecum in this region. So, by criteria of CT scan, this patient does have appendicitis.

Transcript B: The is the same CT scan (as Video 2.3A) in a coronal cut that shows us liver, bladder, and then again, our fecalith. Importantly, it also shows behind that fecalith, is an appendix. A normal appendix is 7 or 8 mm in diameter, maybe 10 or 11 mm long. It is the diameter—this thickness—that is important. This one is probably 15 mm. This is acute appendicitis. This young person needs an appendectomy now.

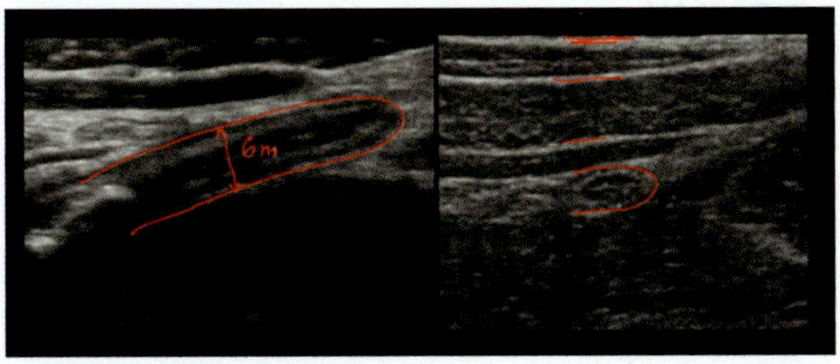

VIDEO 2.4. US for Diagnosis of Appendicitis.
Transcript: We are using ultrasound with the skin on top, muscular layers above, and then we are looking for the appendix. The key for appendicitis is how big the appendix is. I think you can get a sense here on this picture—this is the appendix, and usually it is less than or equal to 6 mm. That is the width of the appendix. The wall of the appendix is 3 mm on either side; there is a small lumen in the middle. So the key is to look at the appendix and then see how big it is.

So here is a picture again: skin on the top, muscle layers, and we are seeing on end, the appendix. Now it has been marked out. Truthfully, this is in a young child, and it looks like it is big but the markings are very small and this could be a normal appendix. Or, if they said it is 15 mm, then we know that is a "hot" appendix. I don't have any numbers here. Same thing here, it looks like we are seeing an appendix and maybe it is swollen. This looks kind of bigger than this side. This is likely acute appendicitis.

Again, what do we see? I think you can get a sense, and we have an arrow here suggesting that maybe that is normal appendix and this is swollen out top. What is this measurement? Normal, 6 mm or less—wall thickness, 3 mm or less.

So let's take a look at the last ultrasound. What do you think? Skin is on top, muscle, this, and this end-on view. We have some echoes, likely a appendacolith, a calcified thing. It changes the way it looks like. The key measurement if this is going to be an appendicitis it needs to be greater than 6 mm, and the wall thickness, what is the number, that is right, greater than 3 mm. If this number came back 9 mm, those are good criteria for this being appendicitis. So, your ultrasonographer, or your tech, that is doing this study really has to label these out and mark them for you.

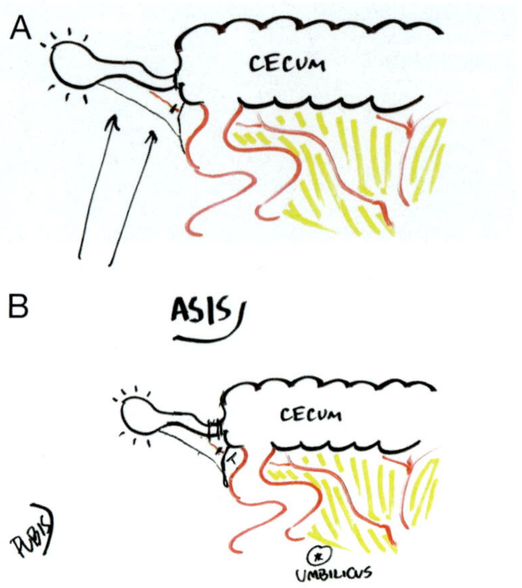

VIDEO 2.5. Surgical Intervention for Appendicitis. A, Laparoscopic. B, Open.

Transcript A: For a laparoscopic appendectomy, the camera port slides in and we look to the right side of the abdomen. We see the cecum, we see the mesentery, we likely won't see the right colic or the ileocolic artery, but we will see the ileum into the ileocecal valve, and this appendix will be down in the right lower quadrant. To take out an appendix, you basically have to divide the base and the appendiceal artery. So simplistically, laparoscopic graspers come in from the side and transect the base of the appendix and the appendiceal artery. That leads to a straightforward laparoscopic appendectomy.

Transcript B: An open appendectomy means that we are going to put an incision on the abdomen, maybe several inches, ideally centered over the base of the appendix. The umbilicus, the anterior superior iliac spine, about halfway in the middle—a curvilinear incision, what is called a McBurney's incision or at McBurney's point. We are going to divide through skin, fatty tissue, external oblique, internal oblique, and the transversalis fascia. Now where is the appendix? Sometimes it is sitting up in the breeze and easy to see and to take out. Other times you are going to need to find the ileum, pull up that ileum and find that little fat pad, the so-called ligament of Treves. It is on the anamesenteric border on the ileum, just before it goes into the ileocecal valve. From there you know where the cecum is and the appendix. Getting a clamp around this, clamp, clamp, cut and tie and look for that appendiceal artery. It will need to be clamped and tied off. The appendix comes out easily at that point. It is a straightforward operation. It is a little bit more painful than a laparoscopic procedure, but sometimes it is truly necessary and an easy operation as well. The most difficult appendectomies become when the appendix is retrocecal, and we have to mobilize the cecum. But when in doubt with an open appendectomy, if you can't find it, find the small bowel, follow the ileum to this fat pad, the ligament of Treves, and that will let you know right where the base of the appendix is.

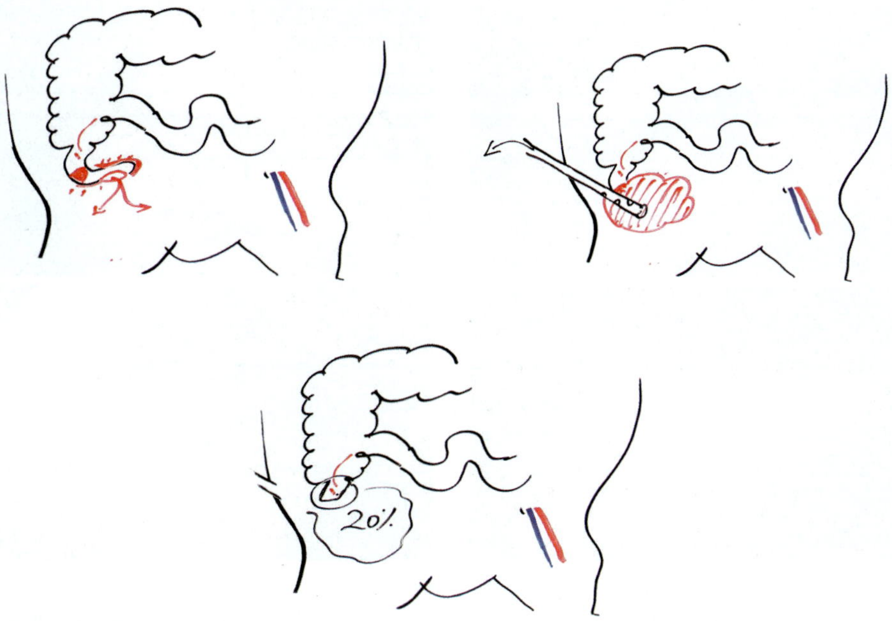

VIDEO 2.6. Interval Appendectomy.
Transcript: Appendicitis doesn't always present with right lower quadrant pain, and people don't know that they have appendicitis. Sometimes the diagnosis is missed. Sometimes stoic people will sit at home for days or weeks. A fecalith blocks things off; the appendix gets inflamed. It inflames so much that the blood supply to the wall no longer exists. If that is the case, it will perforate—so-called perforated appendicitis. There is a hole in the appendix and with that, depending on the communication, there may be stool or succus that is out into the abdomen. When this happens, typically people get what is called a periappendiceal abscess or phlegmon and there is all sorts of material and bacteria. People may actually contain this and feel better over a course of days to weeks. But there are times when people are miserably sick with sepsis. When we see people days to weeks after appendicitis, the treatment for this initially, is percutaneous drainage. We need to get a drainage tube inside of that abscess and let that material come out. This will defervesce folks, the white counts will drop, and they will be fitter and healthier.

At that point, the contemplation becomes that with this abscess cavity now taken care of, do we need to go back in and take care of what is left of the appendix? Historically, surgeons would say yes; 6 weeks later that needs to be taken out. There is more and more data to suggest antibiotics, drainage placement, people get better. Then we sit and watch and try to decide which people need an interval appendectomy. I think as many as 20% of people who have this problem will have another problem with the appendix. So when you talk to your patients you've got to say that there is a 4 chance in 5 that we may never have to do anything with it. In some folks that is good enough and some folks say let's go back and take this out. But, it is never easy after this abscess has been here. The scarring and adhesions make surgery more difficult. So interval appendectomy is a controversial problem and currently treated with IV antibiotics and drainage and then careful assessment between the patient and their surgeon.

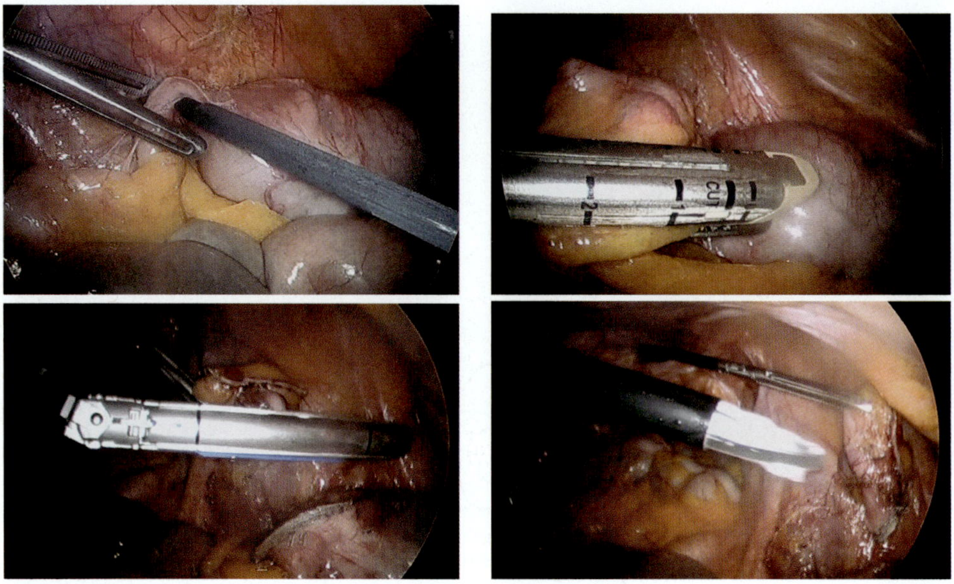

VIDEO 2.7. Laparoscopic Appendectomy: Intraoperative.
Transcript: We have the port in at the umbilicus and we are looking in the right lower quadrant. See the ileopsoas muscle to the top left, we see the cecum to the right, we see appendix sneaking down underneath. Interestingly enough, this patient will have a mass on the tip of the appendix, a benign adenoma, a growth. But right now, bowel grasper in the left hand, hook cautery in the right, trying to find the appendix, the base of it. There it is coming off the bottom side of the cecum, where the taenia coli come together, that will be the base of the appendix.

So now what the surgeon is trying to do is dissect the mesoappendix being careful, there is an appendiceal artery there, but usually it is not right by the base. Trying to create a little hole through here, and it lets us know that now we are through there and we could cut that base and then eventually cut the blood supply and take that appendix out. So we have got the base exposed and then we clean up a little bit more and find out that there is a blood vessel going into that appendix, the appendiceal artery, and the ileocecal vessel.

We have a stapling device that will deploy 3 rows of staplers and cut in between. It is hemostatic and it also transects the mesoappendix. Voila, it is divided. Well almost, there is just a tiny little remnant there at the end. But now with the mesoappendix divided, we can take the base of the appendix. Some people do this in a different order, they take the base first. It doesn't really matter. Here is an articulating stapling device. The surgeon is changing the angle and trying to get straight across that base and they have done a nice job transecting it right at the base of the cecum.

Now we have got an appendix with a little mass in it, it is benign, and we are going to put it in a little bag and pull it out through a little incision. This is the kind of an operation that patients can go home later that afternoon. You need to make sure that everything is a-okay though, for a hot appendix, we do not want to leave pus or bacteria behind and irrigate out; we double check and make sure that there is no bleeding. Look at the stump and make sure that the staples are exactly as we want them. Some extra staples there; we can wash those out and get rid of them.

Appendix Challenge Questions

2.1. When is a right hemicolectomy performed for an appendiceal carcinoid?
2.2. What is the Alvarado score?
2.3. What are taeniae coli? Why are they important?
2.4. What percentage of people have acute appendicitis in their lifetimes?
2.5. In which part of the appendix are most carcinoids typically found?
2.6. What CT findings are important to favor nonoperative therapy?
2.7. What may have been the cause of Harry Houdini's death?
2.8. Is antibiotic therapy useful for appendicitis?
2.9. After drainage of an appendiceal abscess, is interval appendectomy mandatory?
2.10. Who is Reginald Fitz?
2.11. What is an Amyand hernia?

Answers to Appendix Challenge Questions

2.1. When the size is greater than 2 cm or the tumor is located at the base of the cecum.
2.2. Scoring system used to diagnose appendicitis.
2.3. Longitudinal bands (outer muscular layer) that coalesce at the cecum at the appendiceal base; their contraction forms haustra.
2.4. Five percent to 8%.
2.5. Tip of appendix (70%).
2.6. Mild inflammation of appendix and void of a fecalith.
2.7. Perforated appendicitis following a blow to the abdomen.
2.8. Yes.
2.9. No, but appendicitis can recur (20%).
2.10. United States pathologist who first described appendicitis.
2.11. Appendix within an indirect inguinal hernia.

3

Biliary Tree

Embryology

The biliary tree forms in the endodermal diverticulum of the caudal foregut.

Anatomy

The left and right hepatic ducts drain the hepatic sinusoids and join to form the CHD, which joins the cystic duct to form the CBD (Figure 3.1). The CBD joins the pancreatic duct to empty into the duodenum at the ampulla of Vater (Figure 3.2).

Physiology

Hepatocytes produce bile, which passes through ducts and empties into the CHD and into the GB for storage. Cholecystokinin stimulates the GB to contract and push bile out the cystic duct, through the CBD, past the ampulla of Vater, and into the duodenum to aid lipid digestion and absorption.

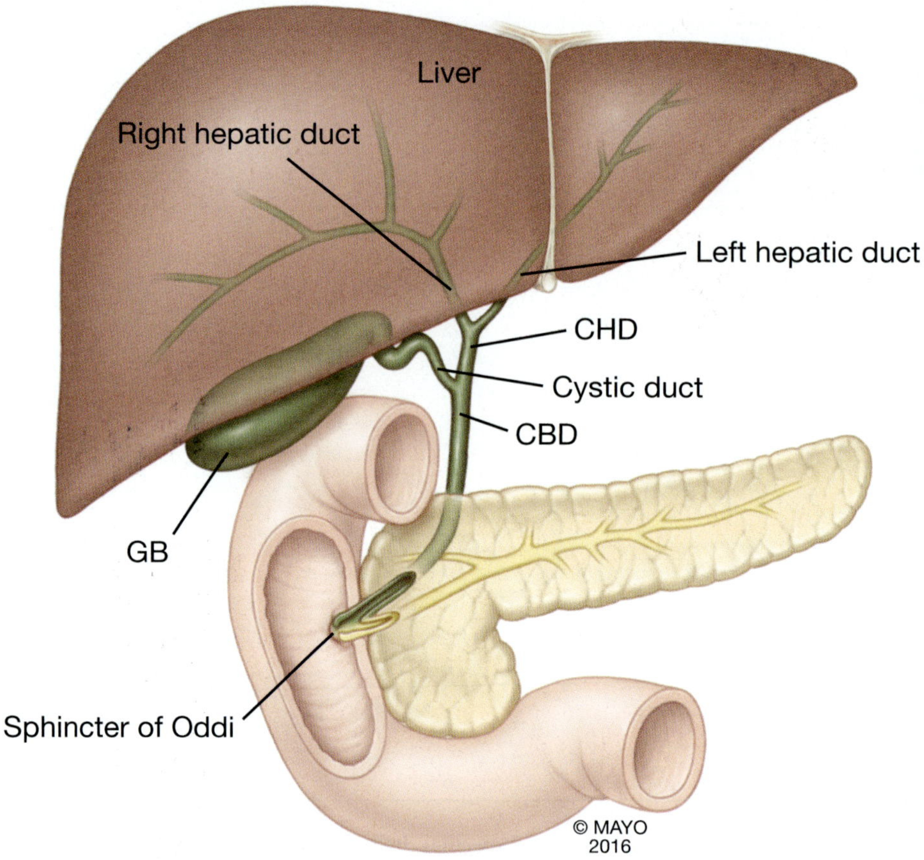

FIGURE 3.1. Anatomy of the Biliary Tree.

Clinical Presentation

Small gallbladder stones occasionally descend into the CBD (choledocholithiasis); if the cystic duct is large, stones can be of any size. Blockage of the CHD or CBD leads to icterus and jaundice (Video 3.1). Cholangitis is likely with RUQ pain, jaundice, and fever (Charcot triad; Video 3.2) and may progress to Reynolds pentad (add hypotension and mental status change). CBD stones result in biliary stasis and bacterial proliferation. Other causes of cholangitis include biliary strictures (usually iatrogenic) or cholangiocarcinoma. Most cholangiocarcinomas occur in the CBD and are ACAs. Conditions predisposing to such rare cancers include gallstones, sclerosing cholangitis, and cystic dilatations of bile ducts. Periampullary tumors (Video 3.3) are usually ACAs; patients often present with painless jaundice.

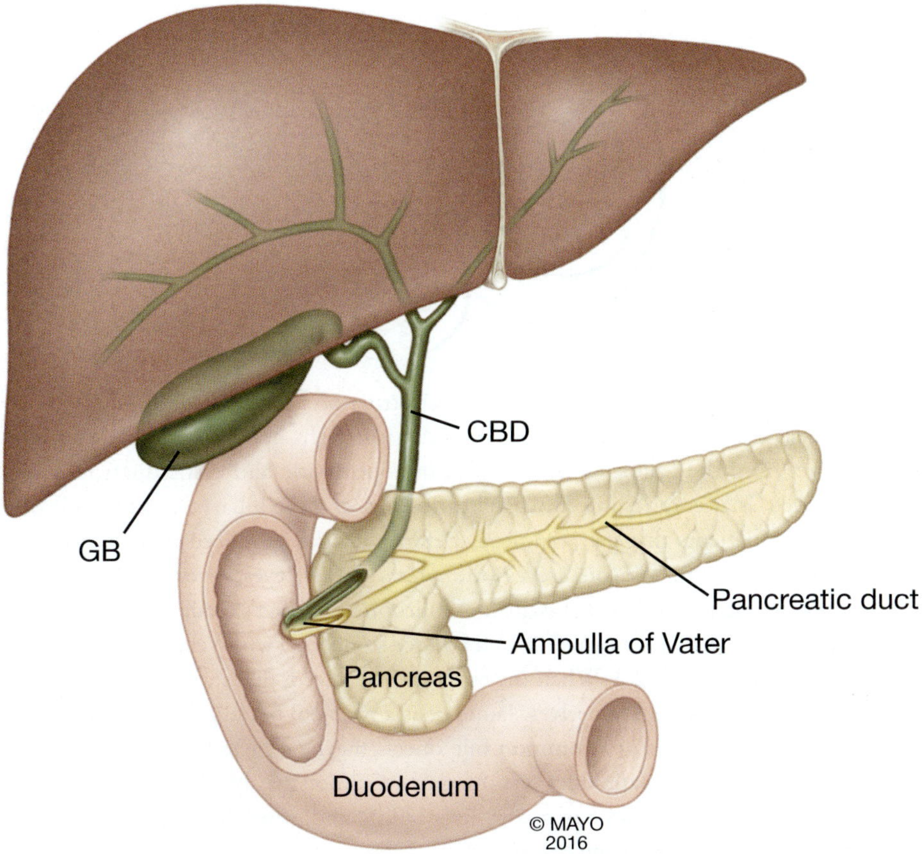

FIGURE 3.2. Anatomy of the Pancreatic Duct and Ampulla of Vater.

Imaging

Dilatation of the CHD (>4 mm) or CBD (>7 mm) is diagnosed with US (Video 3.4). Patients may be evaluated or undergo percutaneous transhepatic cholangiography (Video 3.5) or ERCP (Video 3.6) depending on the level of obstruction. MRI can be used to locate cholangiocarcinomas or further define biliary anatomy.

Operation

Patients with cholangitis should be resuscitated, given broad-spectrum antibiotics, and have the biliary tree drained with ERCP in preparation for cholecystectomy. Gallstones can be extracted using endoscopy with sphincterotomy (Video 3.7) and basket retrieval. The choice of operation for cholangiocarcinoma (Video 3.8) depends on the location: bile duct resection (with or without hepatectomy) with hepaticojejunostomy (Videos 3.9 and 3.10) for proximal tumors or a Whipple procedure (Video 3.8) for distal lesions. Repair of a bile duct injury is required in 1 in 200 laparoscopic cholecystectomies.

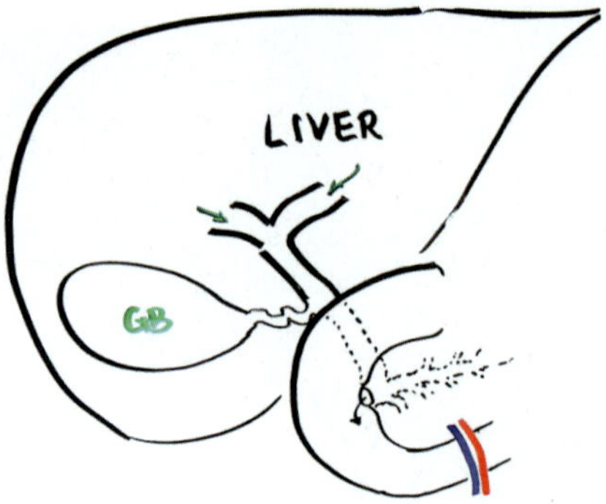

VIDEO 3.1. Anatomy of Biliary Tree and Causes of Its Obstruction.
Transcript: The biliary tree involves the left hepatic duct, the right hepatic duct, the common hepatic duct, the cystic duct from the gallbladder, and the common hepatic and cystic ducts join and become the common bile duct. That empties into the pancreatic duct, and the biliary contents slide out through the ampulla. You'll see patients that get jaundiced. Before they get jaundiced they become icteric; that is a brownish-yellowish hint in someone's eyes (the white of their eyes becomes yellow). The normal bilirubin in a human being is less than 1.0 mg/dL of bilirubin, and that's made up of direct and indirect components; anything less than 1 is normal. When you see somebody with yellowness in their eyes, their bilirubin will typically be 2.1, 2.2, 2.3. When they become jaundiced, that's when you'll see it in the skin, that's when you'll see them itching themselves. Jaundice is a problem because typically it will mean some sort of blockage (for a surgeon) of the common bile duct—maybe a huge blockage or huge stone that swells and blocks the common hepatic duct or some sort of tumor that blocks this pathway. Jaundice is a common problem. It sometimes can occur with liver failure and other disorders, but for surgeons, we have to think about the biliary tree being obstructed.

Complications

ERCP can result in hemorrhage, injury to the duodenum, and pancreatitis. Patients having a Whipple procedure are prone to anastomotic leaks. Bile duct anastomoses rarely leak. CBD injuries do occur with cholecystectomy and require a Roux-en-Y hepaticojejunostomy for repair.

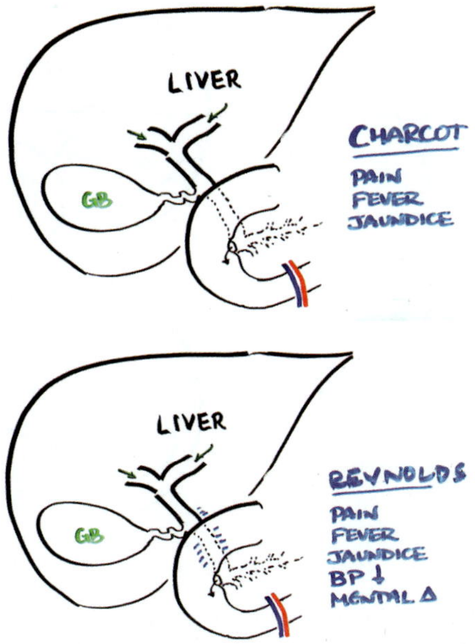

VIDEO 3.2. Charcot Triad and Reynolds Pentad.
Transcript: Charcot was a French neurologist that hypothesized that right upper quadrant pain, fever, and jaundice had to be due to some sort of a stone in the common bile duct. Charcot's triad is a dangerous problem. Basically, stones or tumors in this region back things up. There is swelling, and with infection (with bacteria) people get 3 separate problems. Nowadays, (in modern medicine), when you get right upper quadrant pain, fever, and jaundice, you have to think about Charcot's triad being a source of a biliary problem—what's called cholangitis, inflammation of this biliary tree. It swells and people get septic from this. It's not always due to a stone as it was in Charcot's day in the 1800s. More importantly, there are other things that can happen when people get septic. The blood pressure can drop, and people can get mental status changes, and this is not Charcot's triad—this is what's called Reynolds pentad. So when things go bad with the common bile duct, cholangitis is a serious problem. You need to relieve the obstruction, treat with antibiotics, and carefully assess whether or not surgery is indicated.

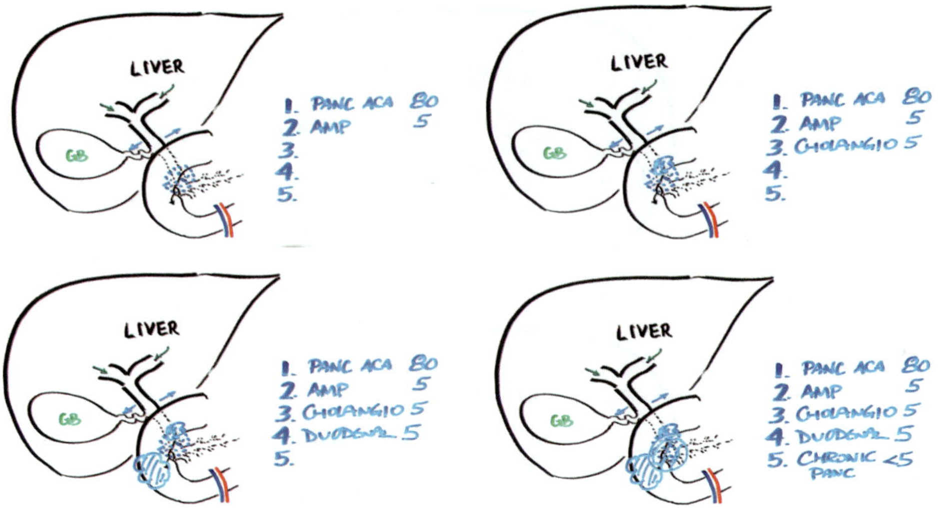

VIDEO 3.3. Periampullary Tumors.

Transcript: From time to time we see patients that come to us with painless jaundice (no abdominal pain, not like cholangitis, but they're jaundiced), and workup will reveal some sort of a mass near the ampulla of Vater. What happens is this mass grows over time and blocks the bile duct, and the bile duct will swell and get big and eventually back up, and now we have someone with jaundice. And so the question is, what is it that's blocking the ampulla? If we had 100 patients with painless jaundice, the number one problem, unfortunately, is pancreatic adenocarcinoma, a ductal adenocarcinoma. I would say roughly 80% of all patients with painless jaundice will have that, maybe even more.

What else could obstruct this biliary tree and pancreatic region? The ampulla itself could be a cancerous spot, so an ampullary tumor or an ampullary cancer. Maybe no more than 5% of patients will have this. This is a good tumor to have because it may be curable and it's right at the ampulla, so people will present sooner with their symptoms. What other structures can block? Well, we've got a bile duct. What if there was a tumor in the bile duct? That's what's called a cholangiocarcinoma, and again, it is fairly rare and uncommon, less than 5% of the time. What else is in this region? A duodenal tumor, a cancer of the intestine itself, could block off this ampulla, and again, probably no more than 5% of the time. What about the rest of the tumors? There are mucinous tumors of the pancreas. Sometimes the tumor isn't cancer, it's chronic pancreatitis and ideally not a great disease to have, but it's not a malignancy, and so if we can get that out of there with what's called a Whipple operation, a mass in the head of the pancreas, and we remove the head, the duodenum, gallbladder, and the common bile duct, that person can be cured from their problems. These are the periampullary tumors that we think about.

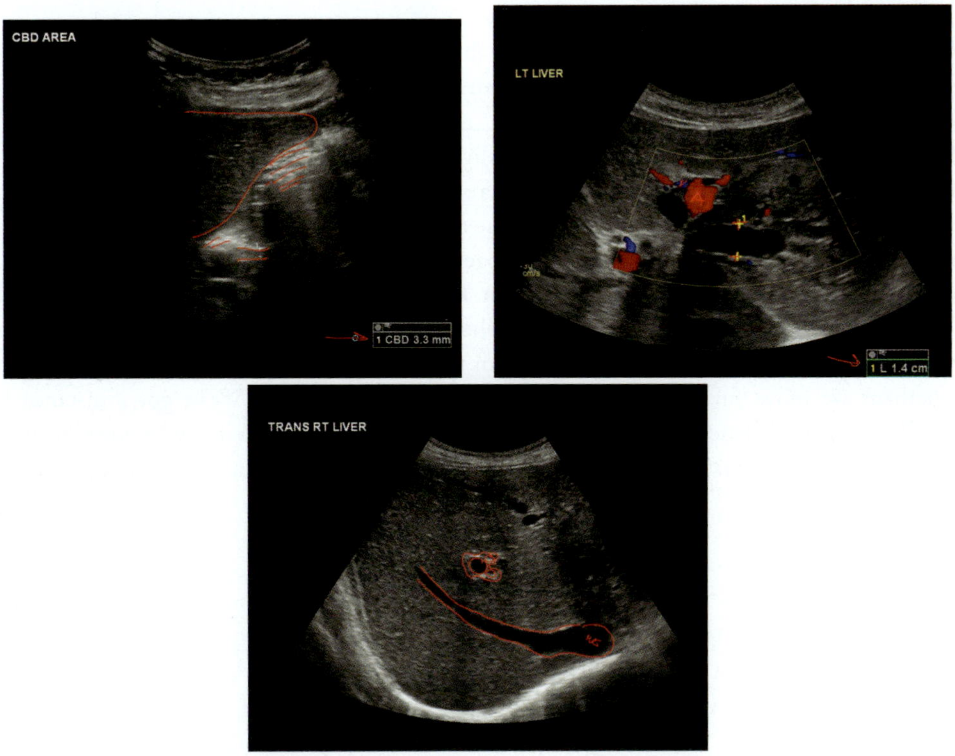

VIDEO 3.4. US of Biliary Tree.

Transcript: One of the best tests we have for looking at the biliary tree is ultrasound. You lay the probe on the skin; sound waves bounce down and they bounce and hit structures. Here they hit the liver; here they hit air. Air is terrible, makes it hard to see. But an ultrasound tech can utilize this and say, "This is a liver. And we can see some blood vessels in here." But they can also put their cursor (and they've got them marked nicely here) and they're measuring it for us—common hepatic duct, 2 mm. That should be 4 mm or less, so this is a normal ultrasound looking at somebody's biliary tree.

Again, we see liver here. Why does it look like it does here? There's probably air, it's hard to see. But there's the bile duct, the common bile duct, and again, the technician has said 3.3. Most everybody's common bile duct is less than 7 mm. Sometimes if you have your gallbladder removed, the common bile duct gets bigger, to a centimeter or so. But these are 2 normal ultrasound pictures.

Let's take a look at some other pictures. Again, the probe on the skin, abdominal wall, and then we see the liver underneath here. This is all liver parenchyma. But what we see on the inside are bile ducts that are far bigger than they should be. Anything inside the liver that's a bile duct should be less than 2 mm. These are actually far bigger than that. This person has a problem. If the bile ducts are big, it's likely blocked downstream, there's something stopping that, and that could be a cancer, a cholangiocarcinoma, a pancreas cancer.

Let's take a look at another picture. Here we see the duct is bigger than it should be. This is a Doppler flow. We see arterial flow and venous flow, but they've measured it out for us here. What is it? It's 1.4 cm. It's way too big. If this is the common bile duct, it's too big. If it's in the liver, it's definitely too big. It's likely obstructed. The question is, from what?

Nice picture here. When you're struggling to look at the liver, any time you see whitish, sclerotic things, that's usually part of the portal triad. Three things go together. What are they? Hepatic artery, portal vein, and common bile duct. They come together and we'll have this little whitish thickening. And so usually

VIDEO 3.4. Continued

when we look inside the liver and we see that, we think about the bile duct because it tends to be obstructed and has the white thing around it. These things are a little bit bigger than they should be. Likely somebody has an obstruction.

Taking another picture. Whitish structure, typically the portal triad; we've got a couple different things that run together—artery, bile duct, and vein. There is also another structure in the liver, and this is a normal picture of what is likely the vena cava and the right hepatic vein. You don't have quite that whitish material around it because the 3 things don't run together.

Another picture; another sense of what's going on. Liver, looks fine up here. This, without any obvious sclerotic thing around it, is likely the hepatic vein. They've measured for us the distance, common hepatic duct, 5 mm. It really should be 4 or less. I'm nervous there's an obstruction somewhere along the line.

And perhaps we move further downstream and our tech says, "Yep. We've got a distance here of 7.8 mm." There is an obstruction, and we get a sense that maybe there is some backing up inside the liver, there's congestion or obstruction, likely from cholangiocarcinoma, pancreatic cancer, or some other source.

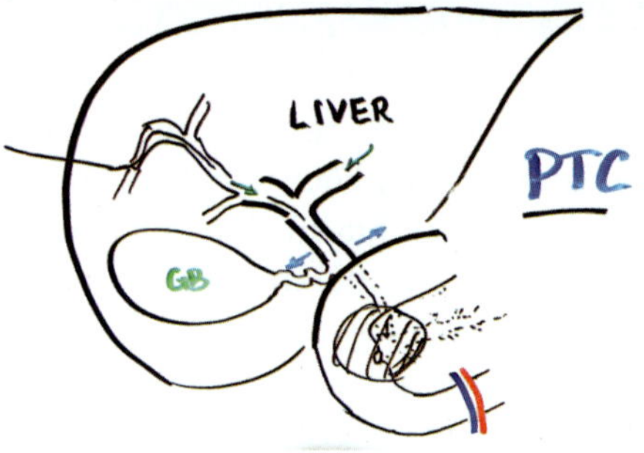

VIDEO 3.5. Percutaneous Transhepatic Cholangiography.

Transcript: Percutaneous transhepatic cholangiography is a diagnostic and useful test that intervenes, with a radiologist typically putting a needle into the liver and sampling it to see if they can find a portion of the biliary tree. They get that little needle in and draw that tissue back, the fluid back, and find bile and then thread a wire down this tree, and they can put a catheter in the biliary tree. This is useful from time to time when people have large tumors that we can't put a scope through or sneak a stent through, to drain and decompress someone that either has cholangitis or terrible jaundice. Getting that bilirubin level dropped down before surgery is useful. Percutaneous transhepatic cholangiography. It means a needle through the abdominal wall, the skin, into the abdomen, into the liver, finding a tiny little bile duct, passing a wire through and then a catheter further along. Sometimes we do this when there's a bile duct injury after a gallbladder surgery or tumors that need to be drained or sometimes palliative to get the bile out of there. PTC.

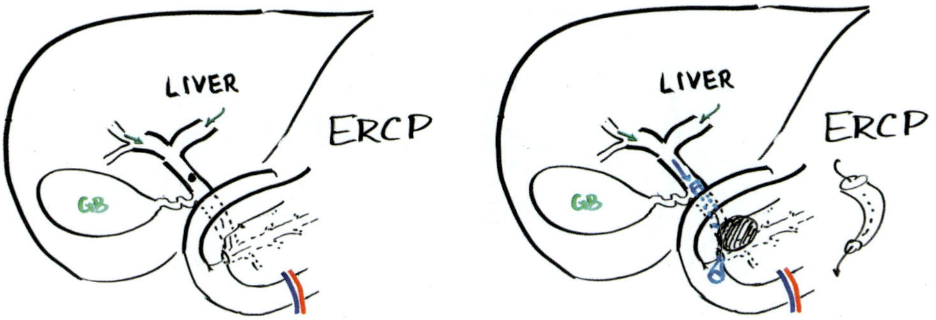

VIDEO 3.6. ERCP.

Transcript: Endoscopic retrograde cholangiopancreatography is a test where a scope is placed through the mouth, down the esophagus, through the stomach, into the intestine, the duodenum, and then with gadgetry sliding in catheters either to the pancreatic duct or, more commonly, the common bile duct. This can be done for a variety of reasons. It can be therapeutic or diagnostic. If you had a stone trapped in the common hepatic duct, you could take the ERCP, the gadgetry, the gastroenterologist and family docs and surgeons can insert a catheter up and basket that and pull the stone out and alleviate that blockage. You can imagine if we have someone with painless jaundice and the start of a tumor here, it's not due to stones but it's due to a cancer, if somebody has a bilirubin of 20 and needs a Whipple operation. A bilirubin of 20 means the liver is not functioning well, they won't clot very well. Their platelets and their ability to coagulate will be off. If you could place a catheter past that, put a stent, a straw if you will, that allows that bile to sneak through the stent and out. This would be very beneficial, so this happens frequently that we put a stent in and it comes out through the ampulla, and even though the cancer is still there, the bile now gets to go through the stent, and someone, instead of having a bilirubin of 20 or 25 or 30, after a few days this bilirubin will drop down to 2 or 3 or 4 and make them much safer for surgery. ERCP has been a fantastic change over the last 20 or 30 years, allowing us to take care of benign problems, strictures, and then tumors in this region.

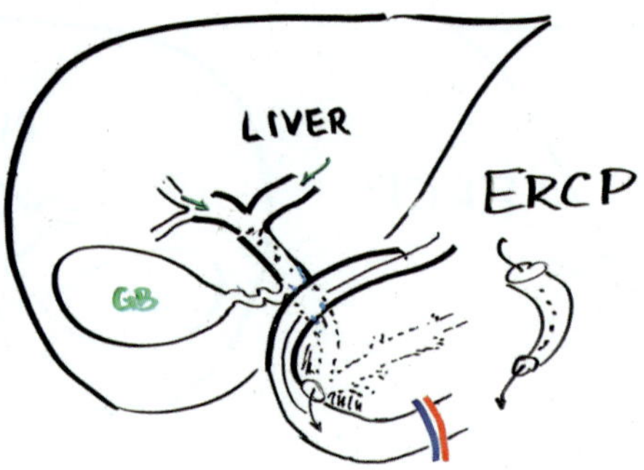

VIDEO 3.7. Sphincterotomy.

Transcript: We've tried putting a stent in the biliary tree. When we put the endoscope in, we can also open this hole, what's called a sphincterotomy. This is the sphincter of Oddi, the ampulla of Vater, and basically cut this open so it's a bigger opening, and whether that helps put the stent in to let bile pass or there's no stent at all, maybe there are a couple simple little stones that we couldn't basket, and if we make this opening bigger, the stones will freely flow out. So this is what's called a sphincterotomy. Now, it has side effects. When you cut this sphincter (this is all pancreas tissue here), when you cut the pancreas, you can develop pancreatitis. Maybe 10% of people get pancreatitis with a sphincterotomy, and a percentage of those, 1%, 2%, 3%, may actually meet their maker because of severe pancreatitis. So we have to think long and hard about doing a sphincterotomy, whether or not that's important, but in some cases it's very nice to open things up and allow the biliary tree to drain. It helps treat cholangitis, it gets rid of gallstones, and it allows stents or other instrumentation through the tree to be done a little bit easier.

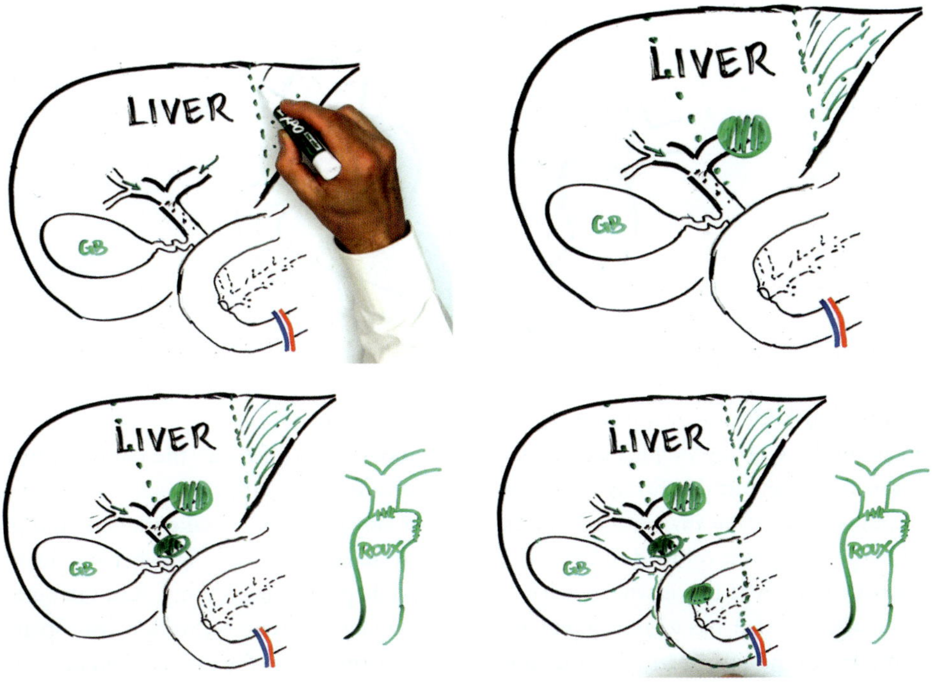

VIDEO 3.8. Roux Limb and Whipple Procedures for Cholangiocarcinoma.
Transcript: Cholangiocarcinoma is, fortunately, a rare tumor because oftentimes it will have metastasis within the liver that makes it unresectable. If it is resectable, several different operations can be necessary to remove the tumor. If it's a peripheral lesion, so-called intrahepatic cholangiocarcinoma, then removing a portion of the liver—maybe the left lateral sector—would be fortuitous to get rid of the cancer if there are no other tumors elsewhere. If we had a tumor within the left hepatic duct that was fairly large but didn't involve the common hepatic or common bile duct, we could do what's called a left hepatectomy; this entire portion of the gland can be removed. The neat thing about the liver is that it will regenerate. We can do the same thing on the other side. If we had a tumor on the right, we could do a right hepatectomy. If the tumor is located in the common hepatic duct, it's possible to remove the common hepatic duct as long as the margins are negative on either side, take out the gallbladder, and bring up a Roux limb. The Roux limb comes up to the bile duct and is sewn in place, and this is what's called a Roux limb. R-O-U-X, a Swiss surgeon from long ago. And this is what's called a hepaticojejunostomy, that anastomosis would be here. If the tumor itself is located in the common bile duct, invariably this involves a Whipple operation; again, if and only if this is resectable. So the gallbladder comes out, the bile duct comes out, common hepatic tumor comes out and the head of the pancreas, and then we're left to put this together (what's called a Whipple operation), but invariably people talk about ideal form—taking part of the liver out—and that's being done with a cholangiocarcinoma. If it's high up in the bifurcation, so-called a Klatskin tumor, we can oftentimes bring up a Roux limb and sew it to the common hepatic duct.

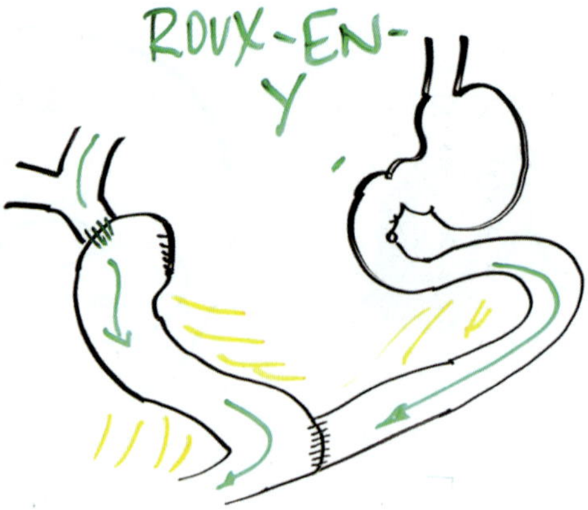

VIDEO 3.9. Roux-en-Y Hepaticojejunostomy.
Transcript: If you look at my esophagus, stomach, and duodenum, normally the common bile duct is here, with the liver here, but this funny little drawing I've made what's called a Roux-en-Y gastrojejunostomy. Basically, what that means is we cut the small bowel downstream, we take that cut and pull it up to this region, but I've got it zoomed in here. This is the left hepatic duct, the right hepatic duct, and the common hepatic duct. And this is what's called a Roux-en-Y hepaticojejunostomy. And so you bring this loop of bowel up here that has a good blood supply with a good mesentery; we sew this opening wide open so that bile can sneak through, and that bile will join the intestine, the gastric contents, the pancreatic juices, that will slide downstream. So a Roux-en-Y hepaticojejunostomy is a clever way that surgeons have put in tissue to drain the bile duct. The problem is the duodenum is fixed, it's retroperitoneal, and you can't just move it up. It's not very far away, just a couple centimeters, but the truth is we need to go downstream, cut the bowel, bring up the limb, and then sew what's called a side-to-side jejunojejunostomy together so that the patient can eat and drink and yet the bile does come down into the GI tract.

Biliary Tree Challenge Questions

3.1. What are the risk factors for developing CBD gallstones?
3.2. Which antibiotic causes sludging and cholestatic jaundice?
3.3. Which bacteria are most commonly associated with cholangitis?
3.4. How should the CBD be incised?
3.5. What is the Bismuth-Corlette classification of perihilar cholangiocarcinoma?
3.6. When do ducts look "beaded" on cholangiography?
3.7. Where are the blood vessels of the CBD?
3.8. Why does laparoscopic cholecystectomy put the CBD at risk of injury?
3.9. Where are the portal vein and proper hepatic artery located in relation to the CBD?
(Answers appear on page 40)

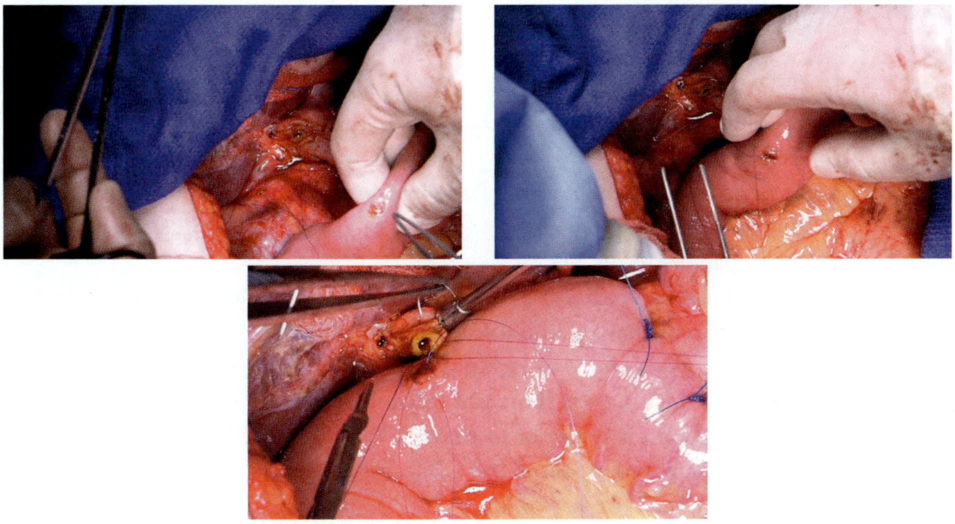

VIDEO 3.10. Hepaticojejunostomy: Intraoperative.

Transcript: This is a hepaticojejunostomy. There's a little hole in the jejunum. The surgeon is going to sew that hole to the hole in the common hepatic duct. It's right in the middle of the screen above where they're working. Fine suture, usually absorbable suture, sometimes Vicryl, sometimes Monocryl, sometimes PDS. The idea is you want something absorbable because the bile duct, if it's permanent, might develop stones and concretions. We can see the portal vein behind where they're working. The liver is underneath that blue towel. There's already been a pancreaticojejunostomy to the right. This is a hepaticojejunostomy. So little bites going inside the small bowel, that's right, inside, coming out through the bowel, and now, as we pull that thing through, we're going to try to get the same bite on the other side and match that up. Outside in, inside out; the idea is so that we're tying here with the knots on the outside. We don't really want knots on the inside. We've got things closer together, nice little bite, healthy bowel. That looks good. Big bite of the outside, but just a little bite of the mucosa. We don't want too much mucosa, but we do want it mucosa to mucosa. That's a nice bite. Fine little sutures magnified here. We want to make sure we sew this anastomosis open. Key thing for a good anastomosis is to make sure it's patent, it has a good blood supply, there's no tension, it's an air-tight seal, and there's no distal obstruction—5 key things.

So again, outside in, inside out. When we eventually tie this knot, that top will flip over the bottom. Sometimes if this hole is really small we'll put a stent into the hole and make sure—it's like a straw—to keep that thing wide open. The surgeon is now training and talking to his residents or his medical students to say, "Be careful now, don't twist that thing. We want to make sure we do it exactly right." He also may be talking about the blood supply. As we think of a clock, the blood on the hepatic duct comes from the 3-o'clock and 9-o'clock positions. So we want to make sure that we don't hurt the blood supply. Beautiful picture. Got gauze up above that's on the liver, probably being pushed by a retractor. That's nice; you don't want to traumatize things. Looks like we need to have another bite or 2 to put this together. That hepatic duct is maybe 3 or 4 mm wide at the most. Sixty-four sutures is too many, but 1 or 2 is too few. With experience, I think this surgeon is going to say, "Yep, I need one between that spot right there and the other two that we have there." If the duct is good enough and the anastomosis is done correctly, oftentimes we don't need a stent, but if we're nervous about how good the patency is, we'll put a little plastic tubing called a stent. This is a nice, safe, tension-free anastomosis. The bile duct tissue is made of good stuff; should be a great anastomosis.

Answers to Biliary Tree Challenge Questions

3.1. Genetics (Pima Indians, Alaskan Eskimos), sex (female), and demographics (obesity, elderly, after bypass surgery).
3.2. Ceftriaxone.
3.3. *Escherichia coli*, *Klebsiella*, *Pseudomonas*, *Enterobacter*, *Proteus*, *Serratia*, and *Enterococci*.
3.4. Incise parallel to the duct.
3.5. It is a classification based on the extent of ductal infiltration (Figure 3.3).
3.6. When patients have Caroli disease (Figure 3.4).
3.7. At the 3-o'clock and 9-o'clock positions.
3.8. The cystic duct may be short and inflammation may obscure the view.
3.9. The portal vein is posterior to the CBD. The proper hepatic artery typically runs along the superior aspect of the CBD (Figure 3.5).

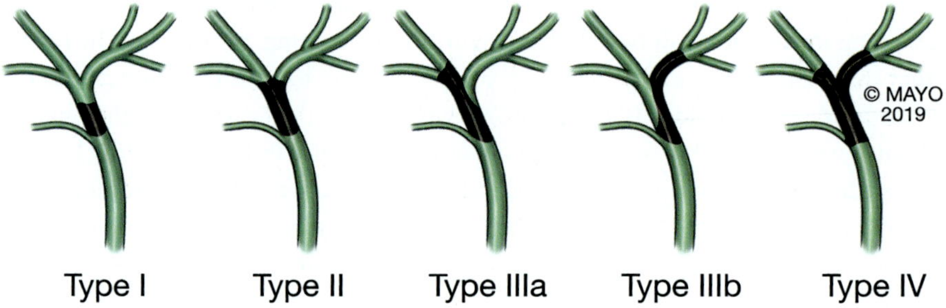

FIGURE 3.3. Bismuth-Corlette Classification.

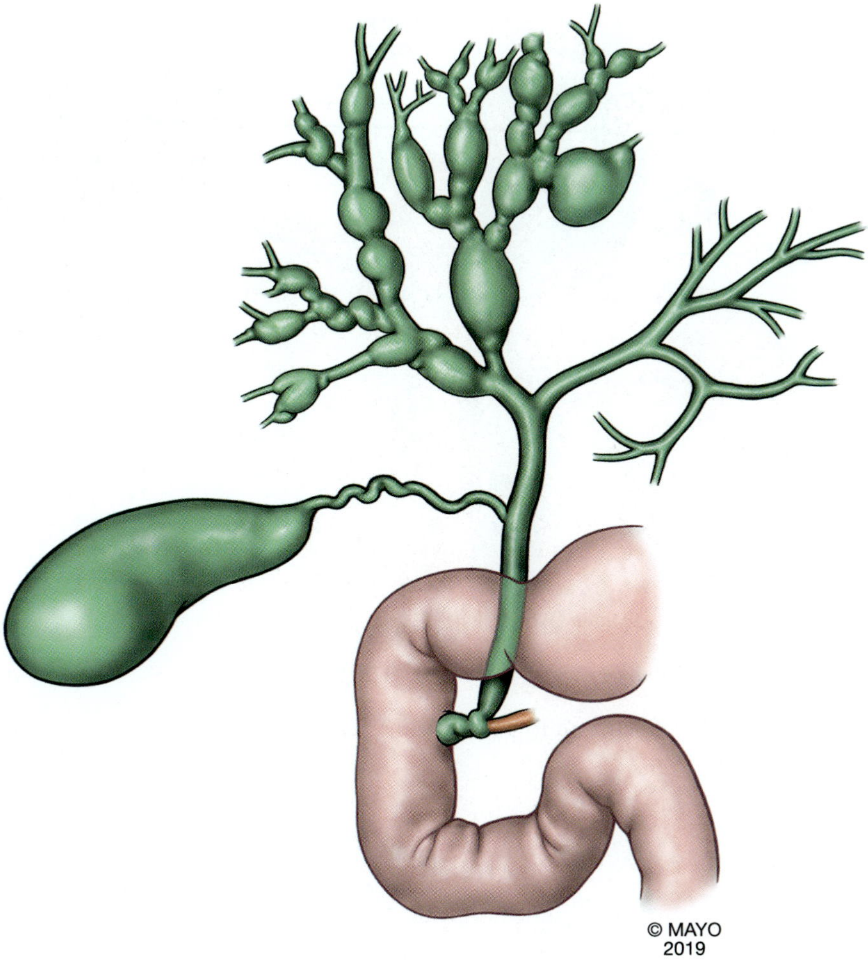

FIGURE 3.4. Caroli Disease.

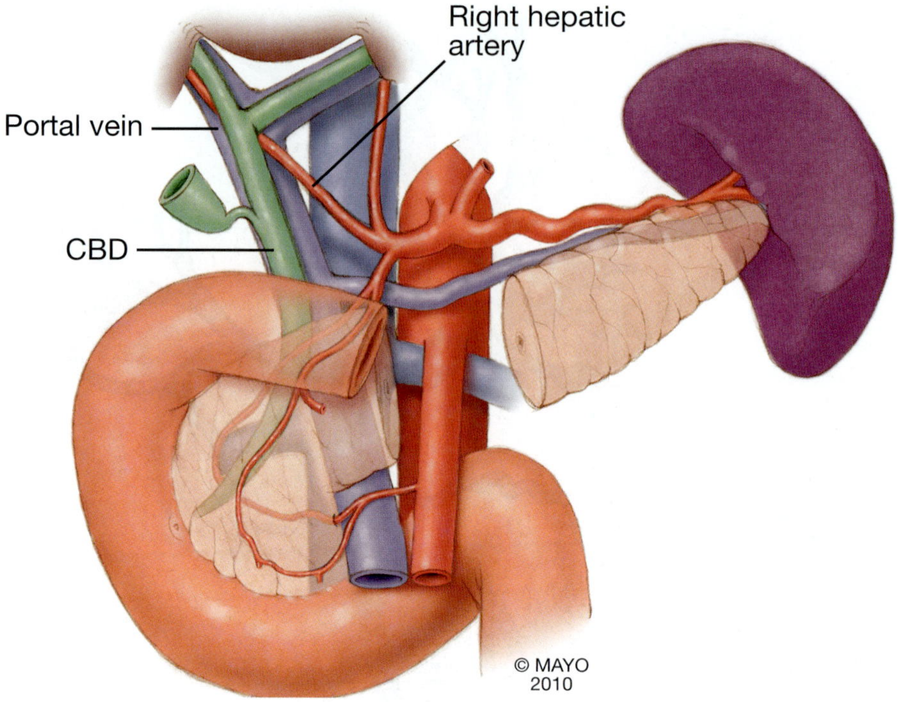

FIGURE 3.5. Anatomy of Portal Vein and Right Hepatic Artery.

4

Breast

Embryology

Breast tissue develops from ectoderm, the primary mammary buds being noted during the fifth week of gestation. Further development occurs as a result of hormonal or biochemical factors after birth.

Anatomy

Glandular epithelium, stroma, and fat receive blood from the internal mammary (Figure 4.1) and posterior intercostal arteries; intercostal, axillary, and internal mammary veins drain the breast. The axillary vein, long thoracic nerve, and thoracodorsal nerves (Figure 4.2) lie within the axilla (Video 4.1). The intercostobrachial nerves (Video 4.2) supply sensation to the upper, inner aspect of the arm; some surgeons attempt to preserve them during axillary dissection.

Physiology

In females, estrogen mediates ductal development. In males, androgen leads to destruction of the epithelial component of the breast bud. Oxytocin controls contraction of myoepithelial cells. Prolactin mediates the synthesis of milk.

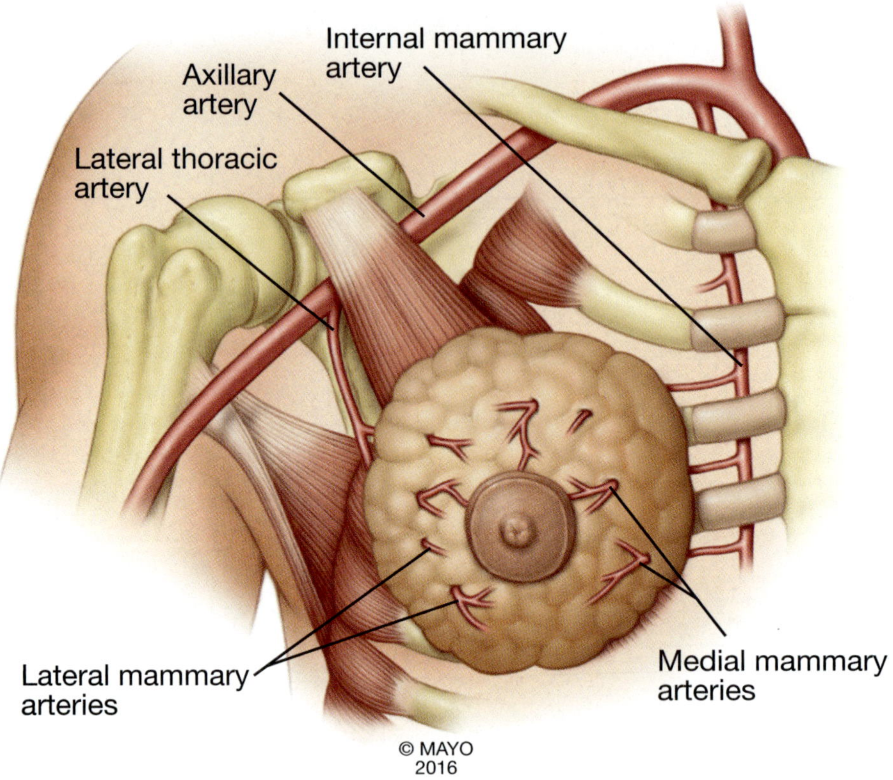

FIGURE 4.1. Anatomy of the Right Breast.

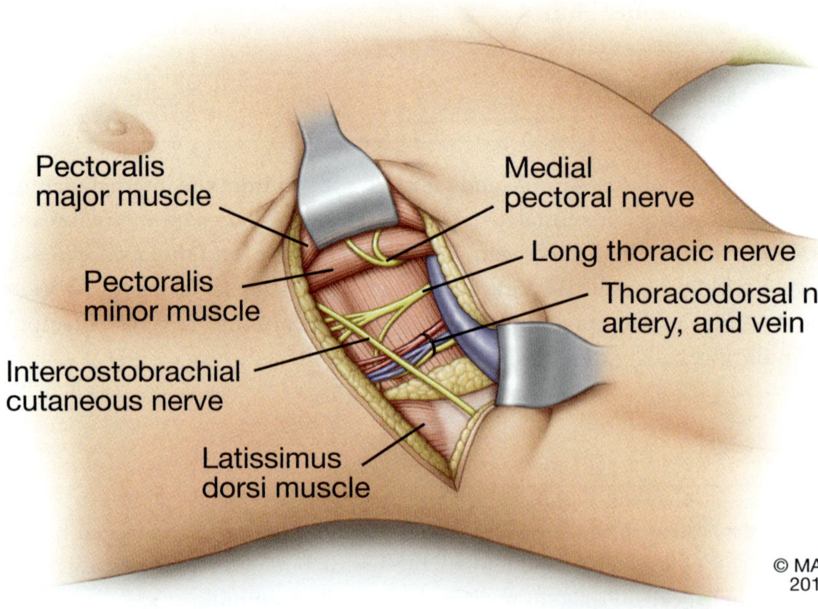

FIGURE 4.2. Anatomy of the Left Axilla.

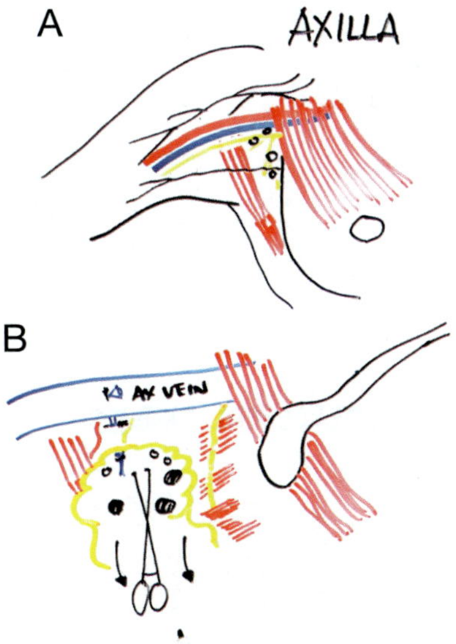

VIDEO 4.1. Anatomy of Axilla. A, Anatomic borders. B, Anatomy during resection.
Transcript A: The picture depicts the right breast and the right axilla with the right arm out. The anatomic boundaries of the axilla are bordered by the axillary vein cephalad. The axillary vein empties into the subclavian vein as the first rib sneaks below it. The latissimus dorsi is the lateral border that comes from the humerus to the attachments of the back and the chest sidewall. This axillary triangle is bordered by the pectoralis muscle, which inserts into the humerus and the chest wall. The axillary confines are axillary vein, latissimus dorsi, and the pectoralis muscle. Within this triangle, are lymphatics and lymph nodes, multiple little blood vessels, and at least 1 nerve, the intercostal brachial cutaneous, it's a sensory nerve to the upper inner arm.

Transcript B: Finding the long thoracic nerve, you need to find the serratus muscle; you need to know where the axillary vein is, putting a little gauze and lightly pulling on the serratus will show you the long thoracic underneath. There is a bit of chest wall fascia or pectoral fascia or serratus fascia that protects that long thoracic nerve. It's relatively hard to injure. The same is not said for the thoracodorsal nerve. That nerve can be consistently found by finding the axillary vein, tying the first thoracic vein, and then finding the second one, the deeper thoracic vein. Invariably that nerve will be right adjacent to it or just posterior to it. So in this little cartoon we're clearing out axilla, perhaps level 1 and level 2 is coming out with some sort of retraction pulling it out with some positive nodes. We've got latissimus dorsi on one side, we've got a posterior thoracic or thoracodorsal artery it's usually out of harm's way from the axilla. But find that second thoracic vein and you'll know where the thoracodorsal nerve is. And you'll want to stay just anterior to that as you peel that off, and you'll keep out of harm's way.

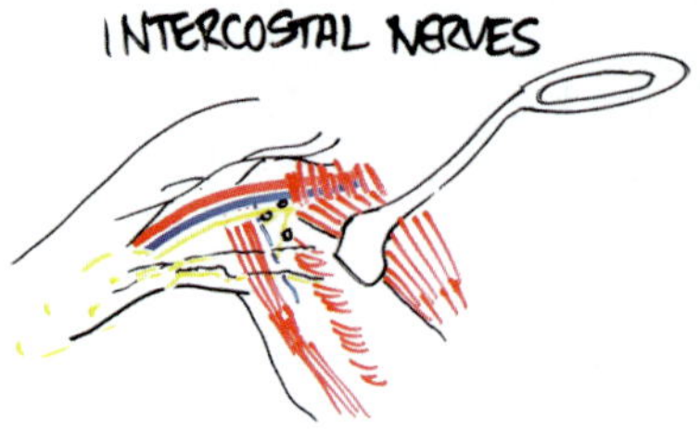

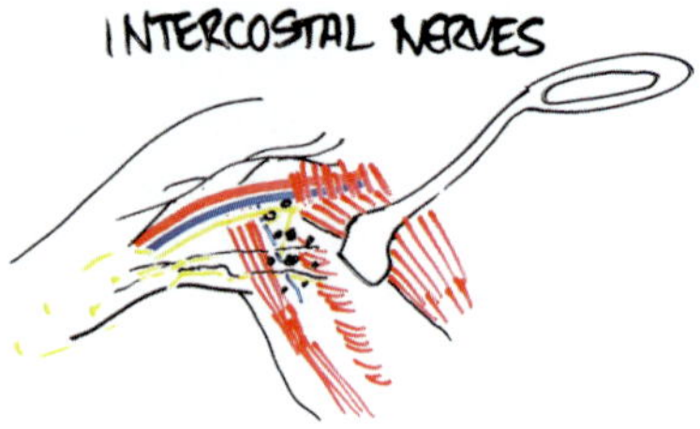

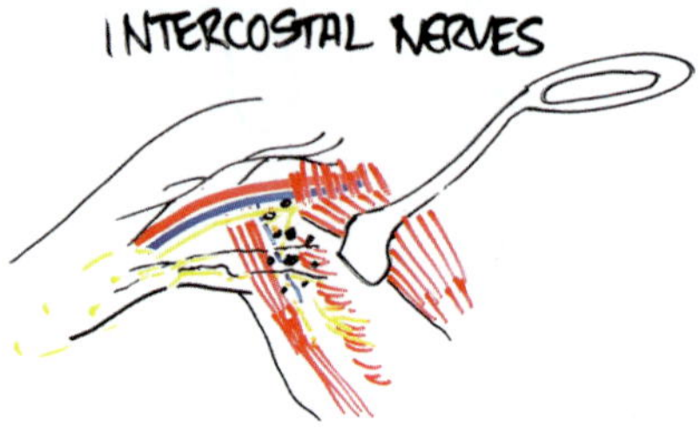

VIDEO 4.2. Intercostobrachial Nerves.
Transcript: Within the wound, a Richardson retractor retracts the pectoralis muscle to the side. We can see the serratus anterior muscle in skinny people. With better dissection we can see the latissimus dorsi muscle. Any nerve that crosses that barrier, going in a left to right manner is takeable; it's a sensory nerve; it's the intercostal nerve or intercostal brachial cutaneous nerve; and it goes by a variety of different forms. But it's this sucker right here and it tends to cause pain and discomfort if you cut it, a burning sensation, if you will, on the upper inner aspect of the arm. It's the medial portion of the arm. So if you can avoid doing that, that's great, but the problem is we find from time to time people, ladies especially, that have lymph nodes that have cancer, and we don't like to leave cancerous lymph nodes behind. Axillary dissection will take out these lymph nodes, oftentimes transect those intercostal brachial cutaneous nerves. The other nerve to be careful of in this region are nerves that run in this direction, the long thoracic which slides into the serratus and thoracodorsal nerve that innervates the latissimus dorsi. Those nerves are typically deeper and not in harm's way, like the intercostal brachial cutaneous nerve.

Clinical Presentation

Most breast complaints are due to a mass (eg, fibrocystic disease [Video 4.3], fibroadenomas [Video 4.4], cancer [Video 4.5]), nipple discharge, or pain. Although the majority of breast disease is benign, breast cancer develops in more than 200,000 women each year in the United States.

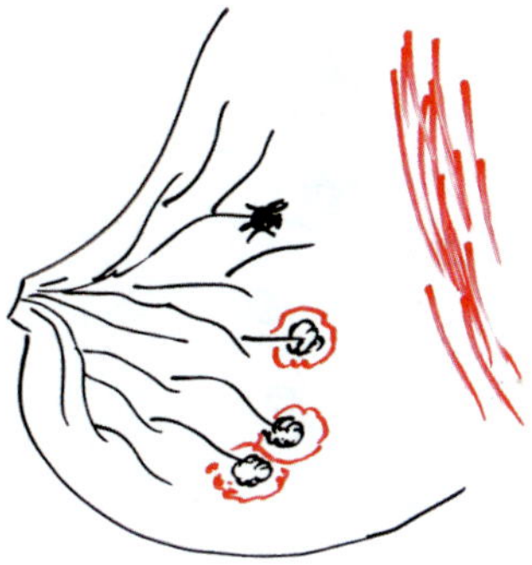

VIDEO 4.3. Fibrocystic Disease.
Transcript: Fibrocystic disease of the breast is very common. It occurs in females, usually ages 30 to 50, and it's mediated by estrogen. Invariably some sort of lobules at some point swell and create lumps and bumps that are palpable. Fibrocystic disease is typically not 1 lump. If there was a cancer, its firm and slowly gets bigger with time. Fibrocystic disease changes through a woman's menstrual cycle and is usually worse just before the menses—more tender and bigger masses. From time to time we find lumps and bumps that are concerning, and palpably so. The best test then would be an ultrasound to take a look and see a cystic mass. If there is any concern, a needle should be placed and tissues removed for cytology—aspirations. Sometimes removing the fluid will alleviate pain and discomfort, but invariably fibrocystic disease is a multiple ductal and lobule problem, and so aspirating each one of those doesn't make sense. Rarely do we use surgery for fibrocystic disease. If we're nervous about an underlying cancer, then perhaps surgical intervention is the treatment of choice. There are medications, including danazol, which helps with severe pain.

Imaging

US (Video 4.6) is useful in young women and as an adjunct to mammography (Video 4.7). Work-up of possible breast cancers may include MRI, positron emission tomography, or bone scanning. Core needle biopsy (Video 4.8) is often performed under US or mammographic guidance.

Operation

Wide local excision, mastectomy, sentinel lymph node biopsy (Video 4.9), and axillary dissection can be useful in men and women undergoing breast surgery. Breast-conserving therapy (Video 4.10) offers equivalent survival to simple mastectomy (Video 4.11) in patients with early-stage breast cancers. Mastectomy (with or without reconstruction) may be useful in women with large tumors, bilateral cancers, or genetic risk factors and in those preferring removal of all breast tissue (Video 4.12).

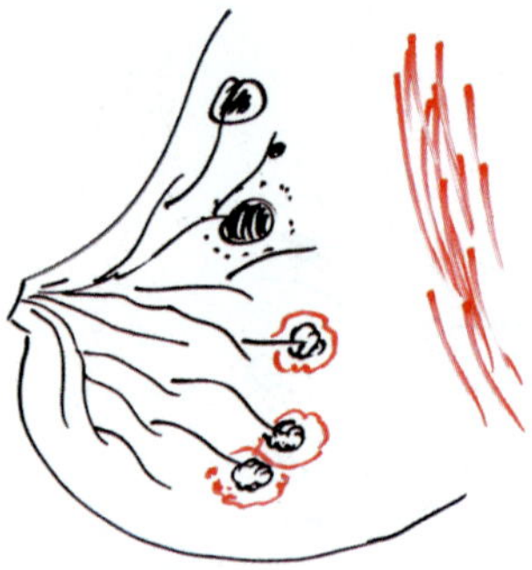

VIDEO 4.4. Fibroadenoma.
Transcript: Unlike fibrocystic disease, fibroadenomas are usually solitary. Having said that, they can come in all shapes and all sizes, but most women will feel them when they get to be 2 or 3 cm. They are palpable. They are typically round. They are firm, and every woman is concerned about an underlying cancer. When we feel lumps or bumps in women that are 15, 20, or 25 years old, fibroadenoma has got to be a number 1 differential diagnosis if it is a solitary bump. If there are multiple, then it is likely to be fibrocystic disease. Usually, the fibroadenoma is mobile. It's nontender; it's round, rubbery, and firm. No treatment is typically necessary, but if there is concern for malignancy, fine-needle aspiration can give us cytology; oftentimes we won't get many cells from these. Usually what mostly happens are adenomas become less problematic with time, or if they get to be 2 to 3 cm in size, we evacuate them with surgical intervention with resection.

Complications

Lymphedema (Figure 4.3) may occur after axillary lymph node dissection (Video 4.13) or radiation therapy (Video 4.14). Mastectomy complications include seroma, hematoma, infection, lymphedema, and nerve damage.

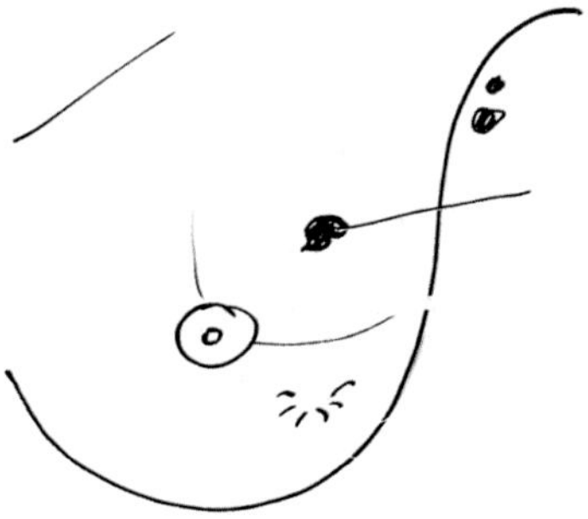

VIDEO 4.5. Breast Cancer.
Transcript: In the United States, 1 in 8 young girls born now will develop breast cancer in their lifetime. That turns out to about 250,000 women this year will develop breast cancer. Most of the breast tissue in a woman is in the upper outer quadrant, perhaps as much as 67% or 75% occurs in the upper outer quadrant. How do we know this lump is a breast cancer? The symptoms are not great. Thus, screening with mammogram is helpful, annual physical exam is helpful, and most importantly, monthly self-breast examination—a palpable mass.

If the mammogram is concerning, or there is anything suspicious, then a needle biopsy can get tissue cells and confirm or give us a sense that this is not an underlying cancer. The risk factor for this lump being a cancer is related to age. The greater the age, the more likely this is to be malignant. A family history, especially if the mother, sister, or daughter has had breast cancer, it increases risk slightly. The BRCA1 and BRCA2 genetic mutations are notorious for causing risks of breast cancer, as high as 70% or 80% in a woman. Families that have BRCA likely should have consideration for removing much, if not most of the breast tissue. A history of endometrial cancer, early menarche, or late menopause, meaning a longer effect of the underlying estrogen, increases the risk of a breast cancer.

As far as symptoms and size, there typically are none. But if the tumor is close to the skin, there may be puckering of the skin and we can see it fixed to the underlying skin. Some women are skinny enough that we can palpate masses that are fixed to the abdominal wall. This would be a sign of concern.

The nipple can become retracted. Ductal cancers occur in the ducts and this is not an infrequent symptom. Having said that, most ladies with breast cancer are asymptomatic.

Later problems might be a palpable node or mass in the axilla, meaning a positive lymph node. Women, ideally at age 50 or younger, should have yearly mammograms, annual physical exam, and monthly breast examination on their own. For those ladies with higher risks, starting mammograms at age 40 or sooner would be prudent.

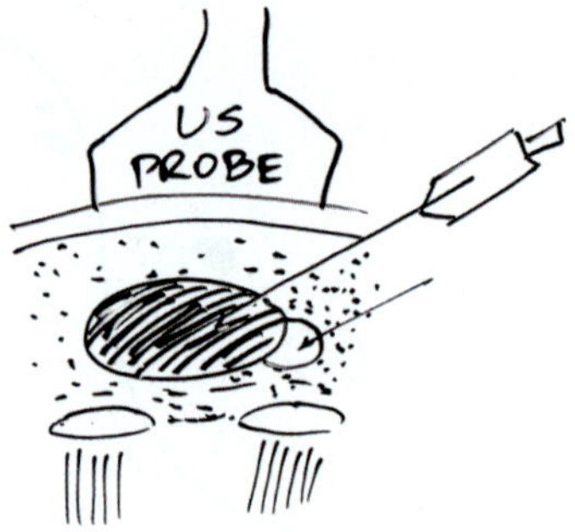

VIDEO 4.6. US to Assess Breast Abnormalities.
Transcript: Ultrasound is common for sampling breast abnormalities and assessing breast abnormalities. Again, ultrasound is based on echogenicity and so fluid or cysts are black, it is basically anechoic, we don't see any signals. This is reassuring that this is a benign process. Fatty tissue or breast tissue, underlying ribs with shadowing, makes this clearly a likely benign abnormality. If it is not, or we are concerned about it, then we can sample it with what is called fine-needle aspiration. This can be ultrasound guided, so the needle goes in safely. If there are concerns for other spots that may be hyperechoic, whitish, when everything else is black or has the same signals or echo as the rest of the tissue, then this is indeed a spot that has to be biopsied. Ultrasound guidance makes this very safe and the yield is incredibly high.

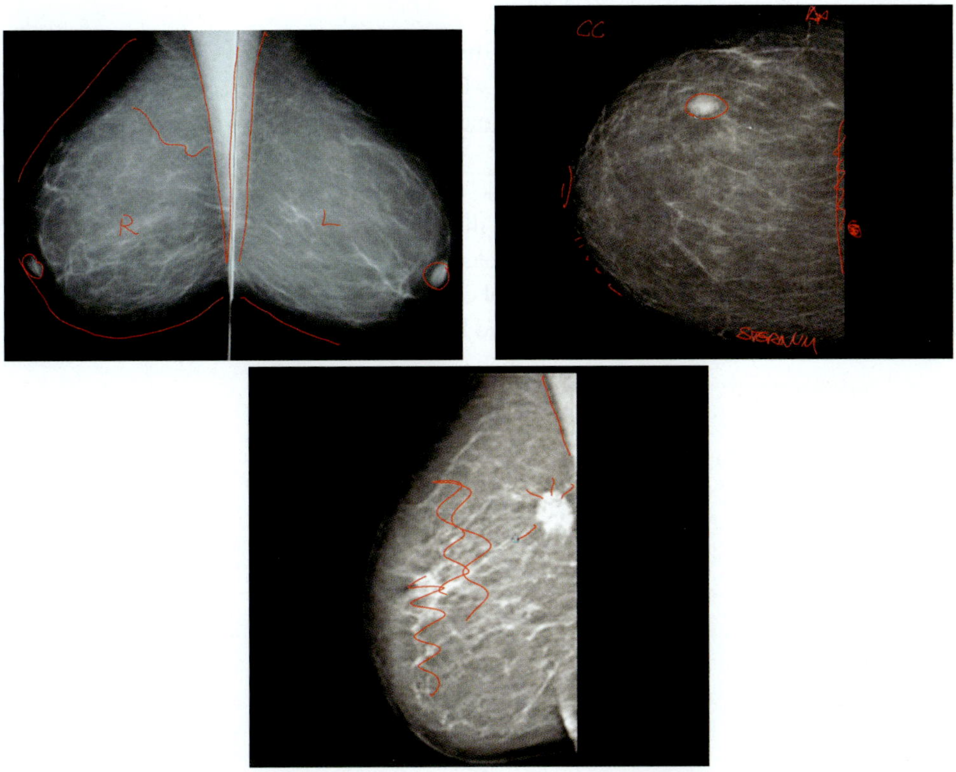

VIDEO 4.7. Mammography.

Transcript: Mammograms are not that hard to read and it is important for medical students to understand it. At some point in time, ladies that are 40, 45, or 50 are going to get an annual mammogram to help look for cancerous problems.

Mammograms come in 2 basic varieties, a mediolateral oblique, which is what this is, you put the film in the armpit and shoot the x-ray into the armpit versus the craniocaudal, putting the breast on the film and shooting from top down.

So, this is mediolateral oblique and a couple of key teaching points: you want to see the pectoralis muscle. So, this is the right breast, this is the left breast and we can see the left pectoralis muscle on 2 separate things, we want to see that muscle. The skin is on the outside, barely visualizable. Cancers sometimes show thickening of the skin and you can see that on a mammogram. The nipple areola complex, more prominent here, and the rest of this tissue is all fatty tissue, blood vessel tissue, and breast tissue. We can see little blood vessels running through and sometimes you will see elderly ladies with calcified blood vessels. But this is a normal mammogram, normal fatty tissue, fatty density tends to be blacker, the more white the breast tissue the more dense it is, in oftentimes younger folks or people taking estrogen.

Let's take a look at another picture. This is the other version; this is a craniocaudal version. Usually there will be numbers or letters up on the side and it will say "CC," craniocaudal, and that will be the axilla. So if that is the case, then this is the axilla and then this would be the sternum down here. What you don't see on this picture and it's really important for medical students and all physicians are that there is no pectoralis muscle. There should be a pectoralis muscle. Ladies don't like mammograms, they tend to be painful when the breast is compressed, but you want to see the pectoralis, if you don't, you are missing breast tissue and there could be a cancer sitting back there. So that is step number 1.

VIDEO 4.7. Continued

The nipple areola in this patient, tougher to see. The skin all looks thin, we can see little fatty tissue, the dark lines, and the rest of the tissue is breast. And what is this abnormality? It is fairly oval, it is round, and until proven otherwise, it is likely a cyst or some benign process. But you need to look at it in the other view, the mediolateral oblique.

Here is another x-ray, I think you can take a look, this is a mediolateral oblique. We see the pectoralis muscle that is good. We see skin and breast tissue, this is sort of normal tissue, but this is not. We get a sense that this is an irregular mass and it kind of looks a little like an octopus. We can get a sense of some arms coming out. This is likely an infiltrating ductal cancer. So this mammogram caught this asymptomatic mass in this woman that can now be treated and likely cured.

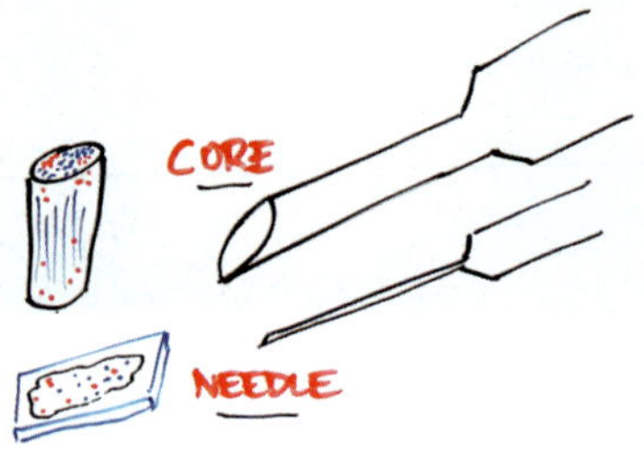

VIDEO 4.8. Core Needle Biopsy.

Transcript: There are multiple kinds of biopsy: surgeon's biopsy, what is called an excisional biopsy, or when we take part of it, it is called an incisional biopsy. But so often common in a breast surgery practice are women with lumps or bumps or mammographic abnormalities, we think about taking a needle biopsy or core needle biopsy.

A needle biopsy is a fine-gauge needle; 27 gauge, 25 gauge, or maybe 21 gauge. Larger than that, I wouldn't call a fine-needle aspiration. What happens is this needle is placed into the mass or the cyst, vacuum is presented, cells get pulled up into the needle and they are eventually squirted out into a drop of water on a slide. We have a pathologist, a cytopathologist, that can look at the cells and sometimes they can tell us that it is malignant, it is benign, it is fibrous tissue, or it is indeterminate, we can't tell.

The advantage of a core needle biopsy is that you get truly that, a core, a cylinder of material because it is larger. If this is 27 gauge, this might be 14 gauge. We can have larger cores or roughly 14 gauge. This gives the pathologist a chance to look at the structure and the architecture. Sometimes certain cells, lobular cells, breast has lobular cells in it, but the architecture may give us a sense that this is lobular carcinoma.

Needle is nice for giving us cheap, relatively painless, and fast information. A core, typically done under local anesthetic, is a bit more painful, a bit more involved, a little bit higher risk of creating bruising or a hematoma, but it gives us far more information and, indeed if it is a malignancy, we can check for hormones, progesterone or estrogen, and test it for a variety of things that will give us a better sense that this is atypical cells or malignant cells. Whereas in the needle biopsy, boy those cells look worrisome, better have a surgeon take more tissue or get a core biopsy.

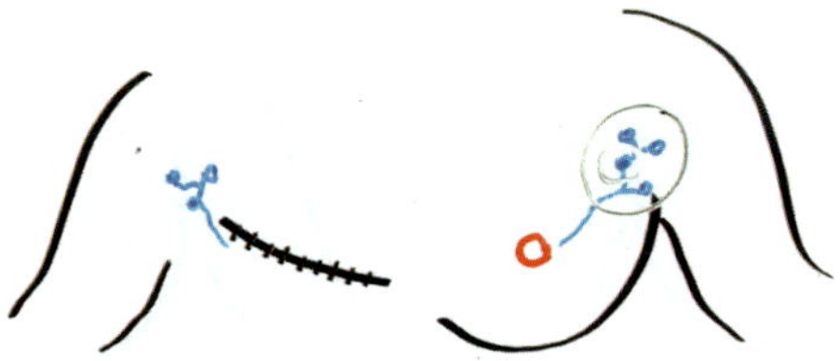

VIDEO 4.9. Sentinel Lymph Node Biopsy.
Transcript: Sentinel lymph node biopsy is a technique that can be used in breast surgery, melanoma surgery, and other forms of cancer detection in lymph nodes. An injection, typically in the breast, is located around that nipple areola complex. It is a region of high lymphatics. The dye that sneaks in there can be radioactive, or it can be a blue contrast material. It is taken up by the lymphatics and taken into the axilla, typically. Sometimes it can go into the internal mammary nodes. But most often it goes to the axilla.

Your surgeon and you will be looking for either a blue node, or if it is radioactive, one that sets off a signal with a gamma counter. And so by this depiction, the dye, the gamma counter, might light up this node as the most likely node to harbor tumor cells. Your surgeon will take this spot out, send it to pathology, and if there are cancer cells, we will remove the rest of those lymph nodes. If that sentinel node does not have tumor cells, that is it for surgery.

The same can be done even for mastectomy. Prior to surgery an injection is performed and then the surgeon goes in and takes out 1 lymph node. If that doesn't show any problems, we don't need to do further dissection.

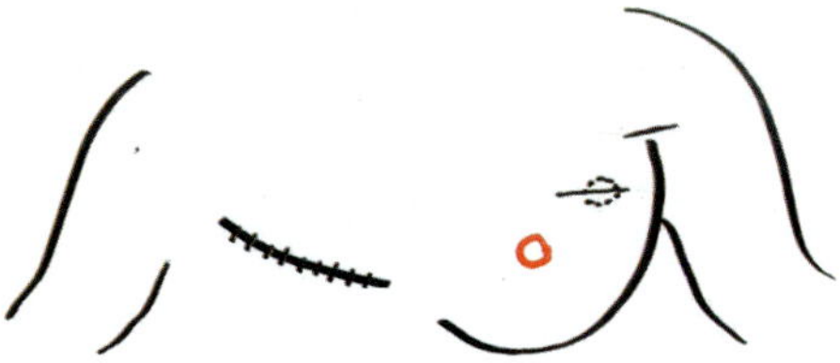

VIDEO 4.10. Breast-Conserving Therapy.
Transcript: Breast-conserving therapy is different than mastectomy. After a mastectomy, without reconstruction, a woman is flat chested with a simple scar on the chest. Breast-conserving therapy for a cancer located somewhere in the breast, likely means a small incision in the breast, removing the lump, and then an incision in the axilla to take out a lymph node. The survival is exactly the same for mastectomy and lumpectomy with breast-conserving therapy. The problem is, or an important difference is, if you preserve the breast, then you need radiation therapy to make sure that that survival is the same for those 2 patients.

Breast-conserving therapy is a nice option, it leaves contour to the patient, but it will require x-ray therapy and 2 little incisions.

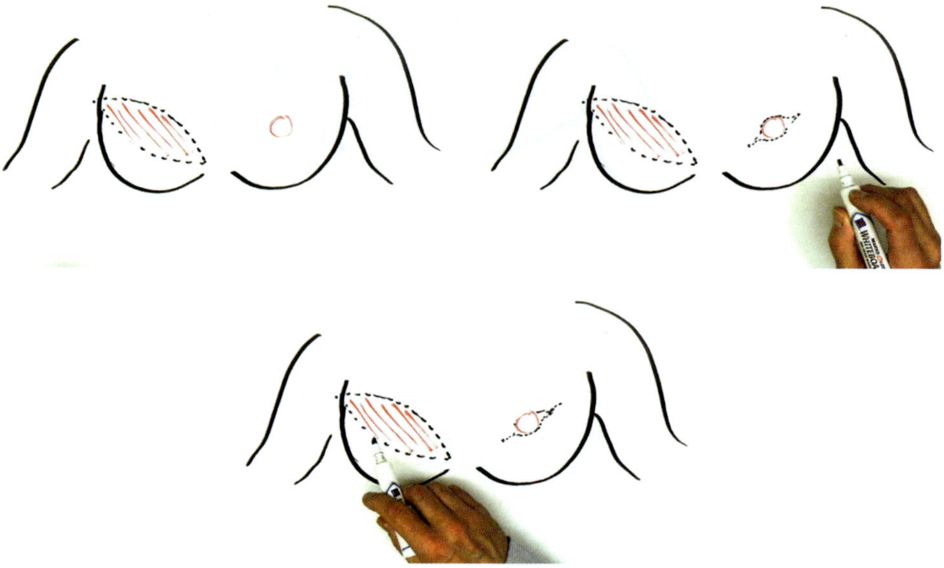

VIDEO 4.11. Simple Mastectomy.

Transcript: Sometimes women need to undergo mastectomy for breast cancer or other breast problems. A mastectomy, simplistically talks about making an elliptical incision on the breast, removing the nipple and the areola, some skin, the breast tissue, and then we are left with underlying pectoralis muscle underneath. So we have just taken the breast off of there.

A couple of other things about mastectomy—there is a variety of other choices, skin-sparing mastectomy that might mean just removing a small amount of nipple, areola, and skin. Another would be nipple-sparing mastectomy. So we leave the nipple behind and just make an incision and take the breast tissue out.

So for simple mastectomy, the entire breast, the nipple and skin is removed. Nipple-sparing means no skin, no nipple, or areola is removed; just a simple little incision. Then a skin-sparing mastectomy means the nipple is basically removed with just a little bit of skin. All are very reasonable options, and it depends on the patient's desire and the type of tumor the surgeon is treating.

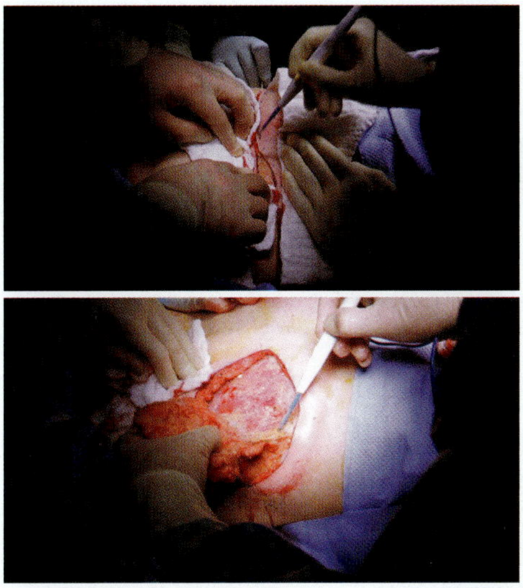

VIDEO 4.12. Mastectomy: Intraoperative.
Transcript: This is a bilateral mastectomy. A simple mastectomy meaning skin, nipple, and areola are widely removed. The patient is not going to have reconstructive surgery, or could have reconstructive surgery. This might be someone with bilateral mastectomy that has a BRCA1 or BRCA2 malformation. So, they want to get rid of the risk of having a cancer. This could be a lady with a cancer in 1 side and says, "I want to be symmetric whether with reconstruction or without, so I would like to have the tissue removed on both sides."

We can see surgeons using the scalpel, some faster, some slower, the key thing is always be safe and be careful. We can see that the electrocautery works well when the surgeons have traction and counter traction. There is a medical student pulling on 1 side hard is a good thing as long as somebody else is going to pull on the other side. Here is a young learner using the tip of the cautery; good, a centimeter flap. When you raise that mastectomy flap, you want to make sure that the blood supply is good. We have got some Murphy rakes, and again our beginner is just slowly methodically moving through trying to keep the fat on the skin and the breast down below. They are pulling hard, the rakes are pulling hard.

Now here is a more expert surgeon, a little bit faster. You can see the whitish, yellowish interface. The fatty tissue above is fat; the whitish tissue is breast below. We try to get exactly in that plane and we can move things along. Cautery works exceedingly well if you use the tip. As you do a mastectomy, you have to think about the pectoralis muscle underneath. When you send off that specimen to pathology, it needs to be marked so in case we find a cancer or there is a close margin, we know where it is. Historically, people would take the pectoralis muscle, we don't do that anymore—that was a radical mastectomy. Now we do what is called a simple mastectomy or skin-sparing or nipple-sparing—trying to take less tissue and leave better cosmesis and outcome for our patients. This is nicely done and typically an hour-long procedure. This will treat somebody with bilateral cancers or risk for cancers very nicely.

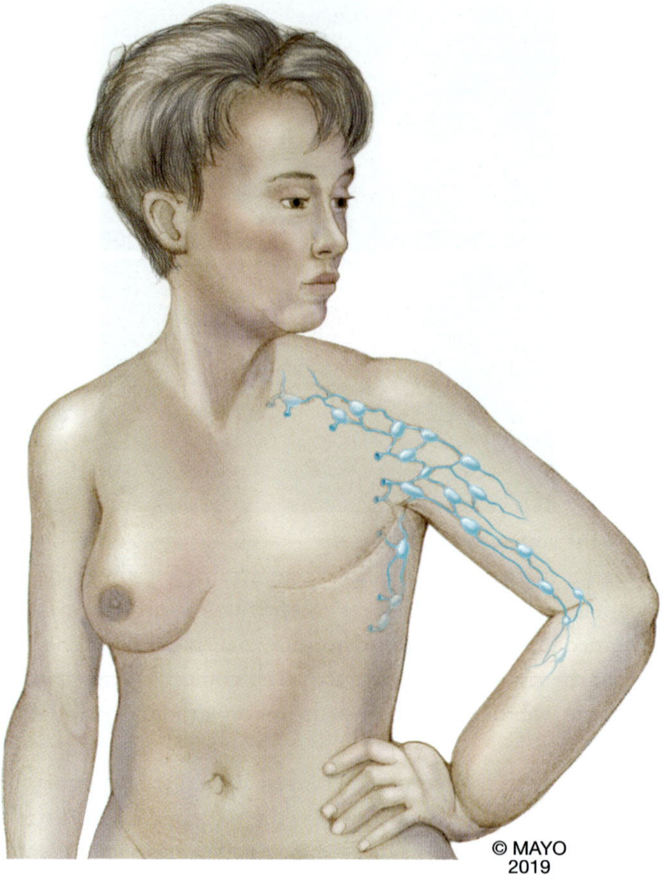

FIGURE 4.3. Postmastectomy Lymphedema.

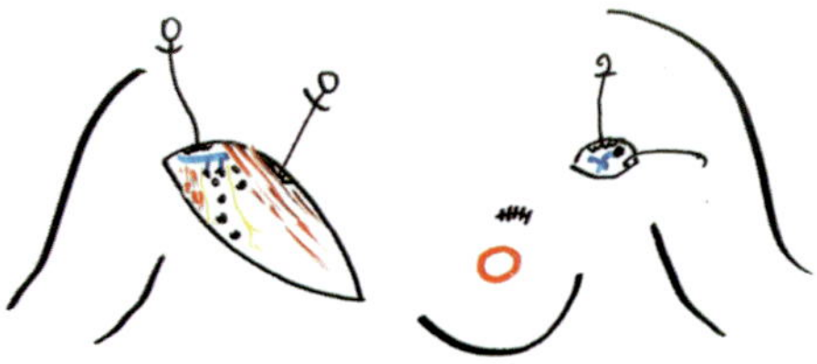

VIDEO 4.13. Axillary Lymph Node Dissection.

Transcript: An axillary lymph node dissection (unlike a sentinel node with a small little incision and perhaps removing 1, 2, or more lymph nodes) involves a formal resection of the lymph nodes that did occupy this region. That region is usually just lateral and deep to the pectoralis major muscle, medial to the latissimus dorsi muscle, and inferior, or caudal, to the axillary vein. Within this dissection you have got to be careful for the blood vessels and, obviously, the long thoracic nerve and the thoracodorsal nerve that innervate both the serratus anterior and the latissimus dorsi. These are important nerves to protect, but when we are doing an axillary node dissection, it likely means that these are not positive nodes. One or more nodes may have cancer in them and we are trying to eradicate cancerous lymph nodes.

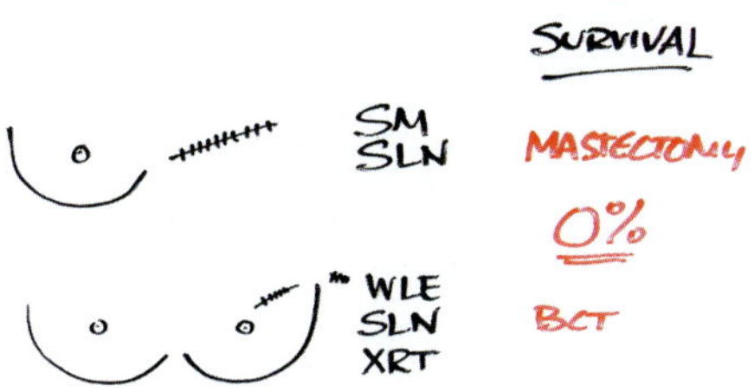

VIDEO 4.14. Radiation Therapy.

Transcript: Women that have a left-sided breast cancer may undergo simple mastectomy with sentinel node removal, or they undergo wide-local excision with sentinel lymph node biopsy and external beam radiation therapy; so-called breast-conserving therapy.

What is the difference between mastectomy and breast-conserving therapy? We have looked at this carefully over the years, and as long as it is stage for stage the same, there is no difference, 0% difference in survival benefit between conserving the breast and doing a mastectomy. Now that implies that the margins are negative and the nodal disease is the same.

External-beam radiation therapy is extraordinarily useful and helpful for decreasing recurrence. Even ladies with mastectomies, if they have multiple lymph nodes, may benefit from external-beam radiation therapy.

The teaching point here more than anything: what is the outcome for mastectomy and breast-conserving therapy? The survival is the same. The cosmetic outcome is different. The need for external-beam radiation therapy of 6 weeks is more than this side. It depends so much on each individual patient and woman, the size of the cancer, size of the breast, and the long-term outlook.

TABLE 4.1. Final Assessment Categories of BI-RADS

Category	*Management*	*Likelihood of Cancer*
0 Need additional imaging or prior examinations	Recall for additional imaging or await prior examinations	NA
1 Negative	Routine screening	Essentially 0%
2 Benign findings	Routine screening	Essentially 0%
3 Probably benign	Short-interval follow-up (6 mo) or continued surveillance mammography	>0% but ≤2%
4 Suspicious abnormality	Tissue diagnosis	4a Low suspicion for malignancy (>2%-10%) 4b Moderate suspicion for malignancy (>10%-≤50%) 4c High suspicion for malignancy (>50%-<95%)
5 Highly suspicious of malignancy	Tissue diagnosis	≥95%
6 Known biopsy-proven malignancy	Surgical excision when clinically appropriate	NA

Abbreviations: BI-RADS, Breast Imaging Reporting and Data System; NA, not applicable.
Modified from Sickles EA, D'Orsi CJ. ACR BI-RADS follow-up and outcome monitoring. In: ACR BI-RADS atlas, breast imaging reporting and data system. Reston (VA): American College of Radiology; c2013; used with permission.

Breast Challenge Questions

4.1. What is the most common cause of bloody nipple discharge?
4.2. What is mastitis, and how is it best treated?
4.3. Where does most lymph from the breast drain?
4.4. What findings make a mammogram suspicious for cancer?
4.5. What is the tail of Spence?
4.6. What is the lifetime risk of breast cancer in women? Risk in men?
4.7. What is a modified radical mastectomy?
4.8. How are axillary lymph nodes defined anatomically?
4.9. What is ductal carcinoma in situ?
4.10. What is neoadjuvant therapy? When is it indicated in patients with breast cancer?
4.11. What is triple-negative breast cancer?
4.12. What is the importance of *BRCA* genes?

Answers to Breast Challenge Questions

4.1. Benign intraductal papilloma.
4.2. Inflammation of breast tissue. Bacterial causes are best treated early with analgesia, heat, and antibiotics.
4.3. Lymph drains to the ipsilateral axilla.
4.4. The BI-RADS criteria are a resource for mammogram findings (Table 4.1).
4.5. Breast tissue that extends into the axilla.
4.6. Risk is 1:8 in women; risk is approximately 1:1,000 in men.
4.7. En bloc removal of breast and axillary lymph nodes.
4.8. There are 3 levels based on location to PMM: 1, inferior to PMM; 2, posterior to PMM; and 3, superior to PMM.
4.9. Ductal carcinoma in situ is an early form of ductal cancer that has not penetrated the basement membrane.
4.10. Hormonal therapy or chemotherapy in advance of surgical therapy. Neoadjuvant therapy is most often used for more advanced breast cancers.
4.11. A breast cancer that is pathologically negative for 1) estrogen receptors, 2) progesterone receptors, and 3) human epidermal growth factor receptors (ER-, PR-, Her2Neu [negative estrogen receptor, negative progesterone receptor, and negative for overexpression of human epidermal growth factor receptor 2]).
4.12. An autosomal dominant gene mutation that is associated with a risk for development of breast cancer (at age 70 years): *BRCA1* = 55% to 70%, *BRCA2* = 45% to 70%.

5

Colon

Embryology

The colon is made up of the midgut which includes the proximal two-thirds of the transverse colon, and the hindgut, which includes the distal one-third of the transverse colon.

Anatomy

The ileocecal junction to the anus is a distance of 1.5 m. The cecum, transverse colon, and sigmoid colon are intraperitoneal; the ascending and descending colon are retroperitoneal; and the rectum (Figure 5.1) is infraperitoneal. Three bands of longitudinal muscularis externa fibers (taeniae coli) (Figure 5.2 letter A) run from the base of appendix to the rectum. Omental (epiploic) appendages (Figure 5.2 letter B) run the length of the colon. Sacculations (haustra) (Figure 5.2 letter C) are characteristic of the colon. Arterial supply (Figure 5.2) is via the SMA (proximal two-thirds of colon) and the IMA (distal one-third of colon). The rectum is supplied from the internal iliac artery. Venous drainage of the colon (Figure 5.3) is by the portal venous system.

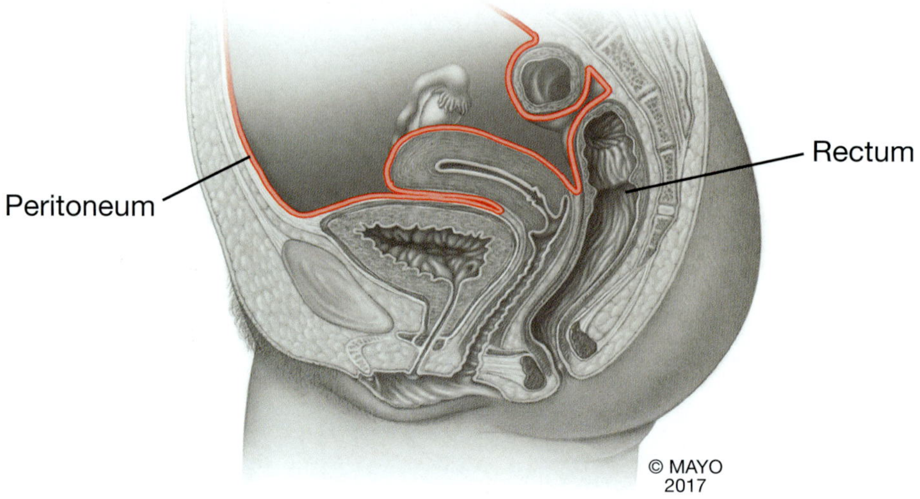

FIGURE 5.1. Anatomy of the Rectum.

Physiology

Digested food (chyme) passes into the colon and is converted to feces by bacteria. Vitamins generated by gut bacteria are absorbed; salts, water, and electrolytes (especially K^+) are reclaimed by the body.

Clinical Presentation

The differential diagnosis of colonic masses includes cancer (Video 5.1), carcinoid, lipoma, diverticular disease, ulcerative colitis (Video 5.2), polyps, and Crohn disease (Video 5.3). Colon cancer may cause bleeding (ascending) or obstruction (sigmoid). Colorectal is the second most common type of cancer in the United States. Lynch syndrome (Video 5.4) is an autosomal dominant genetic condition that poses a high risk for colon cancer. Diverticulitis is common and usually causes left lower quadrant abdominal pain and fever.

Imaging

Diagnostic tests for colorectal masses include stool guaiac, complete blood count, colonoscopy (Video 5.5), CT, MRI, endorectal US, and barium enema (Video 5.6). The liver is the most common site of hematogenous metastases from colorectal cancer. CXRs, liver function tests, and CT (Video 5.7) are helpful for finding metastases of colorectal cancer.

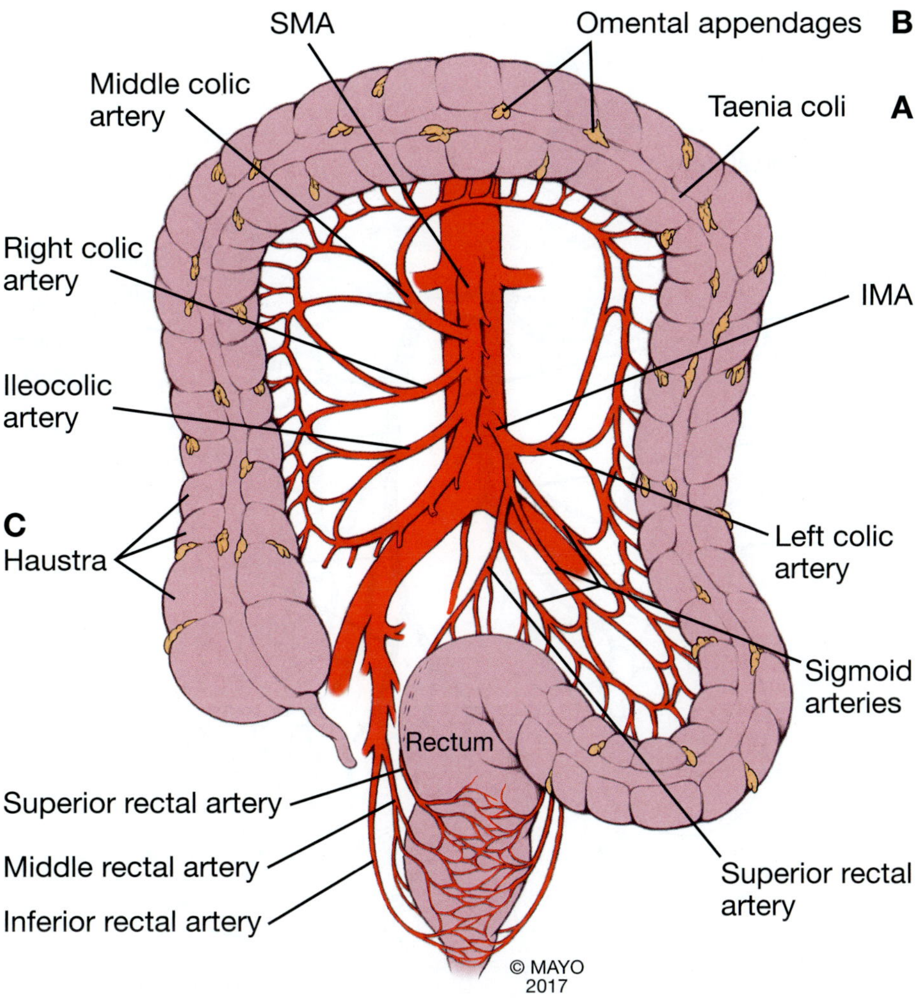

FIGURE 5.2. Arterial Supply and Anatomy of the Colon.

Operation

Treatment of colorectal cancer and symptomatic inflammatory colon disease usually involves wide surgical resection. Operations include laparoscopic, open, or robotic varieties: right, left, sigmoid, and low anterior resections (Videos 5.8 and 5.9). Abdominal perineal resection (Video 5.10) requires an ostomy.

Complications

Complications after surgery may include postoperative bleeding, leakage, and ileus. Colonoscopy may cause bleeding or, rarely, perforations (incidence, 1 in 1,000).

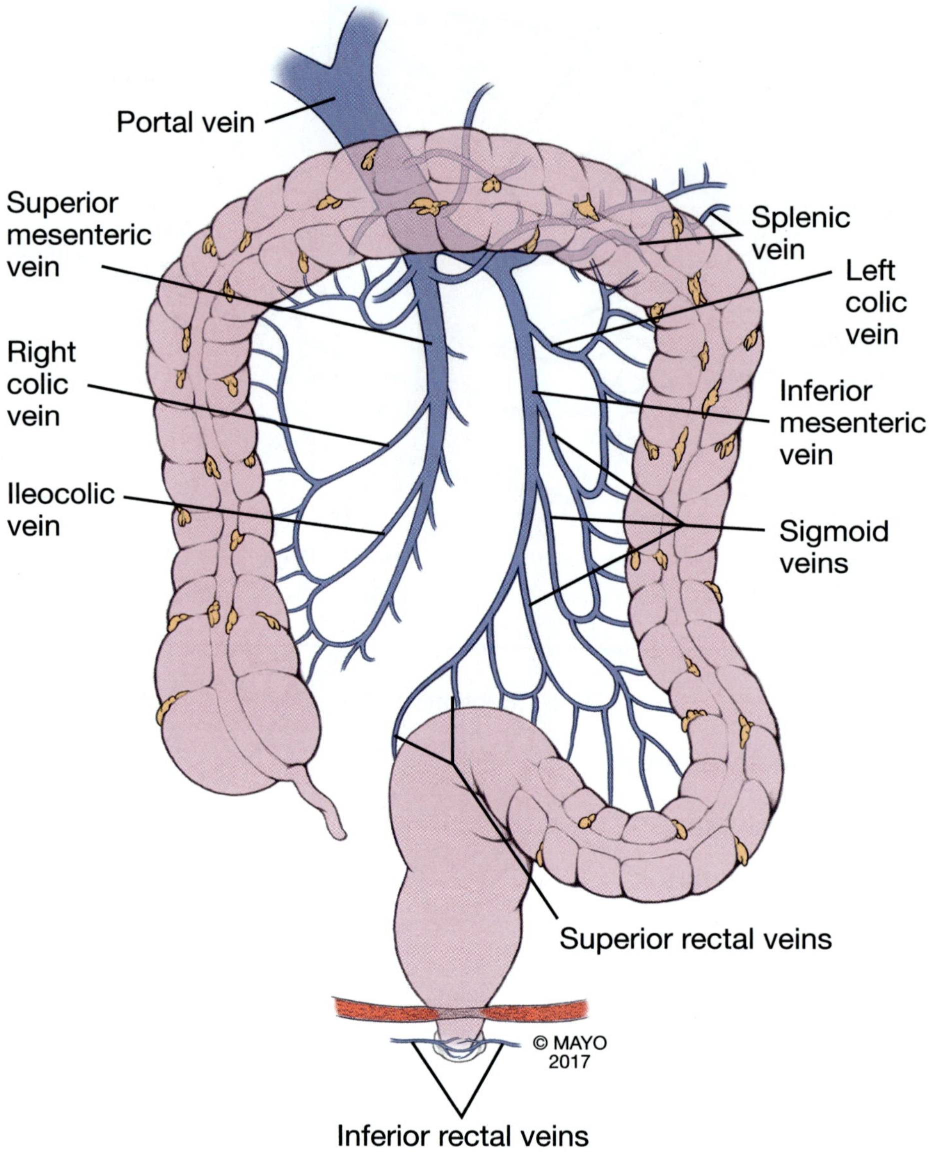

FIGURE 5.3. Venous Drainage of the Colon.

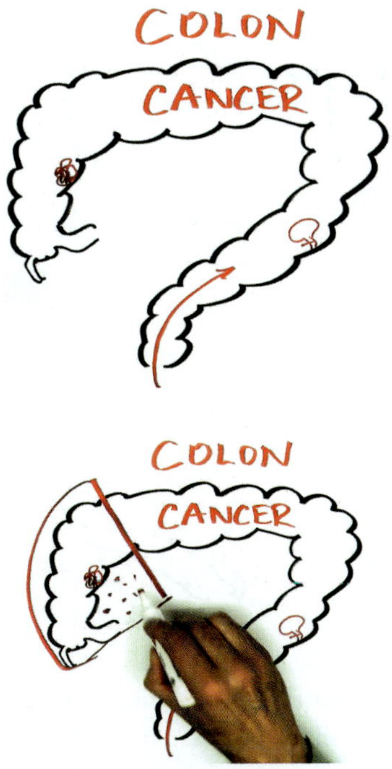

VIDEO 5.1. Cancer of the Colon. CEA indicates carcinoembryonic antigen.
Transcript: In the United States this year, approximately 130,000 people will have a cancer of the colon. It could be in the cecum, transverse colon, descending sigmoid, or rectum. One-hundred and thirty thousand people and half of those people may die from this. Half of the people are probably younger than age 60. That is why colonoscopy looking up inside and finding a polyp that is small and safe and easy to cut out cures cancer. If we have colon cancers, typically what we want to do is resect them. Take out mesentery and a portion of that colon and then put the patients back together again. When we take out these cancers, they will have lymph nodes in it. Surgeons like to have at least 12 lymph nodes to make sure that none of them have a cancer, but many of them do. Many people have lymph nodes and cancer spread to the liver, or the brain, or the lung. Colon cancer is a real problem in the United States and advising patients to get a colonoscopy to find cancers early and eradicated, and then when we do find cancers, to treat those aggressively. Many, many people can be cured of colon cancer. One of the things we look at is the CEA level. Ask your physician and ask your lab people. Colon cancer, a big number there, we are nervous about metastases. When in doubt, colonoscopy by age 50 in the United States.

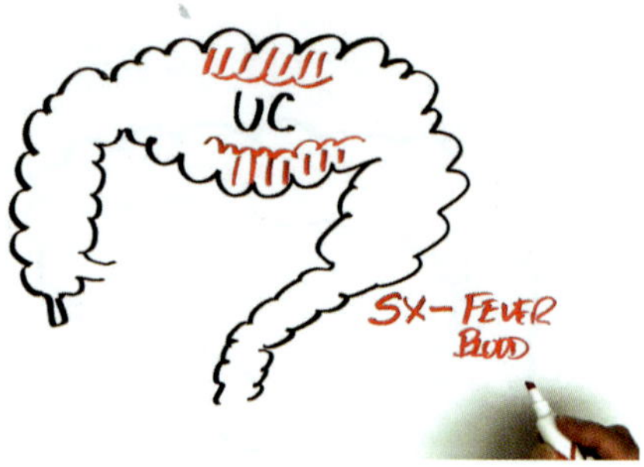

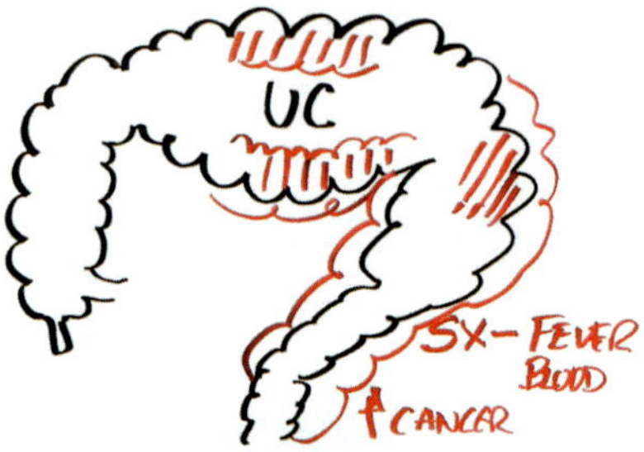

VIDEO 5.2. Ulcerative Colitis. CUC (in narration) indicates chronic ulcerative colitis; SX, symptoms. Transcript: Ulcerative colitis is a huge swelling, an edematous change in the wall of the colon. Oftentimes, it involves the entire colon. Patients get ulcerative colitis; maybe 1 in 10,000 will do that. They will have fever and they will have bloody diarrhea as a major hallmark. This can be a dangerous problem—bloody diarrhea, sepsis, and infection. Ulcerative colitis can lead to higher risk of cancer. Oftentimes people that present with ulcerative colitis will be very sick. Antibiotics, IV hydration, tincture of time, and they get better. The worst things that can happen with ulcerative colitis for a patient is to develop what is called toxic megacolon and that's the colon gets completely swollen and edematous and then there will be areas of necrosis and dying. This can be a lethal problem and for this we usually remove the entire colon.

People with chronic ulcerative colitis, typically we talk about maybe removing the colon because the risk of cancer is so high. In 10 years with CUC, the risk is 5%. But young people can get this disease and over the course of 20 years, the risk of colon cancer maybe 20% or higher. If you get an obstruction or blocking or massive bleeding then surgery oftentimes is the answer. There are folks with chronic ulcerative colitis, not an acute episode, that can be treated with a variety of medications including steroids that temporize things. But folks with chronic ulcerative colitis need to be managed and watched carefully year by year to make sure they don't develop a cancer or ulcerative colitis in an acute episode that can be life threatening.

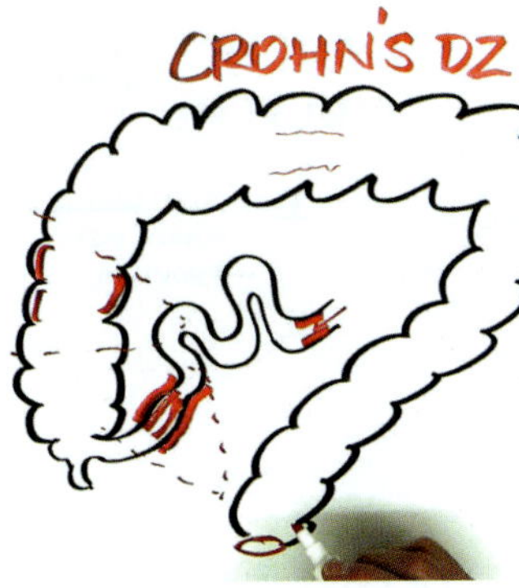

VIDEO 5.3. Crohn Disease.
Transcript: Crohn's disease is a diabolical disease, it makes patients miserable, but some people can live with it just fine. It oftentimes happens in the ileum. The thing about Crohn's disease is it typically involves the entire wall of either the small bowel or the colon. We are not sure what causes this. In ulcerative colitis, the lining is usually the problem. In Crohn's disease it is the entire thickness of the wall and that sometimes means that section of bowel, whether it is the small bowel or colon, should be removed.

Most folks with Crohn's disease can be on steroids or a variety of different medications that quiet this down and they can get through it. But with this transmural involvement over the course of time, people can develop strictures, scarring, and obstruction. It usually means a need for an operation. They can develop bleeding. They can develop fistulas and this can happen in the anus, it can happen in the colon, to the bladder, to the vagina; it is just a diabolical disease. It rarely leads to perforation, but that can happen. There is a great suspicion looking at these patients with a workup that might be a cancer. We are relieved when it is Crohn's, but sometimes cancer is easier to treat. Crohn's disease oftentimes involves younger folks, 20s, 30s, and 40s. Maybe 1 or 2 in 10,000 people will develop it. It is a chronic irritating abdominal disease that can cause pain. In a workup we usually find 1 section of small bowel or colon that is involved. Many of these people will benefit from surgical resection.

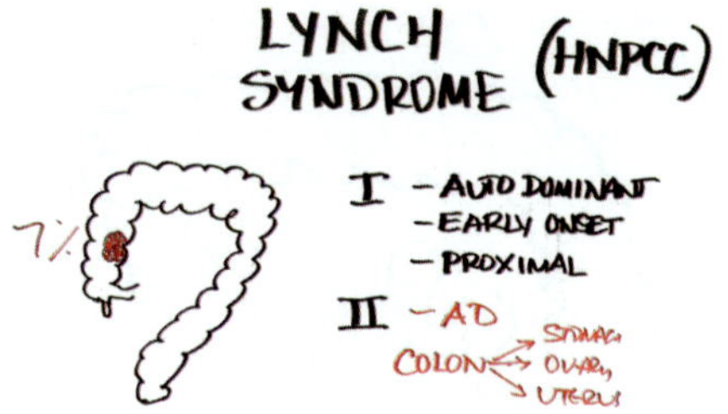

VIDEO 5.4. Lynch Syndrome.
Transcript: Lynch syndrome, named after Dr Lynch, discovered in 1966, familial relationship and autosomal dominant, hereditary nonpolyposis colon cancers. About 7% of our cancers in the United States are Lynch syndrome, cancers of the colon. Lynch I is autosomal dominant, early onset, and oftentimes in the proximal colon. Lynch II is autosomal dominant as well, but these colon cancers also occur with other cancers of the stomach, women of the ovary and of the uterus. The thing to know about Lynch syndrome is it typically happens in younger folks and they need to be screened.

So Mom, Uncle Joe, and Grandma and Grandpa have all had cancer early on 20s, 30s, 40s, 50s, we need to think about hereditary nonpolyposis colon cancer, or so-called Lynch syndrome. And again, colonoscopy is going to be a key test early on for those folks. Genetic testing to find out indeed they carry the gene; they are at a likely high risk of this, of a colon cancer. If that is the case, removing the entire colon eliminates that risk. The problem is now you have to develop some sort of surgery that makes that tolerable and so-called ileopouch anal anastomosis, taking the end of the ileum and sewing it down to the bottom, these patients can still live a very normal life.

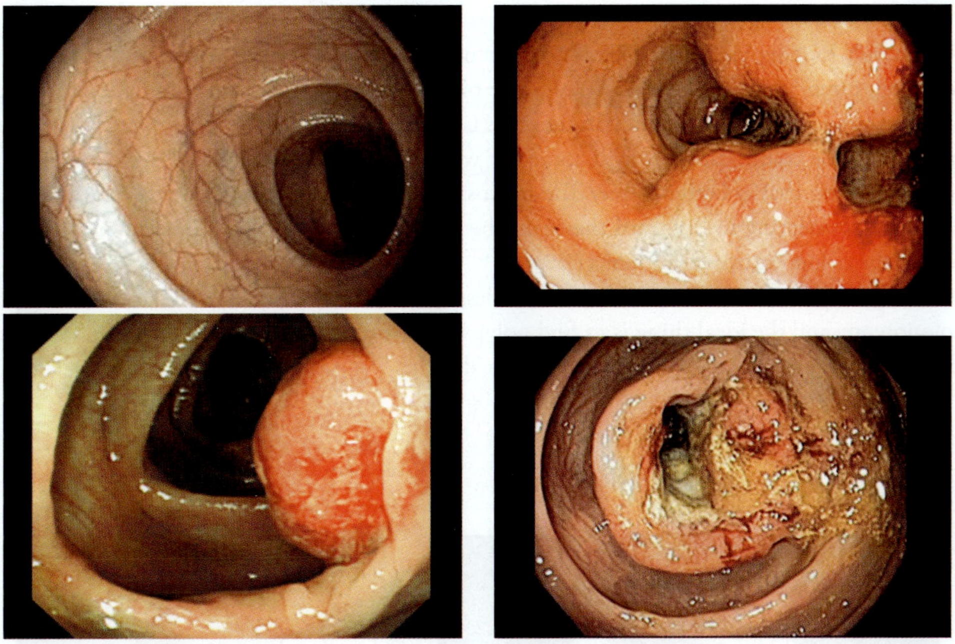

VIDEO 5.5. Colonoscopy.

Transcript: Thousands of Americans get colonoscopy every day. People are nervous about that and they don't talk about it and everybody is nervous that they may need it someday. Truthfully, everybody that is 50 years of age and over should get it.

Here is a picture of the colon. It is a normal-looking colon. This is the cave that we are going to sneak through and take a look at the entire colon. That is a normal sigmoid colon, with normal mucosa, and normal blood vessels.

This is the transverse colon, it kind of looks like a triangle a little bit and that is because there are 3 muscles on the outside of the colon: the taenia coli. The key thing about this is (in the transverse colon), that it's intra-abdominal and it can squish the colon. Other parts of the colon are retroperitoneal. But this is a normal-looking colon and the colonoscope is going to go through that little cave if you will. The colon will sometimes move and contract, but we are looking for polyps and abnormal findings, normal-looking blood vessels, a little bit of stool or fecal material, we see from time to time.

This is the ascending colon. Again, rings of muscular, muscularis layer, and the mucosa looks pretty doggone normal.

We get further along towards the appendix and this is the cecum. It bows out and distends with the gas. A little fecal matter up here but it all looks normal.

What about abnormal findings? This is a sigmoid colon cancer. Everybody can see that it is ulcerated. It looks firm and adenomatous. It is a bad mass, it is a bad cancer. It might be entirely through the colonic wall. If that is the case, it may have lymph node involvement or liver metastasis. This is something that is caught too late. We need to get there sooner.

In the transverse colon, again the triangles in the background, we have a polyp or a mass that could be a cancer. It is bloody and it's inflamed. It might be able to be removed colonoscopically, but I'm nervous as a surgeon that this is a cancer, but it is caught early enough that it can be cured.

VIDEO 5.5. Continued

This is an ugly looking picture. The colonoscope needs to sneak by in the ascending colon. In the ascending colon, oftentimes masses ulcerate and give bleeding and the first sign for someone with a colon cancer is light-headed with anemia and fatigue. This is a bleeding lesion that involves, looks like the entire circumference of the colon. This needs to come out with an operation. Again, caught too late.

This is something that is better to see. The mucosa looks perfectly normal. This is not likely a colon cancer. There is something underneath there, maybe it is a benign polyp or a lipoma or something else outside, but the colon mucosa itself looks normal.

Colonoscopy is a wonderful tool. It has low risk, less than 1 in 1,000 people will have a serious problem from colonoscopy and the ideal thing is to find polyps and remove them and ideally find normal mucosa. If we find cancer, then they need to be treated immediately.

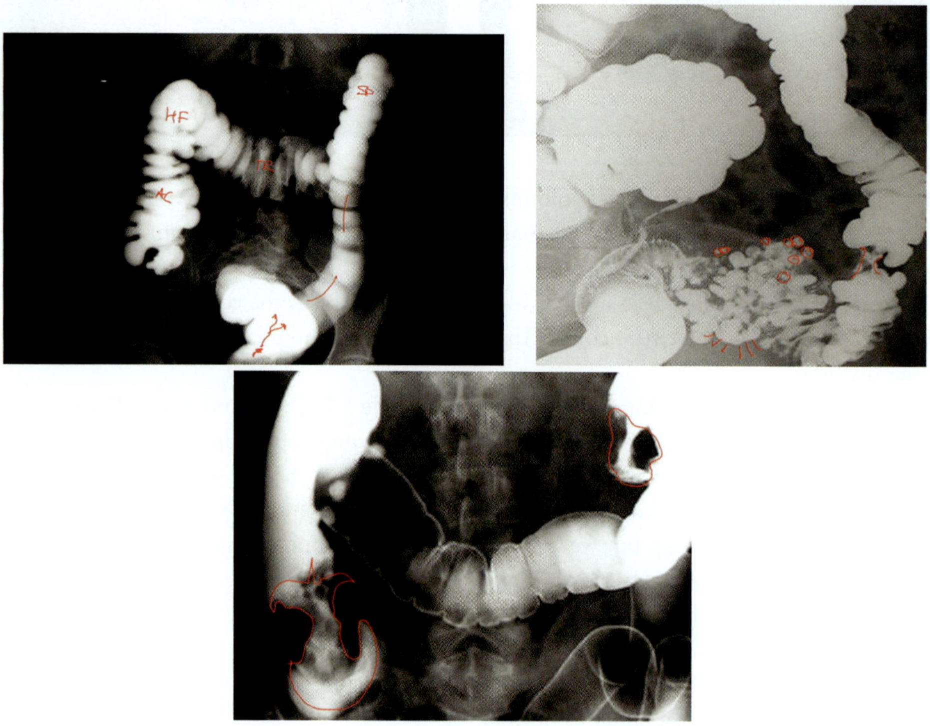

VIDEO 5.6. Barium Enema.

Transcript: This is a barium enema. Barium, a fairly dense material, is placed within the anus, usually with a tube, and the material is injected in under pressure. It slides through the sigmoid colon, up through the descending colon, the splenic flexure, the transverse colon, the hepatic flexure, the ascending colon, and the cecum. This is a beautiful barium enema that shows the outline of the mucosa. It is a test not commonly done much anymore.

VIDEO 5.6. Continued

This is an older fashioned film where you can see the balloon inside the anus and rectum making sure that the contrast goes into the rectum and doesn't leak out onto the table. Again, this is a normal sort of study: rectum down below, sigmoid, descending colon, splenic flexure, transverse colon, hepatic flexure, ascending colon, and cecum. This one you can even see that contrast has snuck back into the ileum.

Let me show you something that is not so normal. You might be able to guess. Contrast is sneaking through here. Look at all these bubbles. The barium is sneaking into diverticulum. Fifty percent, 60%, 70% of Americans have diverticulum. It is not a problem until they become inflamed. It may be diverticulitis which causes pain and fever. But a barium enema is a reasonable test for that. As we look at this barium enema, we also have to be careful—is this normal here? It looks like it is narrowed down and could that be what is called an apple-core lesion. Sometimes you have to wait and distend it up and sometimes it is just a contraction that 1 picture will look like that.

Here is a picture. Can you see something abnormal? Maybe 1, maybe 2. This has got air in it as well as barium. It is easier to see the mucosa, and we can see normal loops of material. But I am hopeful that what you are seeing is on this side, is classically what is called an apple-core lesion. I don't know if my apple is very nice, but we have a couple of bites out of this apple. That is a narrowed lumen and this is likely a right-sided colon cancer. And if we look carefully, we might find something else that is abnormal as well. Three percent of the time, colon cancers will have more than 1 colon cancer at the same time. So, barium enema study, not as common nowadays with colonoscopy being so readily prevalent. But it becomes very useful for some folks. Some people have had so much surgery that the colon is stuck and scarred and this is the best test for them. This is very useful.

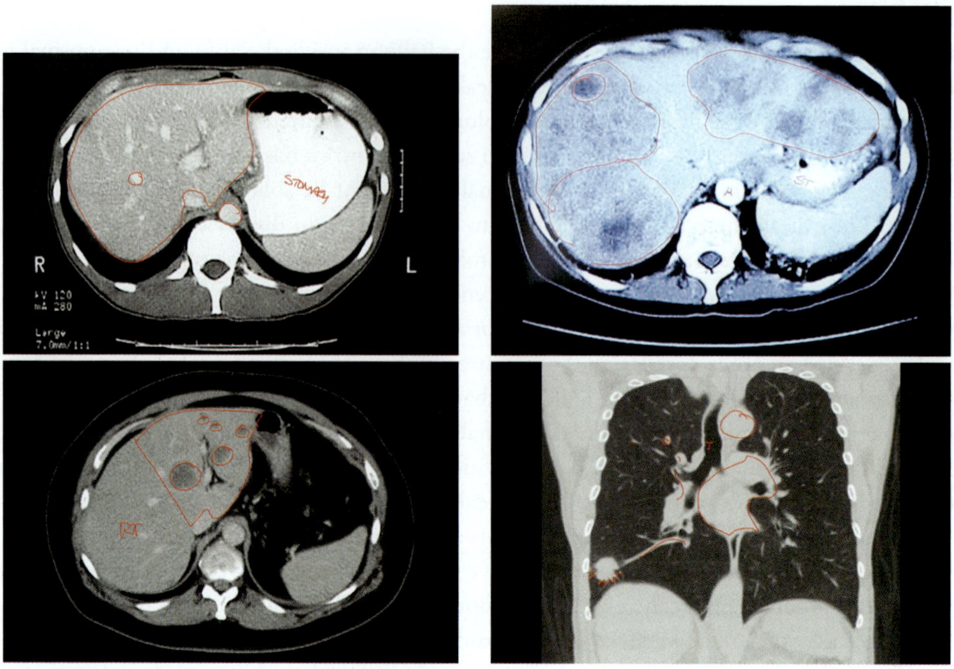

VIDEO 5.7. CT of the Colon.

Transcript: Patients with colon cancer, advanced colon cancer, especially, we are nervous about metastatic spread to the liver. It is the number 1 place that colon cancer likes to go. And for that, we oftentimes use a CT scan. So here is a nice CT scan that shows contrast in the aorta and contrast in the stomach. If we carefully look at the liver, it is this big structure here that is well lit up, and there is a lot of liver mass here. These lesions in the middle here are blood vessels, that is contrast. This is a normal looking CT scan. There is no funny sort of abnormalities.

Let's take a look at some other studies. Here is a CT scan. Same sort of picture, contrast in the aorta, the stomach has contrast that they have swallowed. But now look at the rest of this liver. This is a hideous CT scan. It shows massive metastases, big tumors, with necrotic areas; this is all ugly looking mass. This is liver that is being replaced by cancer.

Another picture, not quite so dramatic. This one might be resectable. A surgeon might be able to take out what is called the left lobe of the liver or a left hepatectomy, because this person has multiple metastases. The right lobe of the liver looks good. It is at least half of the liver or more will allow that patient normal function. But this is someone who will benefit likely from surgery. The other patient, not so much. Chemotherapy would be necessary.

Here is a CT scan with windows cut of the lung and we can see the trachea up above, the aorta, and starting to work into the cardiac region here, but, the important point here is that blood vessels get smaller as they go out, they get smaller. We shouldn't get something that gets bigger and looks spiculated. This unfortunately is a colon cancer that has metastasized to the right lung. CT scan is very good at detecting liver mets and lung mets.

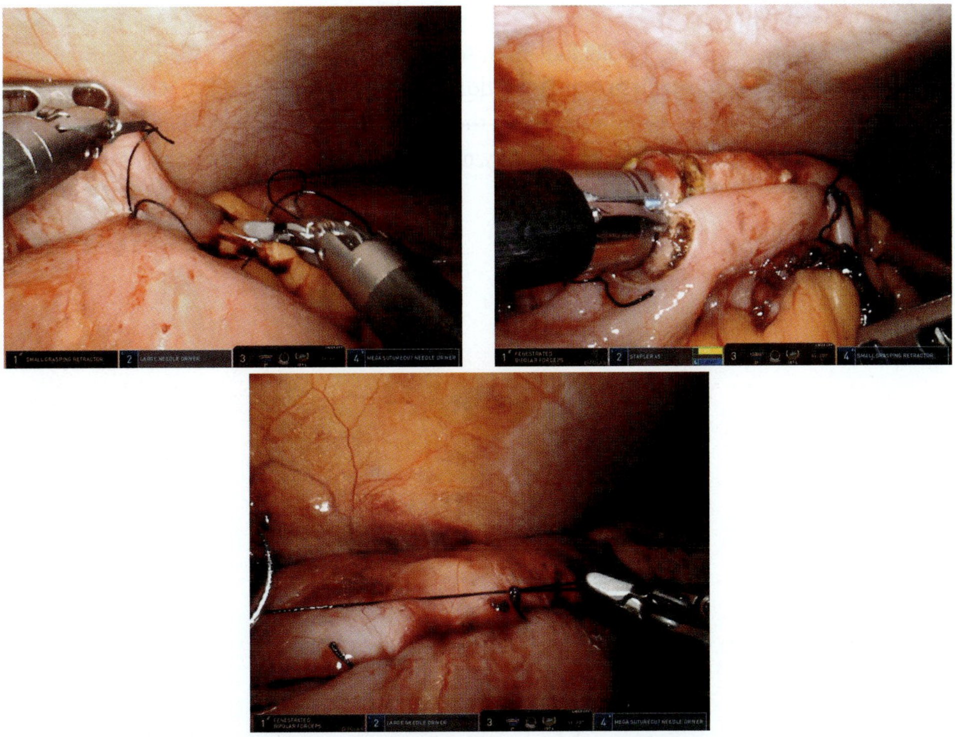

VIDEO 5.8. Right-sided Colectomy: Intraoperative.

Transcript: This is a right-sided colectomy, so-called ileocecectomy and it is done with a robot. The computer is on the side of the room and the surgeon is on the side of the room and a bunch of gadgets are hanging over the patient. The stapling device divides the ileum. And, further downstream we are going to have to divide the cecum or the ascending or transverse colon. The robotic tools are very slick and the staplers work very quickly. You can see how multiple rows of staples are deployed and there is a sharp device that cuts between. It looks like now we have got a little bleeder on the edge of the stapling device and electrocautery can take care of that for us. The stapling device is now going to try to divide the ascending colon. It takes 2 deployments and that specimen has been resected, the bowel has been taken apart. Now it is a matter of trying to sew the ileum to the ascending colon. You can see the robotic tools working very nicely. Now the problem with the robot is that you can't feel anything, you can see amazingly well, but you can't feel it. Although the surgeon sees the needle going through, there is no haptic feedback. You've got to be really careful, and these people are getting really good at this. Tying a knot, if you pull too hard, it will just break. Let's see how they do. They lost it, it slipped. That is a surgeon's knot, 3 throws in it, hoping it will stick. Is it going to hold? Yeah, it is. The nice thing about the robot is that it gives you lots of joints. It is like having your own wrist and hand in there.

So now they have got the ileum and the colon next to each other, and now they are going to make a hole in the small bowel and the colon and sew this together. What is fascinating to me is that for someone who has watched this for 30 years to think that this is being done with the abdomen closed. I would be nervous about spillage of stool and the surgeons are as well. But the more that we do this the more we realize good technique, antibiotics before surgery, good bowel prep. Basically we can do this with little bitty incisions and patients can sometimes leave the hospital the next day. The stapling device into that ileotomy and colotomy deploys and it sews that bowel together and it if it is not sewn, it is interrupted with metal staples. We are left with a little hole that we need to close up and that is a piece of cake for the

VIDEO 5.8. Continued

robot and a good robotic surgeon. Looks like an absorbable suture going in. We have the metal staples on the inside and the key is to make sure that we don't catch the back wall. We want to make sure that this is a nice patent anastomosis. A few stitches on the front and it becomes a 2-layered anastomosis just like we have done historically for 2 centuries. A very nicely done ileocecectomy: a robotic, intracorporeal, "hand-sewn" anastomosis with stapling technique.

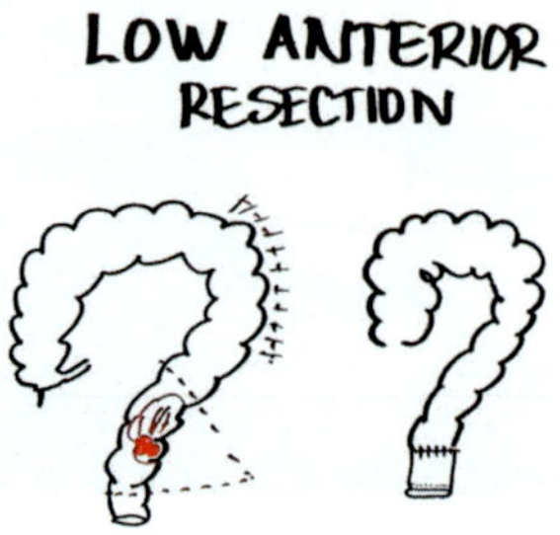

VIDEO 5.9. Low Anterior Resection.

Transcript: Low anterior resection is a colorectal operation that removes problems in the rectum, not at the very bottom, the anus, but the rectum. Usually a colon cancer, a rectal cancer that is big and involves this section can come out. Sometimes, diverticulitis. But what a surgeon will do is mobilize the peritoneal attachments of the colon, pull this down, and then resect the fatty mesentery and the bowel and that piece will come out. Then we can pull this down and make an anastomosis. The nice thing about a low anterior resection for the patient is that they can still defecate through their anus and have control. When you get too close to the bottom of the anus it doesn't work well. But the anal canal is spared in a low anterior resection. And, surgeons are masterful at mobilizing the colon and bringing it down. The colon is beautiful in adapting to removing water and patients with a low anterior resection have the same sort of lifestyle as those that have a normal colon throughout. Typically, for colon cancers in the rectum.

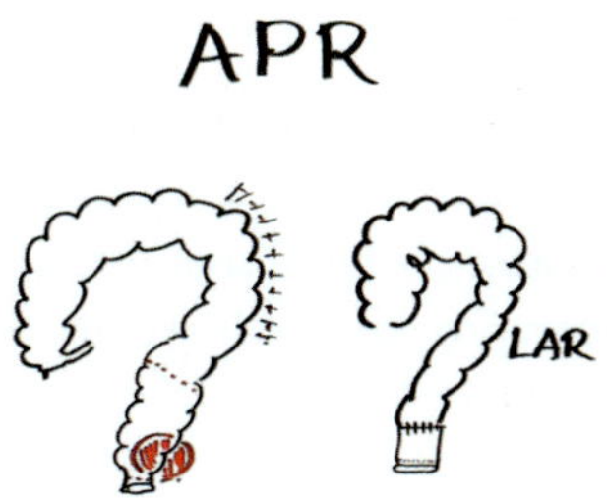

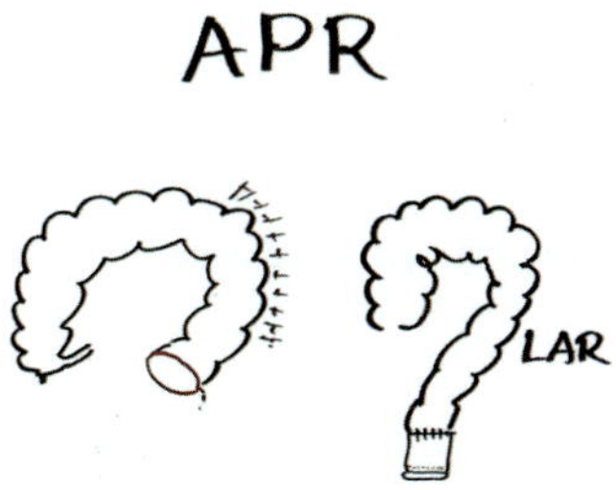

VIDEO 5.10. Abdominal Perineal Resection.
Transcript: Abdominal perineal resection involves resecting tumors very near the anus. The problem with this operation is that if you resect this portion you can't bring this down like a low anterior resection and sew it and let people be able to control their defecation. If you bring this colon down to the very bottom of the anus, stool will leak out with absolutely no control, and that is not a viable alternative or quality of life. But you can remove the entire anus and rectum and then bring out an ostomy, sigmoid colostomy, and a bag over the top; it is not ideal but allows people to have a function of life and a quality of life that is excellent. Abdominal perineal resection, so-called the Miles procedure, removes the entire rectum and anus leaves patients, usually with a left lower quadrant sigmoid colostomy.

Colon Challenge Questions

5.1. What are white lines of Toldt?
5.2. What might microcytic anemia signify in men and postmenopausal women?
5.3. What are the contraindications for hepatic resection of liver metastases from colon cancer?
5.4. What is the diagnostic work-up for colonic obstruction?
5.5. What is the arc of Riolan?
5.6. What is Ogilvie syndrome?
5.7. What is total mesorectal excision?
5.8. What is the most common fistula that forms with diverticulitis?
5.9. Describe a cecal bascule volvulus.

Answers to Colon Challenge Questions

5.1. Avascular peritoneum along lateral edges of ascending and descending colon.
5.2. Colon cancer.
5.3. More than 5 metastases, other distant metastases, or positive portal or celiac LNs.
5.4. Abdominal radiography and sodium diatrizoate-meglumine diatrizoate enema. CT can be considered.
5.5. The arterial connection between the SMA and the IMA within the base of the mesentery. The meandering artery of Drummond is often between the SMA and the IMA, closer to the bowel.
5.6. Colonic pseudo-obstruction (ileus).
5.7. En bloc resection of mesorectum and LNs with the rectum.
5.8. Colovesical fistula.
5.9. The cecum folds upward onto the ascending colon.

6

Duodenum

Embryology

The duodenum develops from endoderm of the caudal portion of the foregut and the cranial portion of the midgut; the ampulla of Vater lies just proximal to their junction.

Anatomy

The duodenum (Video 6.1) is roughly 26 cm (approximately 12 finger-breadths) in length, extending from the pylorus to the ligament of Treitz (Figure 6.1). Proximal to the ampulla of Vater (Video 6.2), the duodenal blood supply (Figure 6.2) consists of the gastroduodenal artery and the superior pancreaticoduodenal artery. Distally, duodenal blood flow comes from the SMA and 1 of its branches, the inferior pancreaticoduodenal artery.

Physiology

Brunner glands secrete a bicarbonate-rich mucus that is protective to the duodenal mucosa and provides an alkaline environment for digestive enzymes to activate. K cells produce gastric inhibitory peptide, which decreases gastric acid secretion. Cholecystokinin (Video 6.3) is secreted by I cells and causes GB contraction. It also causes relaxation of the sphincter of Oddi (Figure 6.3), which allows bile to enter the duodenum. S cells produce secretin, which increases bile flow and pancreatic bicarbonate release.

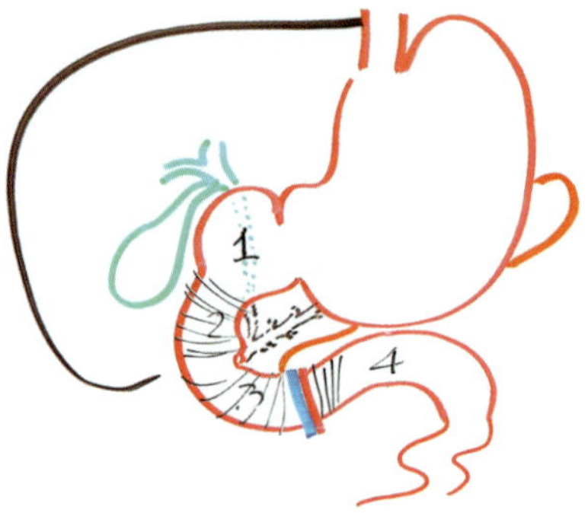

VIDEO 6.1. Four Sections of the Duodenum.
Transcript: The duodenum is the small intestine just distal to the stomach. The duodenum is named duodenum because duodenum means 12, and early anatomists put their hands down and said, "Boy, it's about 12 fingers long," so it became the duodenum, and it's divided up into 4 parts. Part 1 is the bulb, that's intraperitoneal. Part 2 is a retroperitoneal portion that extends down to the ampulla of Vater. This is the second portion of the duodenum. These 2 areas have Brunner's glands that secrete mucus and protect the rest of the intestine from the acid of the stomach. The third portion of the duodenum swings down here to the bottom until it gets to the mesenteric vessels. From there the duodenum actually heads cephalad and truthfully back up underneath the stomach, where at some point this retroperitoneal structure becomes intraperitoneal, so fourth portion, first portion, intraperitoneal; the retroperitoneal is the second and third portions. The ampulla of Vater is important because the foregut is the esophagus down to the ampulla, that's blood supply from the celiac, and then from the ampulla of Vater downstream is supplied by the SMA. This is the duodenum.

Clinical Presentation

Duodenal ulcers, often caused by *Helicobacter pylori*, can cause epigastric pain. Pain occurs 2 to 5 hours after a meal, is relieved by food or antacids, and may radiate to the back. Bleeding occurs with posterior wall ulcers (from the gastroduodenal artery). Some patients present with shock, and others present with chronic anemia. ACA of the small bowel primarily occurs in the duodenum or proximal jejunum and often causes obstructive symptoms. Periampullary tumors (Video 6.4) present with jaundice, GI bleeding, or pancreatitis.

Imaging

UGI (Video 6.5) and EGD (Video 6.6) studies can show ulcers or masses in the duodenum. Jaundiced patients may benefit from US or CT.

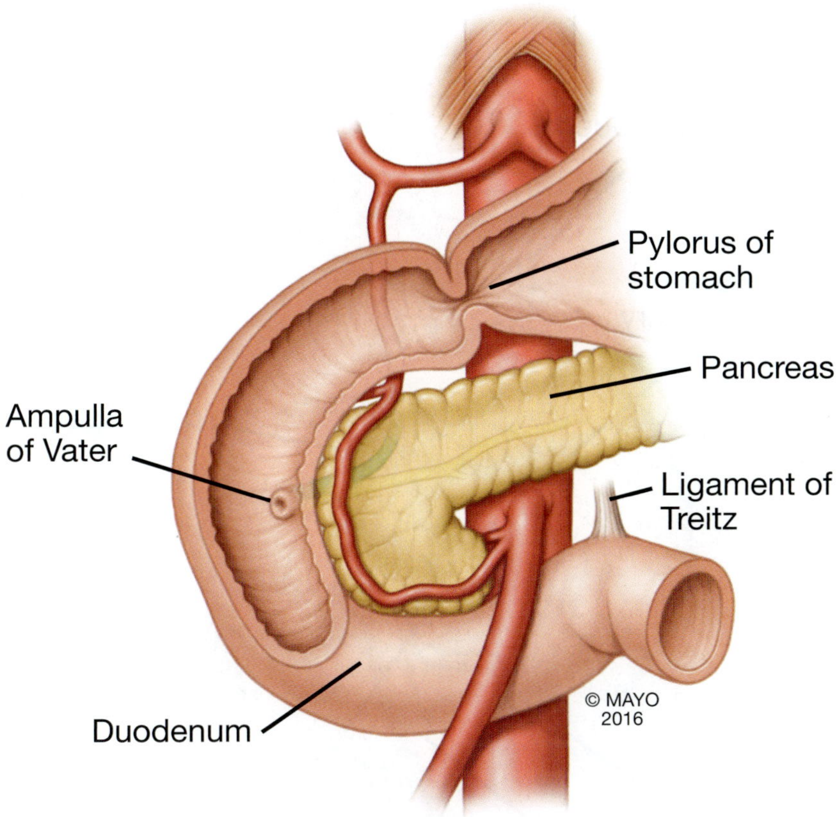

FIGURE 6.1. Anatomy of the Duodenum.

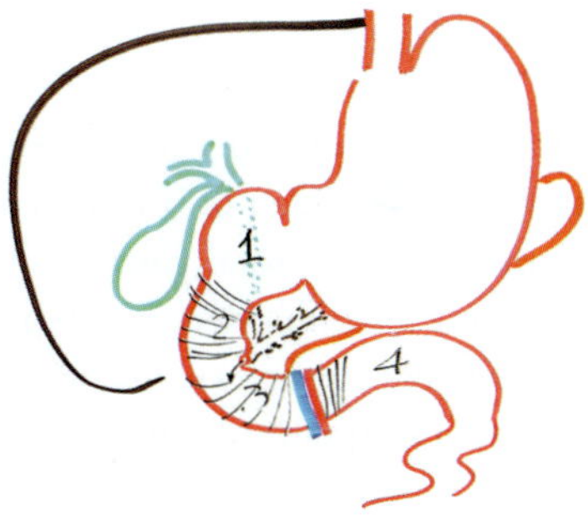

VIDEO 6.2. Location and Action of the Ampulla of Vater.
Transcript: So halfway through the duodenum exists the ampulla of Vater. It's an amazing structure that regulates bile from the liver and gallbladder and the pancreatic juice that sneaks through secreted by the pancreas, and it's responsive to what happens enterally. So people that are eating and drinking and contracting, fluid comes out of the ampulla of Vater. It's regulated by the sphincter of Oddi, O-D-D-I, and it's very complex and it's based on hormones and the pH and a variety of conditions within the GI tract. The sphincter of Oddi is made up within the ampulla of Vater. The common bile duct and the pancreatic duct join together within the head of the pancreas and allow bile to emanate along with the pancreatic juice into the GI tract to help you break down food and food particles.

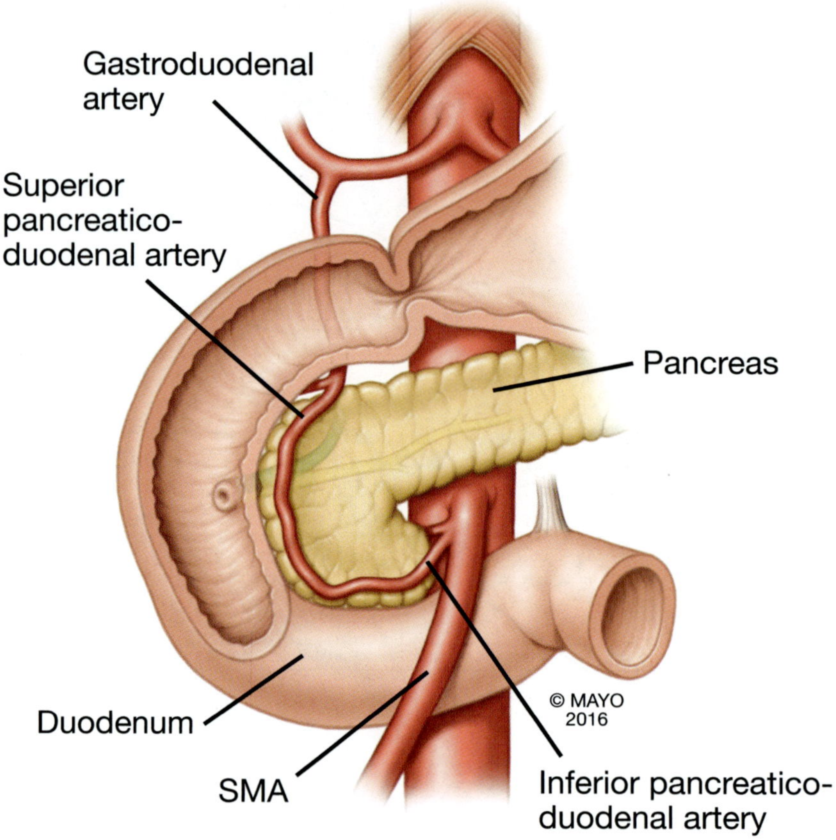

FIGURE 6.2. Duodenal Blood Supply.

Operation

Severe bleeding, perforation, and obstruction caused by duodenal ulcers are managed surgically. The Graham patch (Video 6.7) is a technique used to treat acute perforation. Vagotomy, antrectomy, and subtotal gastrectomy (Video 6.8) may be used to decrease acid secretion. Pancreaticoduodenectomy removes cancers of the ampulla or duodenum in patients amenable to surgery and without evidence of metastatic disease. Ladd band release is indicated for malrotation of the small bowel (Video 6.9).

Complications

Complications of duodenal surgery may include bleeding, anastomotic leak or stricture, bile duct injury, pancreatitis or leak, reflux esophagitis, or dumping syndrome (Video 6.10).

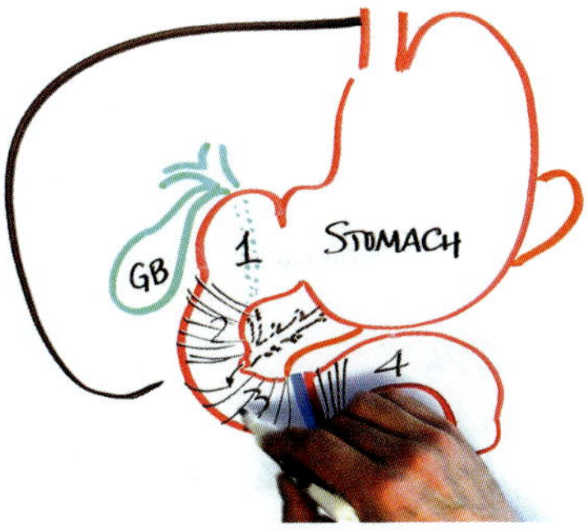

VIDEO 6.3. Cholecystokinin Secretion.
Transcript: Cholecystokinin, or CCK, is secreted by the I cells of the duodenum and the jejunum. They are stimulated by the release of amino acids and fatty acids in the duodenum, so when the body takes food into the stomach and passes that on and breaks it down, cholecystokinin is released from the I cells. The cholecystokinin does a variety of things. It slows down the stomach from emptying so it can help process this, it helps stimulate the gallbladder to contract so more bile comes in and breaks down the fluid in the GI tract, and it stimulates the acinar cells of the pancreas to release pancreatic enzymes to aid in digestion. So cholecystokinin is a crucial hormone that helps increase bile secretion, slows up the stomach a little bit, and then allows the pancreatic juices to break down the protein products within the GI tract.

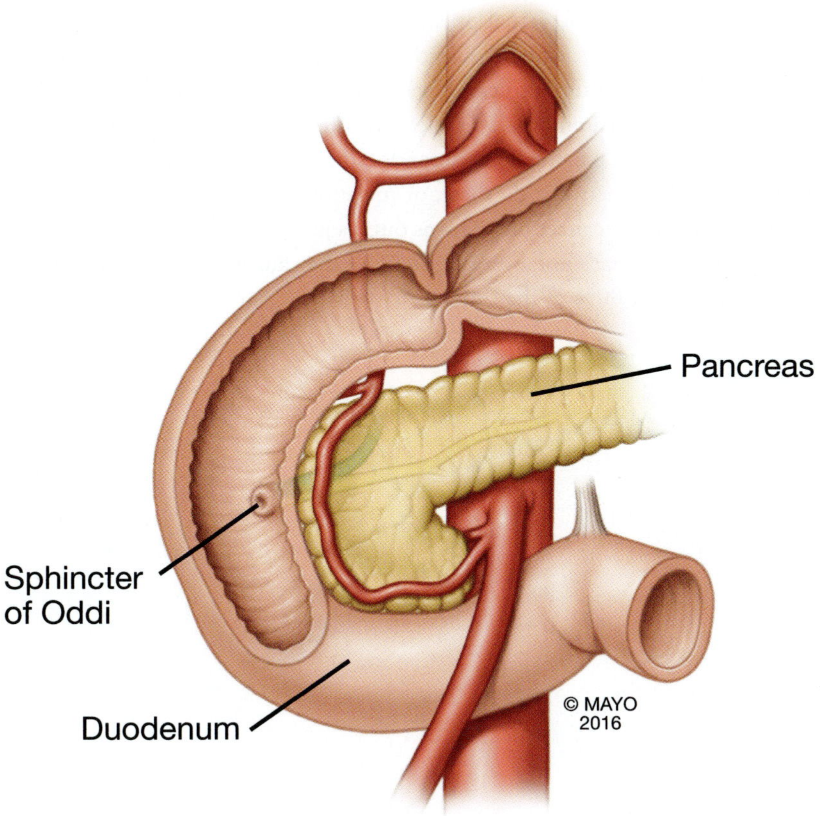

FIGURE 6.3. Location of the Sphincter of Oddi.

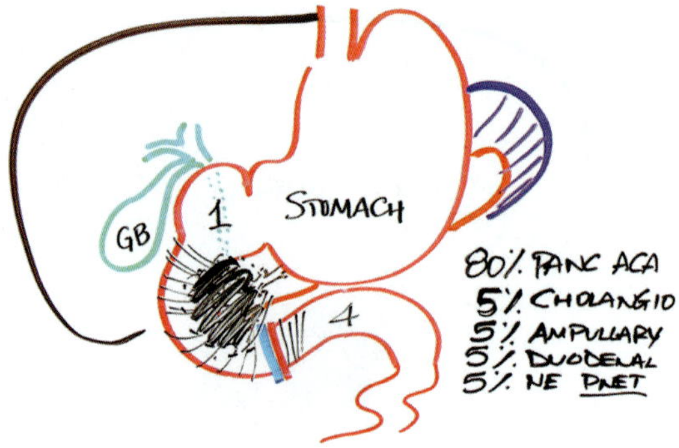

VIDEO 6.4. Periampullary Tumors.

Transcript: Periampullary tumors, that's the region around the ampulla of Vater, so we're talking about tumors at the head of the pancreas, the duodenum, the ampulla of Vater, and the bile duct. These tumors can cause problems, and because they're in this region, they're likely to cause painless jaundice, and that's how they present, with a mass in the head of the pancreas; and so what young trainees need to understand is about 80% of all of these tumors are pancreatic adenocarcinoma. Unfortunately, that has the worst diagnosis. It's sinister, it doesn't show up until the bile duct is obstructed.

Then there are a variety of tumors that make up 5% of the rest of these things, and in no particular order. A bile duct tumor, a cholangiocarcinoma, usually shows up a bit quicker because it's in the bile duct and people get painless jaundice, so maybe the survival is a smidge better than pancreatic adenocarcinoma. The ampulla of Vater, the actual opening there by the pancreatic head, so-called ampullary cancers, probably have the best outcome because the ampulla is the blocking point and people become symptomatic quicker. The duodenum also can have cancers and may cause symptoms earlier such that it's better than pancreatic adenocarcinoma. A variety of other things, so-called neuroendocrine tumors, which some people call PNETs, pancreatic neuroendocrine tumor; sometimes you can have metastatic tumors (especially renal cell cancers can do that), or melanoma. And fortunately, sometimes of this 5% that's left, we think it's a pancreas cancer but it turns out it's just pancreatitis that looks like it. That would ultimately be the best because that's not a cancer. So of all the cancers that are periampullary, think pancreatic adenocarcinoma at least 80% of the time.

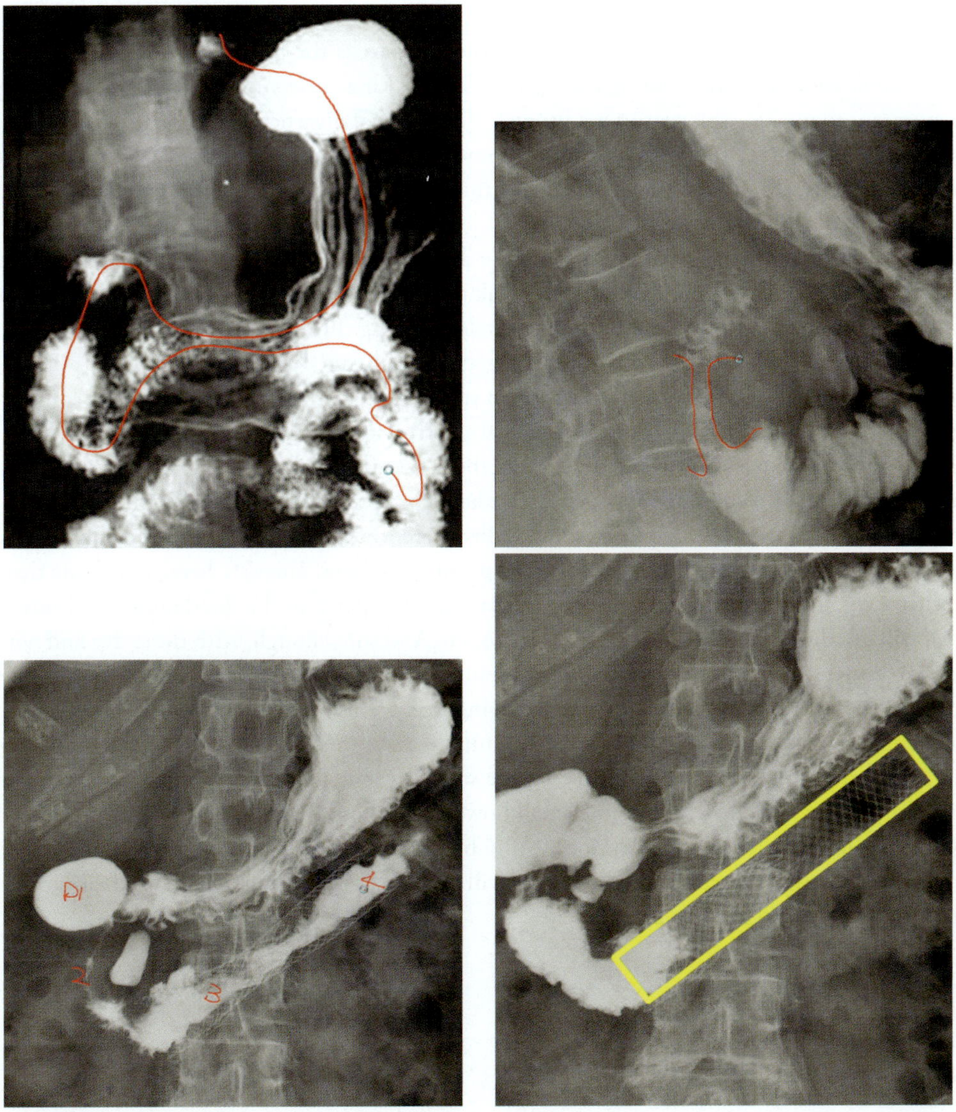

VIDEO 6.5. UGI Radiography.
Transcript: To image the duodenum can be done in a couple different ways, but here's a nice way to do it. Either barium or Hypaque or Gastrografin can be inserted, either swallowed into the stomach, fills the stomach, slides through up into the duodenum, second portion, third portion, fourth portion, and then around it goes. This test, we need to follow it along. This is a still photo of an upper GI/small bowel follow-through.

So let me take you through that if I could just a little bit better. So here's a plain film of the abdomen. I hope you can sense that there's a tube, that's a nasogastric tube. Drinking barium or Hypaque or contrast isn't the most fun thing in the world. So this is a normal little picture.

And now you can get a sense that there's contrast coming out of the tube, and it's filling up the stomach up top and it's sliding down and it's sneaking in through the pylorus, and it becomes the first portion of the duodenum. And then that dye will go into the second portion of the duodenum, and then ideally we'll see more. The third portion of the duodenum, remember that it comes cephalad up, anterior, it comes

VIDEO 6.5. Continued

toward the head, cephalad, or superior. And then the last part is the fourth portion of the duodenum. And as we think about this dye coming through, we'll look for a variety of structures. On this upper GI study, important to note for this person is a funny little duodenal diverticulum. It's benign, usually doesn't cause any problems, but it's funny to note and it sometimes is confusing because D1, the first portion of the duodenum, is usually round and circular, and this is a funny little thing that actually is probably in the third portion of the duodenum.

So the dye has gotten into the third portion of the duodenum. What goes on now? Can you see the dye trickling through? I hope you can. It's trying to sneak through there, and it is getting past it, but barely so. And that's because there's a tumor there, and it's barely sneaking through a duodenal cancer. Again, here's this apple-core lesion. The dye sneaks through, it gets through, and we're into the fourth portion of the duodenum and into the jejunum. So the person can still eat and drink. And we wait a little longer and we see the dye does percolate through, but this is a near-obstructing lesion.

Back to our anterior-posterior view, we can see the stomach and the first portion of the duodenum, and we get a sense that it's cut off here. What do we have for options? Dye sneaking through, it's trying to get through there. We can actually put in what's called a stent. I think you can see that there very clearly. Endoscopists can put in a stent, and there are a couple of them here. There's 1 here, and inside that 1 they put another 1 in, and it actually stretches out the cancer and opens up the duodenum. And now the endoscopist will use the dye to say it's open or it's not open. And sure enough, with more dye and with more contrast we can see again first portion of the duodenum, second portion, here's the third portion, it gets all the way to the fourth portion, and the dye is moving freely. This person, who may have been obstructed and vomiting, now can eat and drink for the remaining days of their life or undergo chemotherapy.

Again, another picture, importantly showing the stent is wide open, and more importantly than that, we know for a fact it's all the way into the small bowel and colon. This is a very successful procedure in somebody that, if we didn't have this option, would be nauseated and vomiting the last days of their life. As it stands now, they can eat and drink, and they will meet their maker but at least on their terms; it adds a great quality of life, and this is a patent stent.

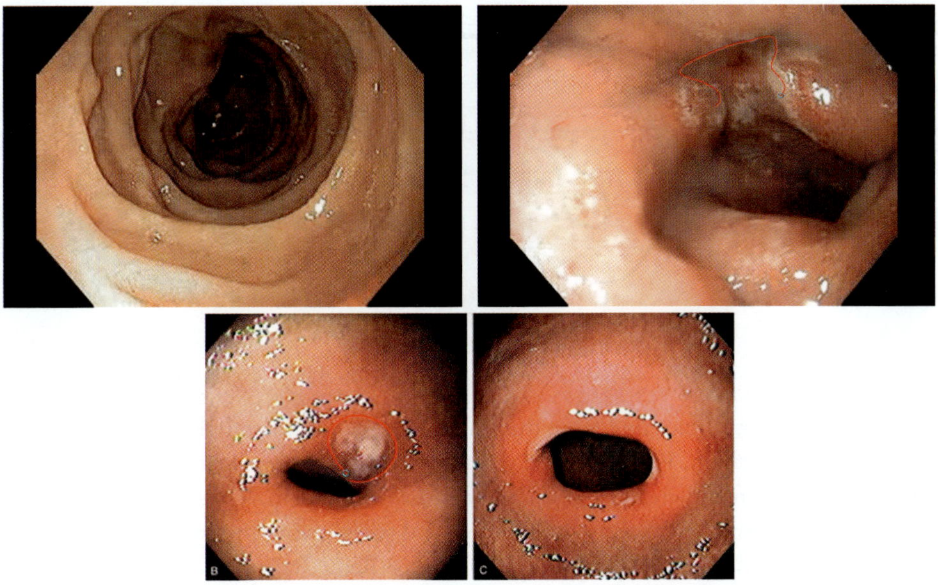

VIDEO 6.6. EGD of the Duodenum.

Transcript: The best way to image the duodenum is to directly look at it, and that's best done and easiest for the patient with an endoscope placed down through the mouth, into the esophagus, into the stomach, and then into the duodenum. This is a normal-looking duodenum, normally about 12 inches long, and most endoscopists can see the whole thing. It's a little tougher in the third and fourth portions, but this is the first and second portions of the duodenum. We see these concentric rings, very normal-looking duodenum.

Things change as acid increases, ulcerations can happen. We see a little bit of erythema and a little ulcer. It's a start, it's a minor little thing. Things like this can actually happen with the trauma of the scope, passing it down, so when you go in and look, look carefully first, because when you pull back the scope, you may have caused some trauma, some erythema, some bleeding, but this is a small little ulcer.

As we progress along, we can see serious ulceration. This has been here a while for that to happen, and this is excess acid, *H pylori*, typically more common in men than in women, more frequently in people that smoke or drink. The better your health, the less likely it is you'll develop peptic ulcer disease. But you can see the swelling, the edema in this duodenum. We no longer have these concentric rings.

Here's a smaller little ulcer on the side, looking downstream. Maybe over the course of time it gets better and heals up; if you eradicate *H pylori*, give antibiotics, give some sort of antacid, the body can heal itself up.

Something like this, looks like we've got an ulceration, and maybe we come back a couple days later, it's still red and inflamed, and maybe the ulcer is healed up, maybe not. We need to slide through the next concentric ring and make sure there isn't other trouble downstream. Duodenum and duodenal ulcers are best imaged with an endoscope.

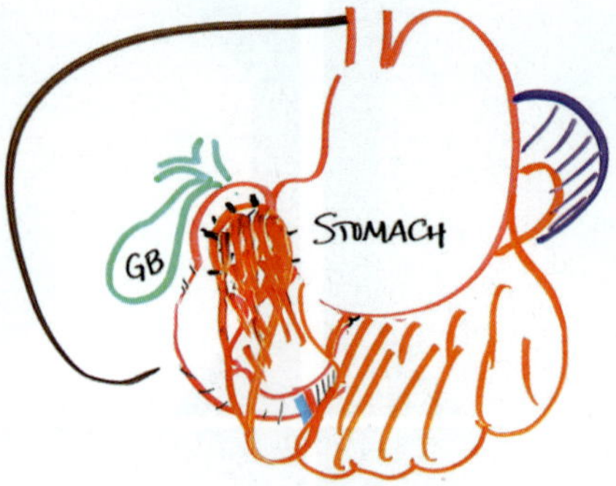

VIDEO 6.7. Graham Patch.

Transcript: A Graham patch is nothing more than taking the omentum and placing it over a hole, which is oftentimes in the duodenum. People with ulcer problems, high acid output—the acid comes into the duodenum, it breaks down and creates a hole, a perforation, acute pain. It's usually a tiny little hole—2, 3, 4, 5 mm in size. Oftentimes the tissue is inflamed, and when trying to sew it together, it won't hold together, so what surgeons have done (first done by Roscoe Reid Graham in 1937) is took part of that omentum and brought it up and actually sewed it over the top. They took some silk sutures and said the tissue isn't very good but the omentum is good, and we'll sew this over the top and see what happens. And low and behold, the omentum, which is the policeman of the abdomen, basically scarred this thing shut, patient got better, they treated him with antacids, and the patient did just fine. The other choice is to remove the duodenum or remove part of the stomach—those are big operations. So when you hear surgeons talk about a Graham patch, it's kind of a simple little band-aid over a hole in the first portion of the duodenum. It works exceedingly well, and nowadays, with less and less problems with ulcer disease, we treat people for *H pylori*, lower acid content, and if they need an operation, this can be done laparoscopically or even endoscopically at times. The so-called Graham patch.

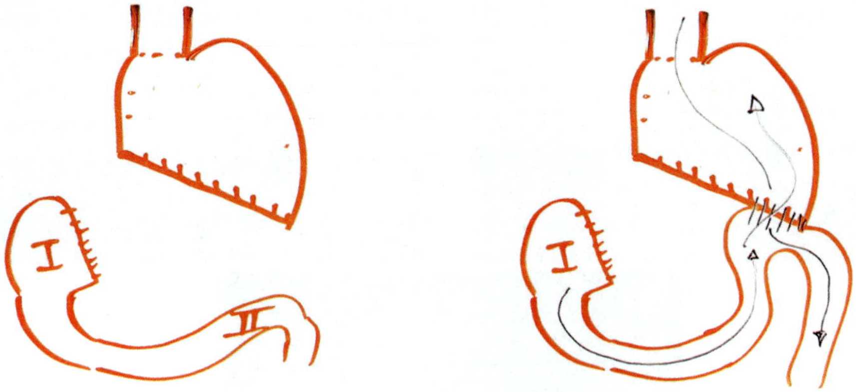

VIDEO 6.8. Subtotal Gastrectomy. I indicates Billroth I anastomosis; II, Billroth II gastrectomy. Transcript: Removing a portion of the stomach is called a subtotal gastrectomy, and usually that's at least half of the stomach or more, a near-total gastrectomy, versus total gastrectomy. So as we think about subtotal gastrectomy, which is probably the most common operation—fortuitously less common now than it was in the 1910s, 1920s, and 1930s, when stomach surgery was far more common and acid was more problematic—we talk about doing what's called an antrectomy, and that means removing the antrum and maybe a portion of the body of the stomach. If that was simply the case, it would look something like that, with a cut edge, and the duodenum would be cut. So now what you need is to somehow hook the stomach, without the antrum, either back to the duodenum or to the jejunum. If you hook it to the duodenum, that's called a Billroth I anastomosis, in honor of Theodor Billroth, who did this in the late 1880s in Germany. If you take the jejunum and sew it to the stomach, that's called a Billroth II gastrectomy. It's rare that we put the stomach to the duodenum anymore. So what typically it looks like in the end (pardon my drawing), but it looks something like this (that's a little easier than it really is), but now we have a side-to-side or end-to-side gastrojejunostomy, so now the food comes down the esophagus and through and it's smart enough over time to head downstream. Unfortunately, we also now have bile and pancreatic juice that sneaks up, and because there's a hole there and not a pylorus and it's not controlled, it can come up. So these operations give great bile access to the esophagus and can cause heartburn; but simplistically, a Billroth II gastrectomy, gastrojejunostomy after an antrectomy.

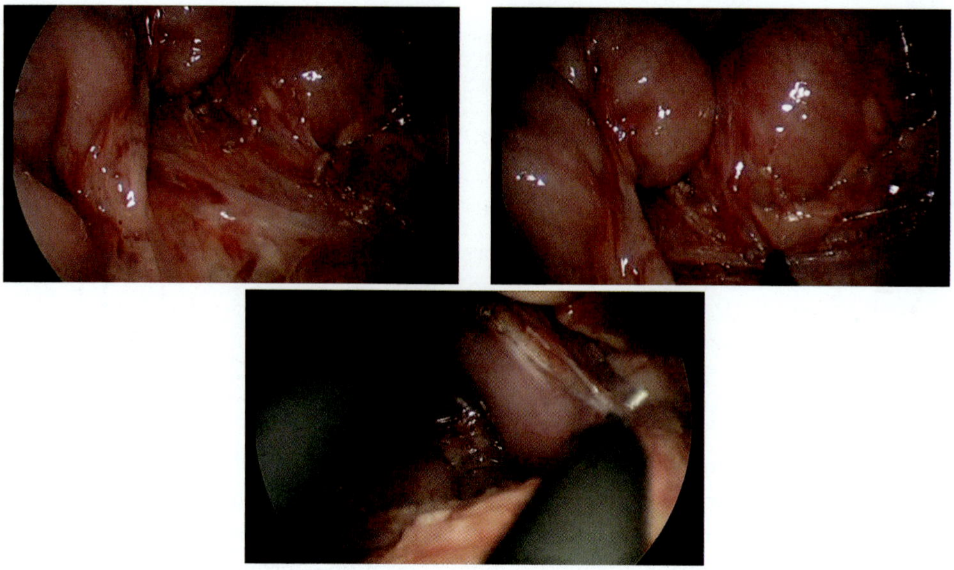

VIDEO 6.9. Ladd Band Release: Intraoperative.

Transcript: Surgical correction of malrotation is an operation pediatric patients oftentimes need, and we do what's called a Ladd's band release. That's the appendix, and it's actually sitting up underneath the liver here, and we've got some pediatric surgeons working hard on a young patient, maybe a couple months old, maybe a couple years old, but the appendix doesn't belong in the right upper quadrant, and that's because there was malrotation. So what needs to be done is this band that sort of crosses the duodenum to the right upper quadrant needs to be released. Beautiful, healthy-appearing liver here. Tough to know what's colon, what's duodenum, and being there for the whole procedure, we get a sense of where we are. The duodenum is up above, the small bowel is to the left, and we've got some bands that are going across left to right, and so with the hook cautery, our surgeon is going to release that and allow the mesentery of the small bowel to open up.

The problem with malrotation is the mesentery gets tethered with these little fibrous attachments; I think you can get a sense they're going left and right. The surgeon needs to lift up a little bit and be careful not to burn anything below it. That little hook cautery, a little pulse, a little teasing, and a little pressure will eventually release, and so the duodenum, behind it the small bowel, can open up and we can get a sense that it will be better perfused and there won't be a kink, there won't be an obstruction. People go from symptomatic to somebody that has a nice life if we can get this done safely, and especially with little bitty incisions, a patient like this, a pediatric patient, might go home within a day or 2.

Historically this would have been something in the hospital for several weeks. Teeny little bands again off the backside of the duodenum; that's being held up. You can see that whitish mark—that's a char mark. We've got to be careful that we don't burn the bowel. This is dangerous surgery. You really have to be extraordinarily careful. You need a great team. Somebody's running the laparoscope to make sure that we can see what it is that we're doing. At this point those Ladd's bands have been released, and we get a sense that we can move the bowel pretty much wherever we want, and if we can't, we've got a little bit more to do.

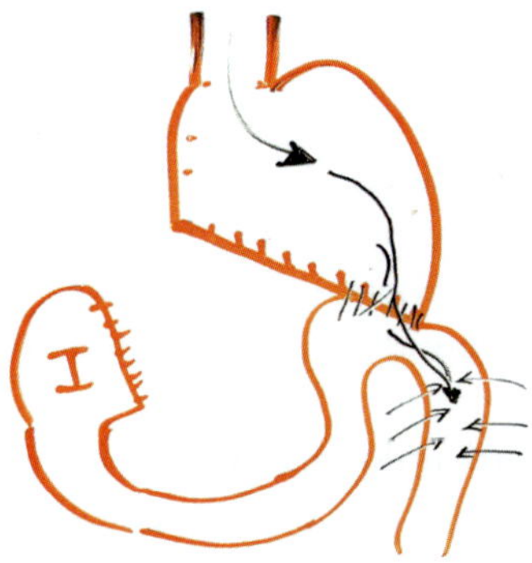

VIDEO 6.10. Dumping Syndrome. I indicates Billroth I anastomosis.
Transcript: Dumping syndrome is related to the fact that we eat food and it sneaks into the stomach. Folks that have an early connection from the stomach that goes to the small intestine, the jejunum, are set up for dumping syndrome. Without this stomach and pylorus that slows things down, we can have hypertonic food, and that could be a milkshake, that could be potato chips, that could be a variety of structures, that sneak in and gain quick entry into the jejunum. Because of that, the jejunum is not prepared, it's not ready for all that material, and it will oftentimes dilute that hypertonic food bolus; it will throw water or mucus in there, and actually people get dehydrated, get light-headed, get nauseated, can pass out. The symptoms are fairly common after an operation like this—an antrectomy or subtotal gastrectomy—where we gave access to the small intestine. Most of the time it will resolve with time.

The body is pretty doggone smart, and the patients are smart themselves. They'll start to eat smaller meals, lower fat, lower carbohydrates, and higher protein. Protein doesn't seem to be the problem; it's the carbohydrates that cause the problems. They're careful about how much liquid that they race through. So a dumping syndrome is an unusual syndrome that happens after stomach surgery where there's easy access into the small bowel and the body has a tough time adapting.

Duodenum Challenge Questions

6.1. Why is the portion of the small intestine just distal to the stomach called the *duodenum*?
6.2. Who was Dr Roscoe Reid Graham?
6.3. What is a parietal cell vagotomy?
6.4. Describe a marginal ulcer.
6.5. Who gets SMA syndrome?
6.6. How is a Billroth I reconstruction different from a Billroth II?
6.7. Describe the treatment for duodenal diverticula.
6.8. What is the most common malignant tumor of the small intestine?
6.9. What is the treatment for *H pylori* infection?

Answers to Duodenum Challenge Questions

6.1. Anatomists noted that this portion of the intestine was approximately 12 finger-widths long, the measurement *duodecim* in Latin.

6.2. A Canadian surgeon who developed the omental patch repair (Graham patch) for perforated duodenal ulcers.

6.3. A selective vagectomy that removes innervation to the body and fundus of the stomach.

6.4. An ulcer that occurs at the anastomosis, just on the distal side.

6.5. Thin people. The SMA may compress the third portion of the duodenum.

6.6. Billroth I: end of the stomach to proximal end of the duodenum (gastroduodenostomy). Billroth II: side of the stomach to side of the jejunum (gastrojejunostomy).

6.7. First, observation (most common); next, invagination; and last, resection.

6.8. ACA.

6.9. Combinations of 3 antibiotics: metronidazole, omeprazole, and clarithromycin, or ampicillin, omeprazole, and clarithromycin.

7

Esophagus

Embryology

The esophagus develops from the tracheoesophageal septum of the foregut.

Anatomy

The esophagus is a hollow muscular tube approximately 25 cm in length, extending from the cricopharyngeus muscle (Figure 7.1) to the gastroesophageal junction at the gastric cardia. Blood supply (Figure 7.2) to the cervical esophagus is through the inferior thyroid arteries, to the thoracic esophagus through aortoesophageal branches, and to the abdominal esophagus through the left gastric and inferior phrenic arteries (Figure 7.3). The esophagus enters the abdomen through the esophageal hiatus (Figure 7.4) at roughly the level of T10.

Physiology

The esophagus is the only organ that uses peristalsis (Video 7.1). The lower esophageal sphincter (Figure 7.5) relaxes as the peristaltic wave travels downward, allowing a food bolus to enter the stomach.

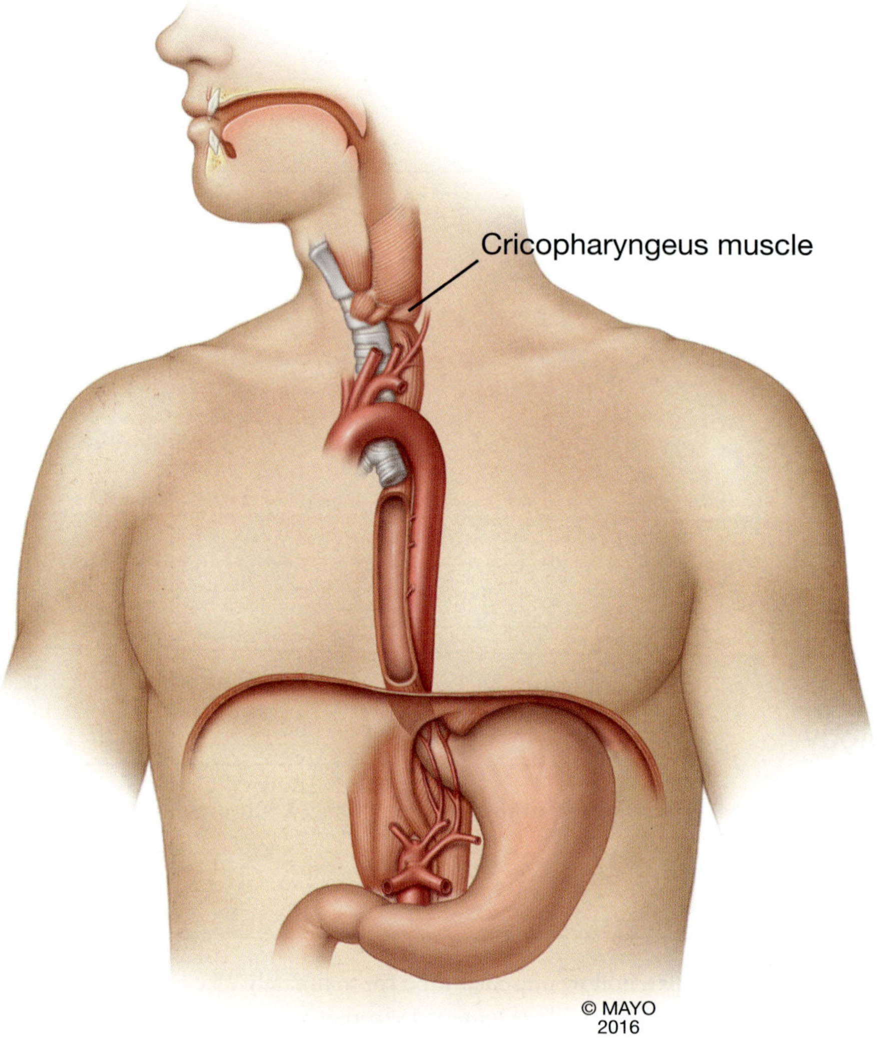

FIGURE 7.1. Location of the Cricopharyngeus Muscle.

Clinical Presentation

Achalasia (Video 7.2) is defined as failure of lower esophageal sphincter relaxation with concurrent esophageal aperistalsis; achalasia causes dysphagia to solids and liquids, regurgitation, and weight loss. DES is characterized by uncoordinated contractions resulting in chest pain and dysphagia. GERD is the most common disorder of the esophagus and presents with heartburn, regurgitation, dysphagia, chronic cough, hoarseness, or asthma. Long-standing GERD may lead to mucosal metaplasia. Diverticula of the esophagus (Video 7.3) are rare. Progressive dysphagia for solids and then liquids with weight loss raises concern for esophageal cancer.

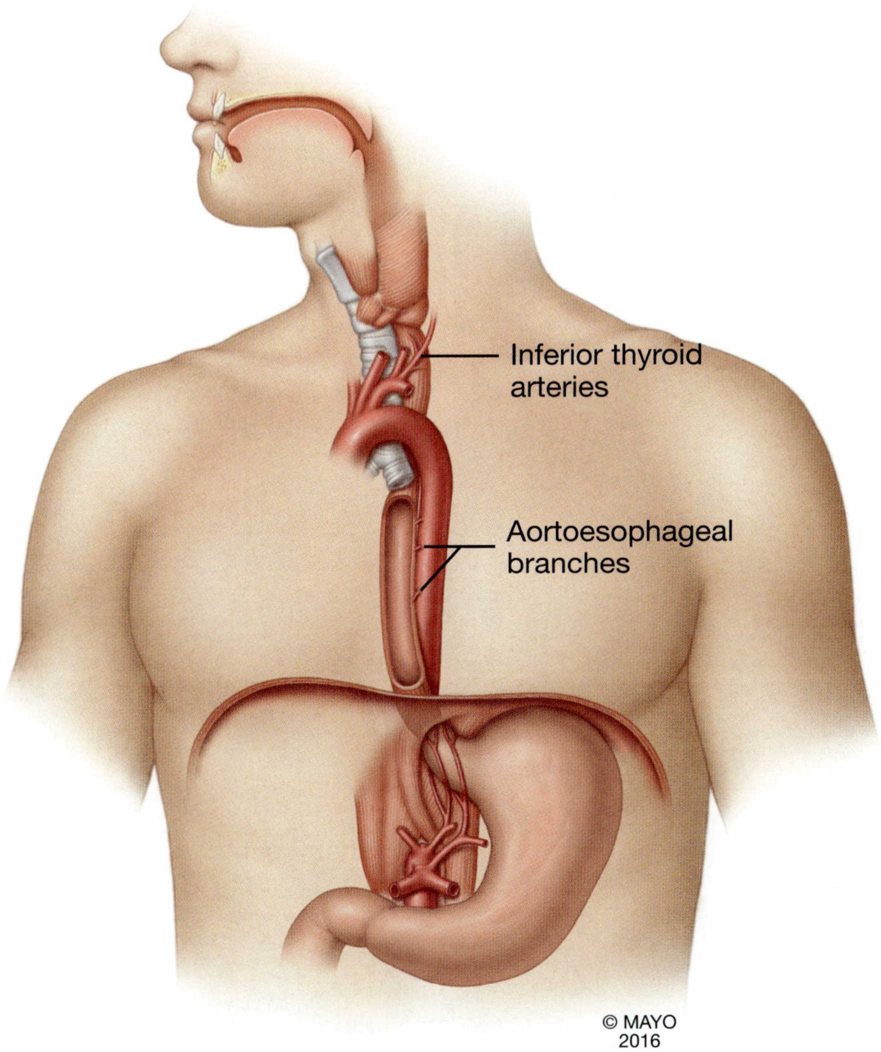

FIGURE 7.2. Blood Supply to the Cervical and Thoracic Esophagus.

Imaging

Esophageal manometry (Video 7.4) is the standard for diagnosing achalasia and DES. A barium esophagram (Video 7.5) identifies structural and functional abnormalities. Esophageal endoscopy (Video 7.6) helps to identify cancer (Video 7.7), strictures (Video 7.8), esophagitis, and mucosal metaplasia (Figure 7.6). CT is used to stage esophageal cancer.

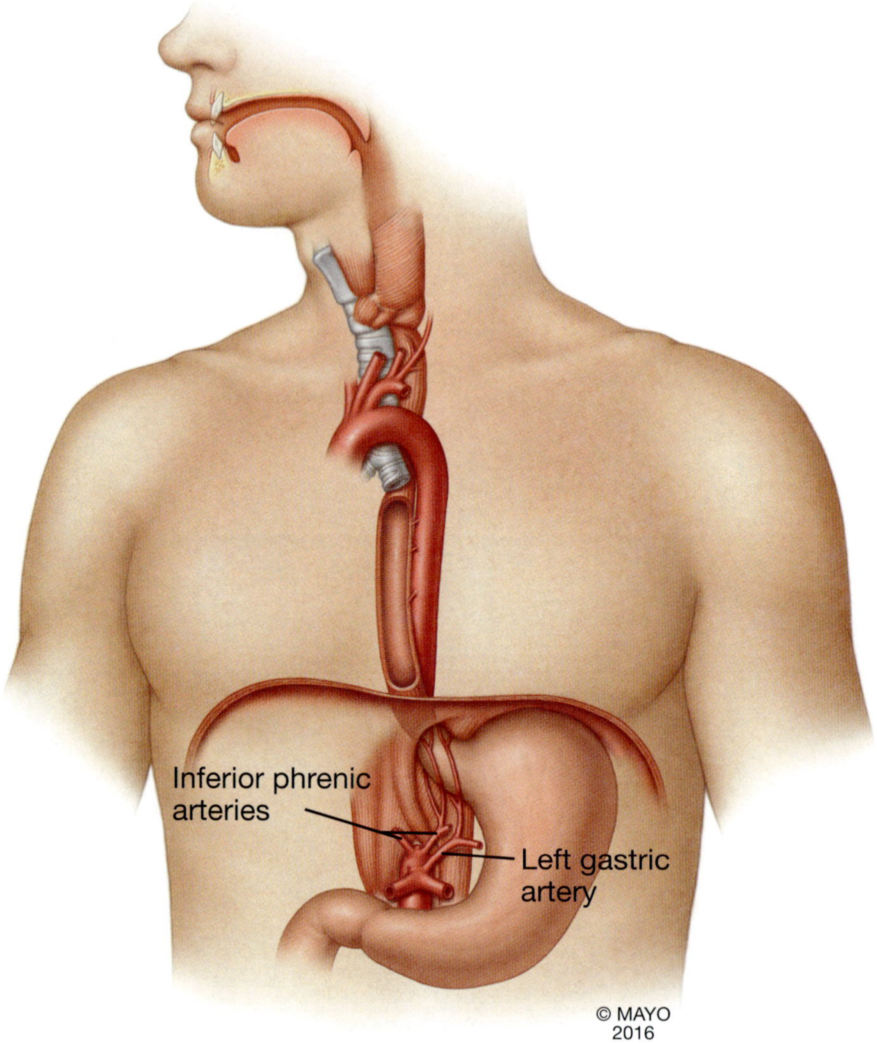

FIGURE 7.3. Blood Supply to the Abdominal Esophagus.

Operation

Achalasia is managed surgically with a Heller myotomy (Video 7.9). If medicine fails for DES, a long esophagomyotomy may relieve pain. Zenker diverticulum (Video 7.10) is treated when larger than 2 cm (diverticulopexy vs diverticulectomy). Esophageal cancer is resected with an Ivor Lewis esophagectomy or transhiatal esophagectomy (Video 7.11). GERD is often treated with a Nissen fundoplication (Video 7.12).

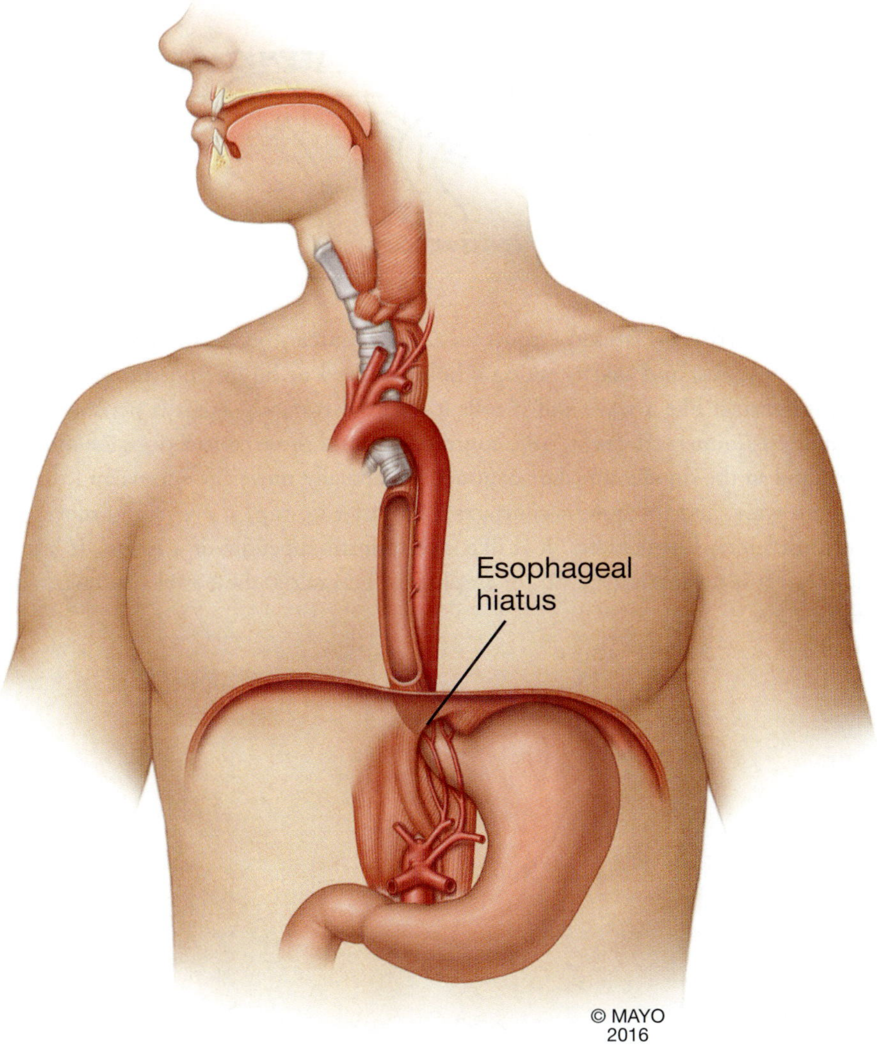

FIGURE 7.4. Location of the Esophageal Hiatus.

Complications

Esophageal surgery may result in an iatrogenic perforation (Video 7.13), thoracic duct injury, or anastomotic leak. A Heller myotomy may result in postoperative acid reflux and therefore is usually combined with a partial fundoplication (Video 7.14).

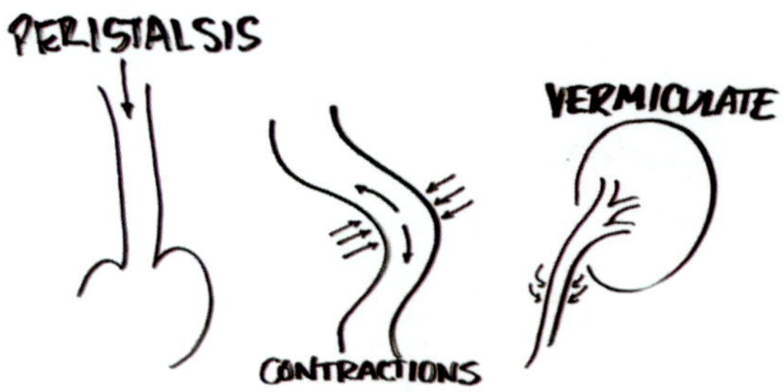

VIDEO 7.1. Peristalsis of the Esophagus.
Transcript: The term peristalsis is used erroneously in the human body. The only organ that truly has peristalsis is the esophagus, and that is taking a bolus of food or liquid and running it the entire way that the muscles contract like a wave and it rolls it into the stomach—that is peristalsis—where small bowel, duodenum, jejunum, and ileum, have contractions, and those contractions are more common up in the stomach and in the duodenum, but contractions actually move the succus and the milieu inside the intestine both ways, and (because it contracts a lot faster up top) it eventually moves things to the bottom. Lastly, the ureter vermiculates. It is like a vermiform appendix or a worm. It has a funny sort of contraction, but it is not peristalsis. So, in esophagus, peristalsis; the bowel contracts; and the ureter vermiculates.

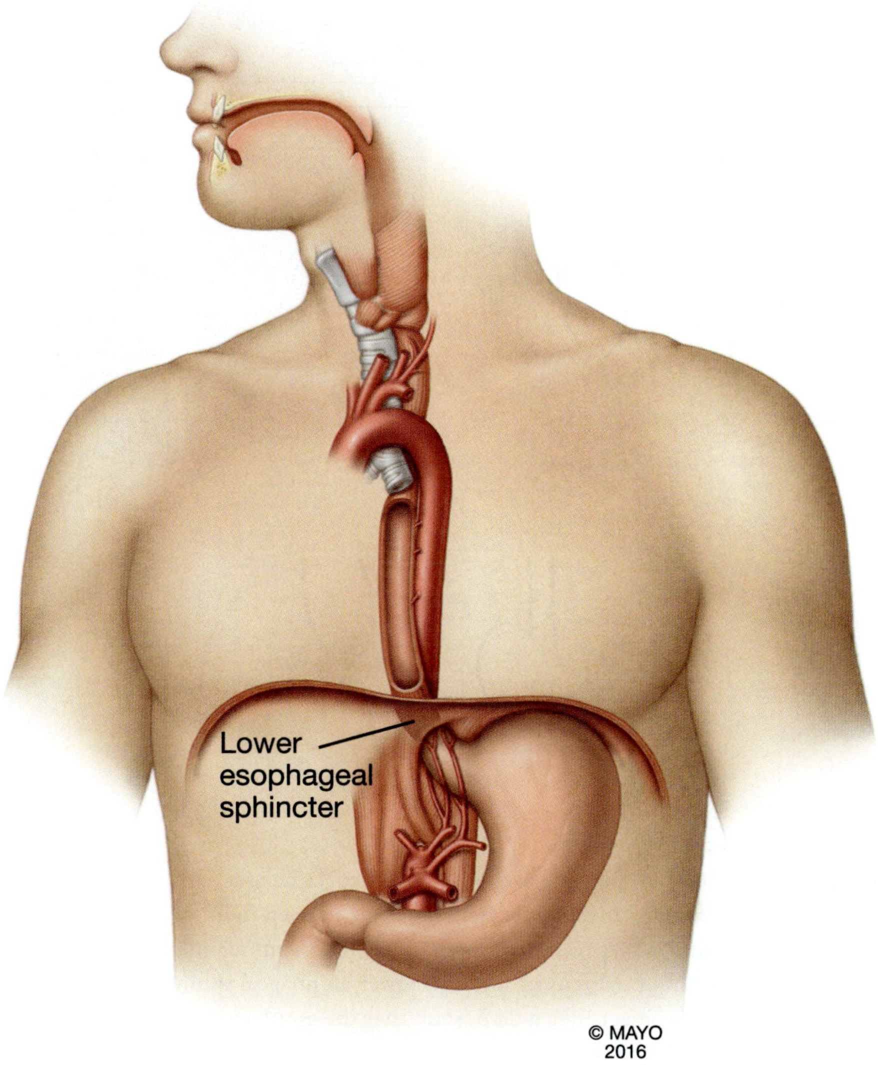

FIGURE 7.5. Location of the Lower Esophageal Sphincter.

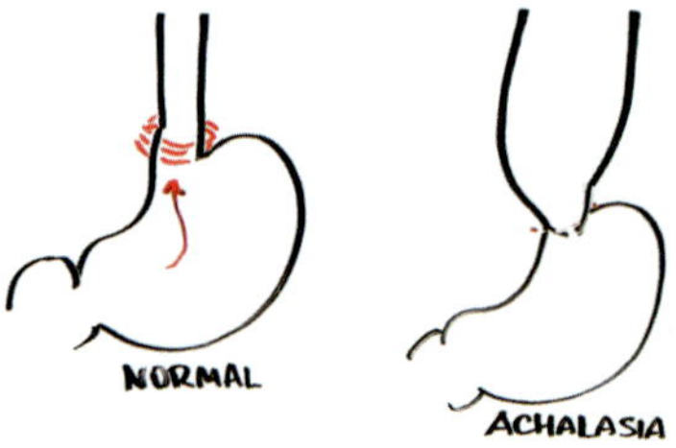

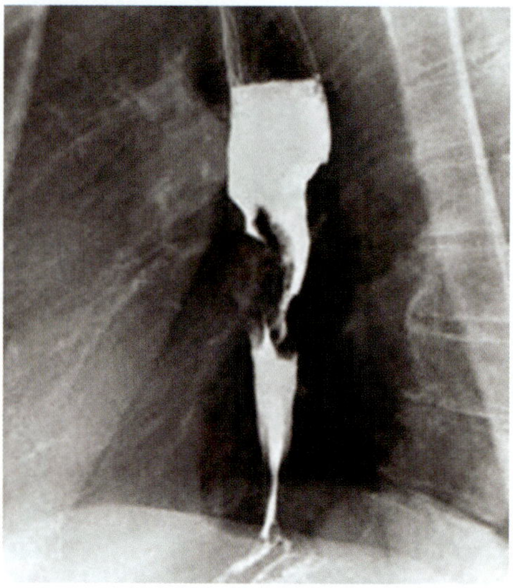

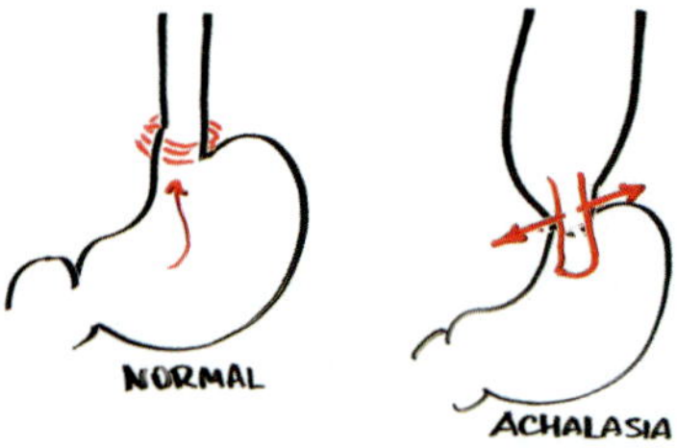

VIDEO 7.2. Achalasia of the Esophagus.
Transcript: Roughly 1 in 100,000 people have what is termed "achalasia." In the normal esophagus and stomach, there is a lower esophageal sphincter that allows us to keep food from coming back up, and it allows food to slide through when it relaxes properly. If there is a tumor there or the ganglion cells are not working, over time this thing tightens up and this lower esophageal sphincter doesn't allow things to move through. Because of that, it acts like a dam, such that the esophagus enlarges and it narrows down to something that looks like a bird's beak.

We will show you a barium esophogram which shows you that bird's beak. Indeed, that is what it looks like. It is a rare problem, and ideally surgeons fix this problem by dividing this lower esophageal sphincter in what is called a "Heller myotomy." You could also put a tube down and dilate with a balloon and stretch this out; that sometimes is very useful. People have used botulinum toxin to also to work on these nerves and what not, and relax things and allow things to slide through. It is a functional obstruction, people can have this backed up, there will be food in the esophagus, and they will typically have bad breath. They will typically have to have a lot of fluid to kind of wash it down. People have a lot of problems with this, so this is an important diagnosis to make and it is also a premalignant condition and it sets people up for what is called "squamous cell carcinoma." So, achalasia is a problem with the lower esophageal sphincter. Some way, 1 of 2 or 3 ways, surgery, botulinum toxin, or dilatation to alleviate that obstruction is important.

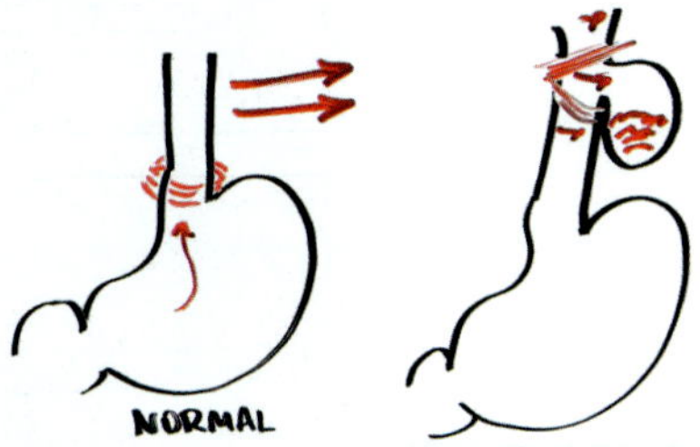

VIDEO 7.3. Diverticula of the Esophagus.
Transcript: The normal esophagus is this nice hollow tube and looks like a garden hose with no out pouches or bubbles. Outpouching, so-called diverticula can happen. More commonly in the colon, far more commonly, but 2 reasons for it to happen in the esophagus: 1) If something is pulling on the esophagus, inflammation, lung or cardiac, or pericardium, there is something on the outside of the esophagus pulling. In tuberculosis, you can get an outpouching of diverticula. 2) The far more common reason is there is muscular contraction narrowing and there are higher pressures. The pressure wants to push out and it pops out and creates a diverticulum. It isn't a true diverticulum because only part of the wall is out of there, so this is what is called a "false diverticulum"—this is called a Zenker diverticulum; it can be treated by a variety of things including resecting it or endoscopically opening this thing up. But they are fairly common, food fills up in these things and people have bad breath and sometimes pain in the neck or the upper chest. They regurgitate food later in the day, and it is a problem that people don't like, and they like to get it fixed up. Invariably, the larger they get (>3 cm in size), the more Zenker diverticulums are repaired with surgery.

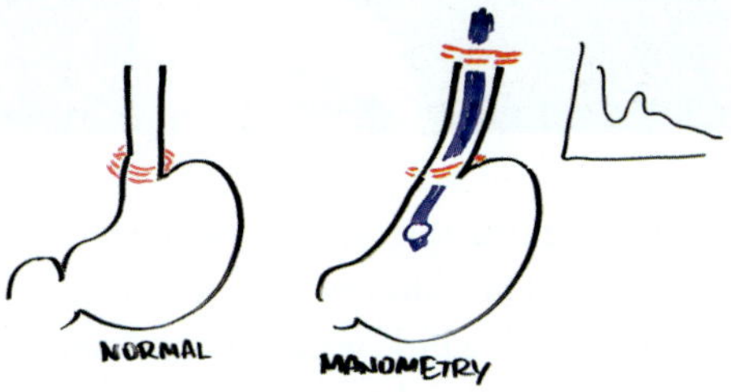

VIDEO 7.4. Manometry of the Esophagus.
Transcript: From time to time, people will have upper GI endoscopy and things look perfectly normal; but, they may not be perfectly normal, and 1 of the tests that we use is manometry. Patients can swallow tubing that has the ability to assess the pressures. So you can imagine if you are in the stomach, there is basically no pressure on this manometry, and the tubing that goes through the lower esophageal sphincter will have pressure, there should be a resting pressure there. In achalasia would be much higher and in some other disorders, it may be far too low. The normal esophagus will have a pressure, typically not high while it is resting, and then where the cricopharyngeus and other musculatures of the upper esophageal sphincter that will contract. Now you might imagine when water is sipped or fluid, this peristalsis will happen, relax here, relax here, and relax here, this wave of peristalsis will slide through and that will give us an opportunity to see the pressures in the esophagus. And the manometry picture shown to you here shows some evidence of a normal manometry, and those that might happen with achalasia or other disorders.

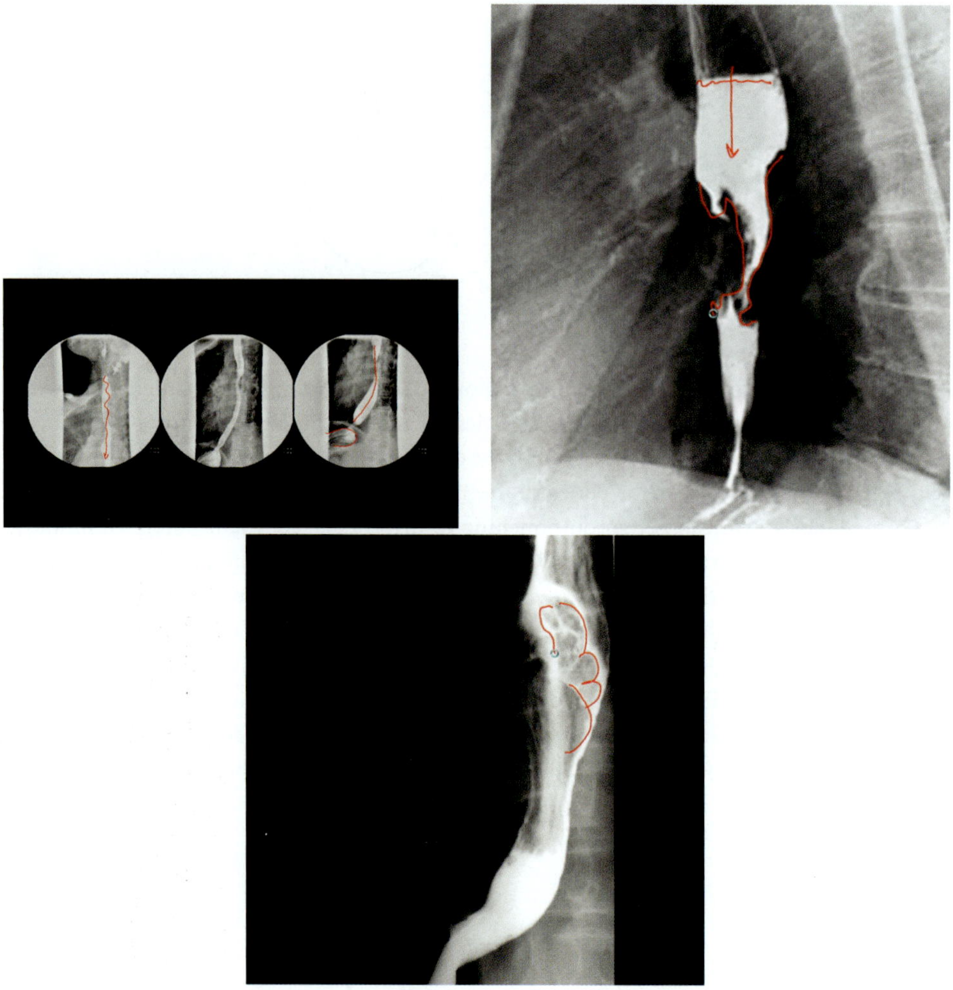

VIDEO 7.5. Barium Esophagram.

Transcript: The esophagus is an amazing structure. It takes foods and liquids from the pharynx down into the stomach. And how do you evaluate and how do you look at it? In the old days, we started with barium study, an element that we can see, mix it with a little water and have somebody swallow it. You could actually get a video recording from top to bottom watching this or you could shoot separate pictures. These are barium esophagrams. They are pictures, it is not an active video but we can get a sense of the material that is sneaking down through here. The heart is in the way and pushes things. We can look at it from the side, a lateral view, and look at it with the dye into the stomach. But this is the esophagus. These are normal pictures.

Let me show you what an abnormal esophagram would look like. So this is an abnormal esophagram, and I think you can sense that the barium sneaking down, that it is actually sitting there and not going anywhere. The esophagus allows peristalsis and pushes this material through, but not so much for this one. We can see that there is an abnormal filling defect here. Some people talk about an apple-core lesion or narrowing down. This is somebody with an esophageal cancer. This is grossly abnormal.

This is a different sort of an esophagram, a different patient, and we get a sense that the dye is moving through, but I am hopeful that you can get a sense that maybe there is something in there. That would be fine if it was a little food or something, but this is actually a mass, a tumor, mucosal cancer, an adenocarcinoma, or squamous cell cancer of the esophagus. This is not a good sign. This is something that needs to be taken out.

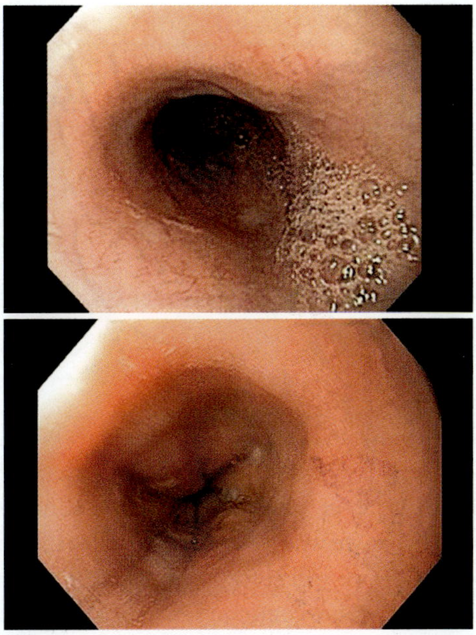

VIDEO 7.6. Esophageal Endoscopy.
Transcript: As medicine has progressed over the last century, we went from x-rays and barium esophagrams to gadgetry that can actually look at, biopsy, and treat endoscopically. This is an esophageal endoscopy. This is what the esophagus looks like: it is pink, it is round. You put a little air in there and it blows up and we can see that it is nice and smooth. This is a normal look at the esophagus.
If we sneak closer down to the stomach, you can almost get a sense that it is puckering there, waiting for the peristalsis to move tissue through. Again, normal looking mucosa. This is a normal esophageal endoscopy.

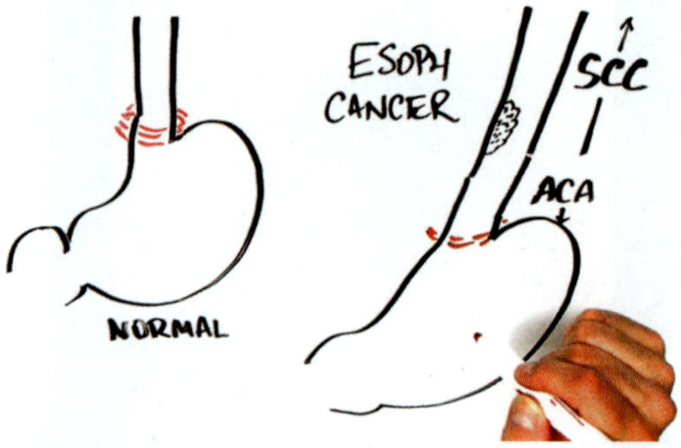

VIDEO 7.7. Cancer of the Esophagus.

Transcript: The normal esophagus is pink and red and healthy tissue. When we get esophageal cancer that is far from the case. Sometimes it can be subtle to start out, but eventually we will see erosions, ulcerations, masses within this tubing. The closer we are to the stomach and the intestine, which tends to be glandular, adenocarcinoma, that is what we will see down in the distal portion of the esophagus. Further up toward the jaw, toward the mouth, we will see what is called "squamous cell carcinoma." So, more common for adenocarcinoma here, and more common for squamous cell there.

Causes of adenocarcinoma are bile refluxing up through the lower esophageal sphincter, increases the trauma to the cells there and they can develop cancerous cells. The squamous cell cancer tends to be associated with alcohol, achalasia, and esophagitis. Somebody that swallows lye might be at an increased risk for squamous cell cancer. Smokers have a higher risk of squamous cell cancer.

Typically what happens in any sort of a cancer, people present with dysphagia, difficulty swallowing. With this difficulty and pain and discomfort, they tend to lose weight. The unfortunate thing, no matter which kind of esophageal cancer it is, roughly 50% or more patients will have distant metastatic disease, and it is theoretically incurable at that point. When people have symptoms of pain and difficulty swallowing or weight loss, doing an EGD, endoscopic gastroduodenoscopy or esophagoduodenoscopy allows us to look at the area, biopsy the area, and maybe even treat the area either stenting it or putting in a balloon to dilate things up and allow people to eat. But esophageal cancer is not an uncommon cancer in the United States. It would be nice to see it early on so we can treat it. Certain countries around the world have high evidence of esophageal and stomach cancer and will do prophylactic endoscopy. In Japan, Finland, or other places with higher risk, they will look for this cancer. The risk is not so high in the United States.

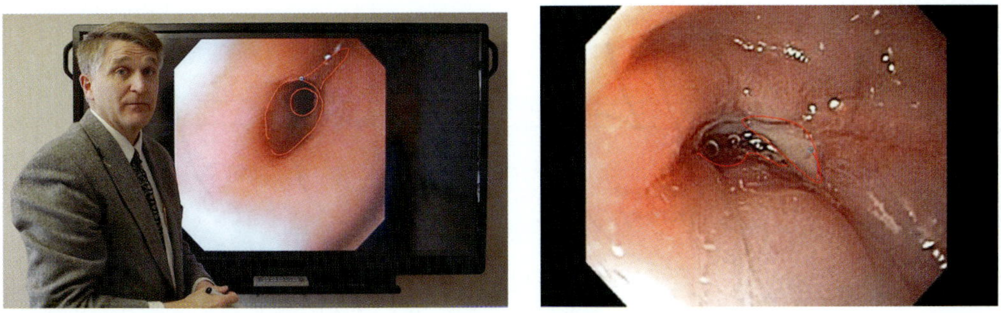

VIDEO 7.8. Strictures of the Esophagus.
Transcript: Taking out the endoscope and looking at the esophagus here we see an abnormality. Number 1, if we try to blow this up with some air, it doesn't look like it is blowing up as much and in fact, it is narrowed down, and we see some scarring here. This is likely a stricture. Somebody can swallow acid, can have bile reflux, radiation, a variety of different things can cause it. But there is an abnormality there.

Now we are taking another look at a different patient. It is pink on the outside but you get a sense that it is narrowed, it is scarred, and in this region here it is white and scirrhous. Is it a cancer? Is it scarring? Not sure. The nice thing about the endoscope is that you can biopsy and take a little bites of that and get some tissue. But, this is an abnormal esophagus study using the endoscope.

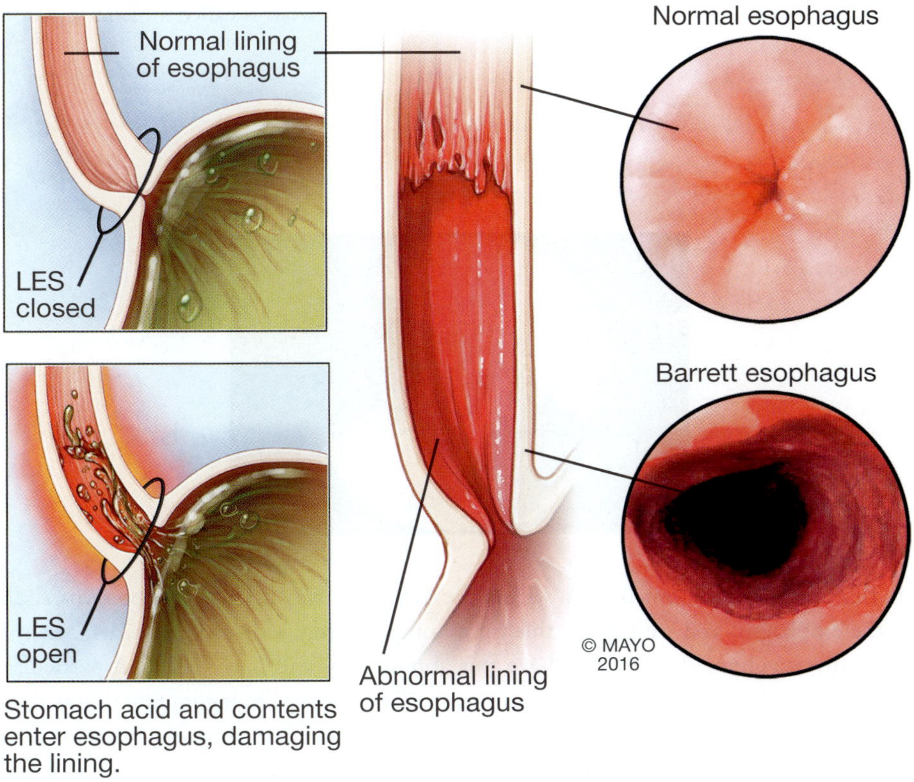

FIGURE 7.6. Barrett Esophagus. LES indicates lower esophageal sphincter.

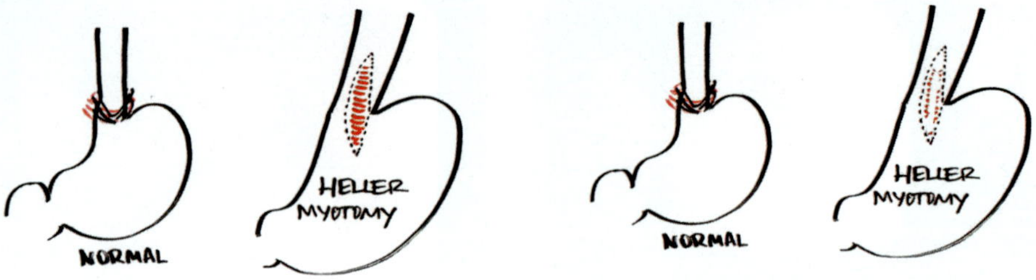

VIDEO 7.9. Heller Myotomy.

Transcript: If patients have the bird's beak of achalasia, esophageal achalasia, the muscle is too tight. So what surgeons do to counteract this is do is what is called a "Heller myotomy." This is typically done laparoscopically through the abdomen. The esophagus is up in the chest and the diaphragm sits over the top and we mobilize things up, and looking up underneath the diaphragm, we find the esophagus and stomach. We incise the peritoneum and the outer layer, the serosa if you will, and see the underlying muscle. And, usually with cautery or harmonic scalpel, we divide the bands of the muscle and this pops open and if we do it right, we don't cut through the mucosa and that may pouch out up at us and it breaks this achalasia wide open and it makes it a nice huge path. And, if anything, it pulls apart too much and so invariably what people will do at that point, just because it is a simple layer of mucosa, we will take the fundus of the stomach and lay it over the top and stitch it. This is termed a variety of different things, a Nissen fundoplication, or a Dor fundoplication. There is a variety of different things that people can do to buttress this, so the funny thing is to incise the layer of the muscle and patch it over so that it is not completely exposed to things popping and breaking loose. This is what is called a Heller myotomy.

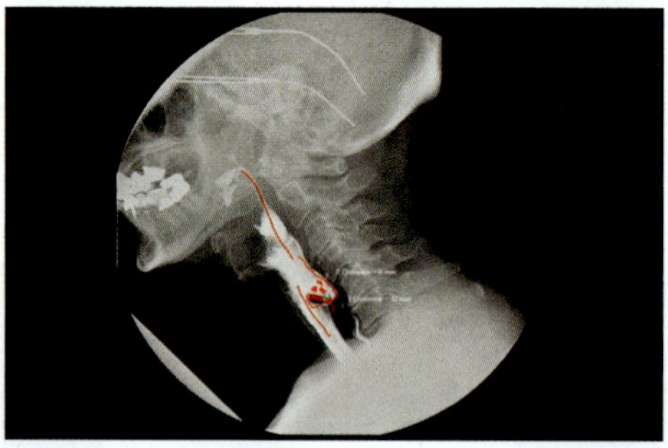

VIDEO 7.10. Zenker Diverticulum.

Transcript: This esophagram shows barium within the esophagus way up high, the pharynx sliding down to become the esophagus, and we can see this funny outpouching, a diverticulum. It goes by a special name, Zenker diverticulum. Patients that have this abnormality will have food and particulate matter that will sit in there. They will get halitosis, bad breath. They sometimes regurgitate things that they ate 2 days ago. The cricopharyngeus muscle is just overactive and squishing things down and this outpouching happens. It can be fixed endoscopically or surgically. It is a benign condition, but it is a problematic one, Zenker diverticulum.

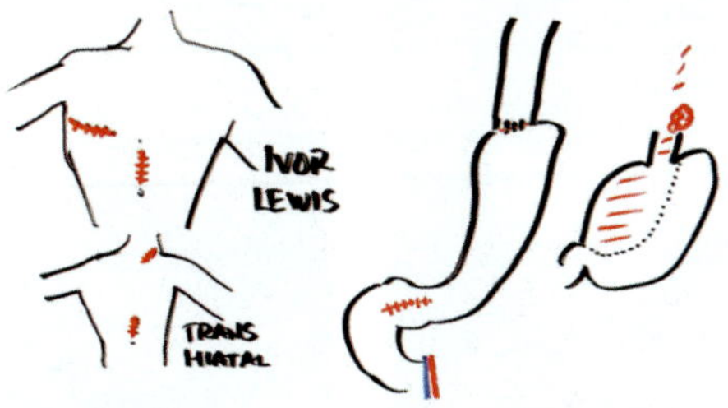

VIDEO 7.11. Ivor Lewis Esophagectomy.
Transcript: When patients have a cancer of the lower esophagus or upper stomach, there are a couple different strategies for taking that out and then putting people back together. Ivor Lewis, the only name of a surgical operation that is named after a first name and a last name; he is a real person, his first name is Ivor, and last name is Lewis—he talked about an incision in the chest and the abdomen; usually a midline laparotomy and a right thoracic approach. Another choice would be to make an incision in the abdomen, free things up from the bottom through the diaphragm, do what is called a transhiatal approach, and make an incision in the neck. This discussion is on Ivor Lewis so laparotomy, thoracotomy.

The normal stomach looks like so and perhaps we have an esophagus tumor here and what surgeons will do is cut this stomach and create a conduit, keeping the blood supply intact here and this part of the stomach, as well as the esophagus, will be removed. Because you have got that conduit you can pull it up and sew the esophagus that is above that tumor to the stomach, an esophagogastrostomy, a tubing connection. Because this nerve innervation of the stomach and the duodenum and pylorus is no longer intact because of this operation, we have to do what is called a pyloromyotomy, and open this muscular layer up and relax the pylorus, so food can slide through nicely. So an Ivor Lewis operation involves a laparotomy, a thoracotomy, and a patient with likely esophageal or very proximal gastric cancer, named after 1 surgeon using a gastric conduit to sneak up into the chest. And that anastomosis is performed through the thoracotomy.

Esophagus Challenge Questions

7.1. What is the Killian triangle?
7.2. Define the 4 types of hiatal hernia.
7.3. What parts of the esophagus do SCC and ACA affect?
7.4. Boerhaave syndrome is a rupture in which part of the esophagus?
7.5. What is the most common benign tumor of the esophagus?
7.6. How is it treated?
7.7. Who was Ivor Lewis?
7.8. What are the 7 "birds" of the thorax?
(Answers appear on page 109)

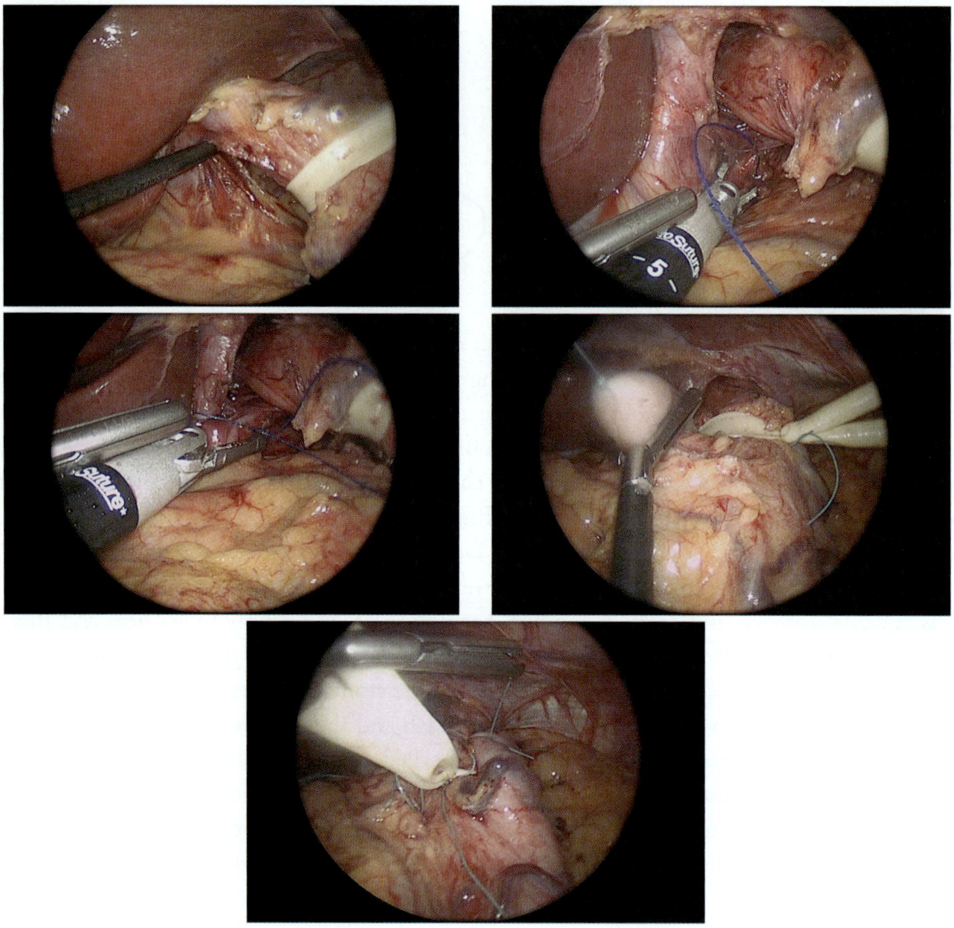

VIDEO 7.12. Nissen Fundoplication: Intraoperative.

Transcript: Nissen fundoplication is good to help patients with reflux. We see the liver up above, we see the GE junction. The esophagus joins the stomach up near the diaphragm. You can see a beating heart. We are working on the backside of the GE junction, a little blood in this section there, trying to sneak through, yes, we are back free on the other side, and we have got a Penrose drain around the top. We have to be careful here with bleeding vessels around the GE junction and we have to be careful of the vagus nerves, blunt dissection, a little traction and little teasing things through.

We are now going to use an endostitch, or an endosuture. We are going to close the crura of the diaphragm. Instead of having a big hiatal hernia, we are going to take bites of that muscle and close that gap so instead of having something as big as maybe a fist could go through; we are going to have something much smaller. So here the surgeon is going to do some laparoscopic knot tying and cinch down the crus of the diaphragm together—the right and the left crus, making the hole around the esophagus and the stomach much smaller. With the idea of trying to minimize the chance that gastric acid or bile can sneak up and get into the esophagus, which is painful. We have got to be careful with these bites that you are just taking muscle. The aorta and vena cava are not that far away. There have been times when surgeons have injured both of those structures with this procedure. So knowing how big of a bite to take is important.

So if the crura are closed, now typically what happens is, we take the top part of the stomach, the fundus if you will, and wrap it around the esophagus; what is called a Nissen fundoplication, and stitch that back together again. This is tough to see on this picture but the idea is that we are wrapping the stomach

VIDEO 7.12. Continued

around the top of the stomach, that extra stomach we can slip it around. So here comes this stomach from the back side and we pulled it through. So now we are going to wrap it around and stitch the stomach, there is a bite of the stomach, we are going to think about stitching the esophagus, we have got to switch the stitch, there we go, take a nice bite of the esophagus, but not too deep, and then we will take a bite of the stomach on the other side. Again, much like the crura of the diaphragm, we are going to try to narrow this down a little bit so fluid does not want to sneak up and back into the esophagus. This is what is called a wrap. This is a Nissen fundoplication and we put a stitch, putting the fundus to itself on either side. Multiple stitches, eventually allows us to close this down nicely. We don't want it to be too tight. So here the surgeon is letting go of that Penrose, taking a bite, nervous about big blood vessels, the stomach has wonderful blood supply. We have to be careful that we pull this thing together nicely. Now we are going to take a little bite of the diaphragm and the idea is to take tension off those lines of suture holding the stomach in its place. Don't let it sneak up into the chest, and again, be careful with these bites because the heart, the esophagus, and the diaphragm are right there and can all be easily injured.

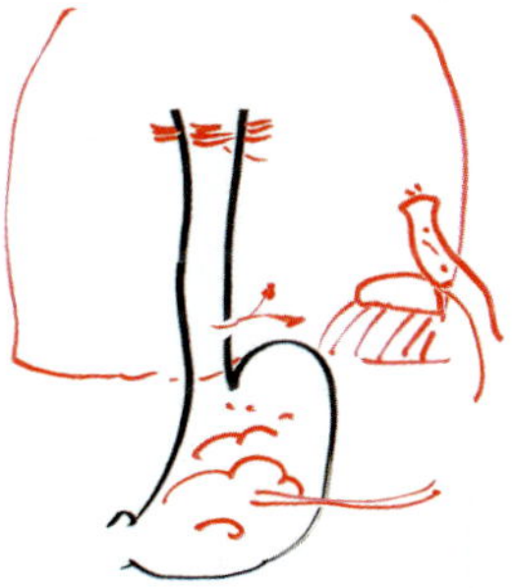

VIDEO 7.13. Perforation of the Esophagus.

Transcript: Perforation of the esophagus is fortuitously not terribly common. If it is going to occur, it occurs near the cricopharyngeus muscle, somebody swallowing a potato chip or a needle and choking on things, or somewhere else in the esophagus. There is a famous syndrome called "Boerhaave syndrome," where people eat massive amounts of food, retch and vomit, and pop a hole, and material comes out. The problem with the esophagus when material comes out is it goes into the chest and that sets up mediastinitis, pericarditis, and pneumonitis; structures that you cannot live without and people get bad sick when there is a perforation in the esophagus. Usually people will get pain in the neck, because it is more common to have a perforation up high. If the perforation is down low, the story will be, boy I was doing fine and was eating a-okay, but I had chicken and maybe swallowed a chicken bone, and then I didn't feel so well—it pops through—and people usually get a heart rate that goes up, the blood pressure goes down, a fever that happens. Those are classic signs for trouble, and oftentimes the chest x-ray will show fluid in the chest. We are sitting here looking at the x-ray, there may be fluid and we may actually see air, because air is leaking out. In the operating room we might find peas or beans or some other food product in there. Esophageal perforation is a dangerous problem and it will typically happen swallowing a chicken bone, a massive food intake, or some other traumatic instrumentation. In can happen with an endoscopy or other medical interventions.

A chest x-ray is a good choice. The next best choice at this point would be to swallow some material, either Hypaque or Gastrografin. Barium is also useful, but when barium gets out, that causes a problem. We don't like to use barium if we think there is a hole in the esophagus. In general, we like to operate on these people within 24 hours of putting a hole there. If it is after 24 hours—maybe it is 5 days in an

VIDEO 7.13. Continued

older gentleman, or in a nursing home and it pops out—typically, all we can do is get a chest tube and put it in there, drain out the material, and then support the patient with usually intubation, fluids, and try to settle this out. At some point, we sometimes put a tube in the stomach or a tube in the neck, an NG tube, anything to keep more material coming out of the chest. Esophageal perforations are rare, but deadly.

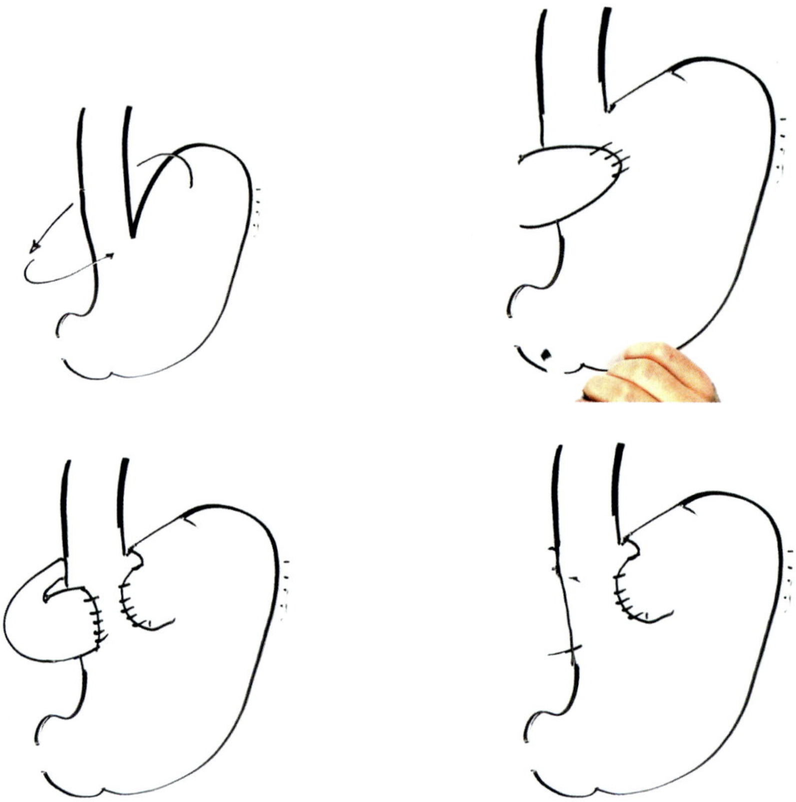

VIDEO 7.14. Types of Fundoplication.

Transcript: Surgically when it comes to buttressing or wrapping around the esophagus, sort of creating a lower esophageal sphincter, there are a couple different strategies to do it. There is a Nissen fundoplication, a Dor fundoplication, and what is called a Toupet fundoplication. But basically you can imagine if you cut the short gastrics and mobilize the stomach, the fundus if free and floppy, and we would slide this thing underneath the back side of the esophagus and wrap it around, such that if that were the case, then we could take this stomach and wrap it around the esophagus. It is going behind, it comes around, and this esophagus, depending on how tight we stitch it, may get completely wrapped, that would be a Nissen fundoplication. If we did a Toupet fundoplication, we might put a little bit of the stomach from this side, and a little bit from the back side, and we have tightened it, but we haven't completely crimped it off like a Nissen fundoplication typically does. A Dor fundoplication is usually even less restrictive and it just takes the front and flops it over and it is based on how much of a wrap. So the Dor fundoplication usually wraps it about 180° around, the Toupet, 270°, and the Nissen, 360°. This helps for reflux esophagitis and people with bad heart burn, or people after an operation from myotomy, Heller myotomy, achalasia, wrapping, and buttressing a cover. This is a fundoplication.

Answers to Esophagus Challenge Questions

7.1. The Killian triangle is midline of the inferior pharyngeal constrictor between the thyropharyngeus and cricopharyngeus muscles.

7.2. Type I, gastroesophageal junction slides into chest (most common). Type II, paraesophageal hernia, in which the stomach herniates into the chest and gastroesophageal junction remains in abdomen. Type III, stomach and gastroesophageal junction are in chest. Type IV, stomach and gastroesophageal junction are in chest and, also, another organ (eg, spleen, bowel) is in chest (Figure 7.7).

7.3. SCC affects the upper two-thirds of the esophagus; ACA affects the lower one-third.

7.4. Distal.

7.5. Leiomyoma (66%).

7.6. Leiomyoma is treated with surgical enucleation.

7.7. Ivor Lewis was a distinguished thoracic surgeon who pioneered the right-sided surgical approach to treating esophageal carcinoma.

7.8. "Esophagoose," "vagoose" nerve, "azygoose" vein, hemi-"azygoose" vein, thoracic "duck," "swallow," and accessory hemi-"azygoose."

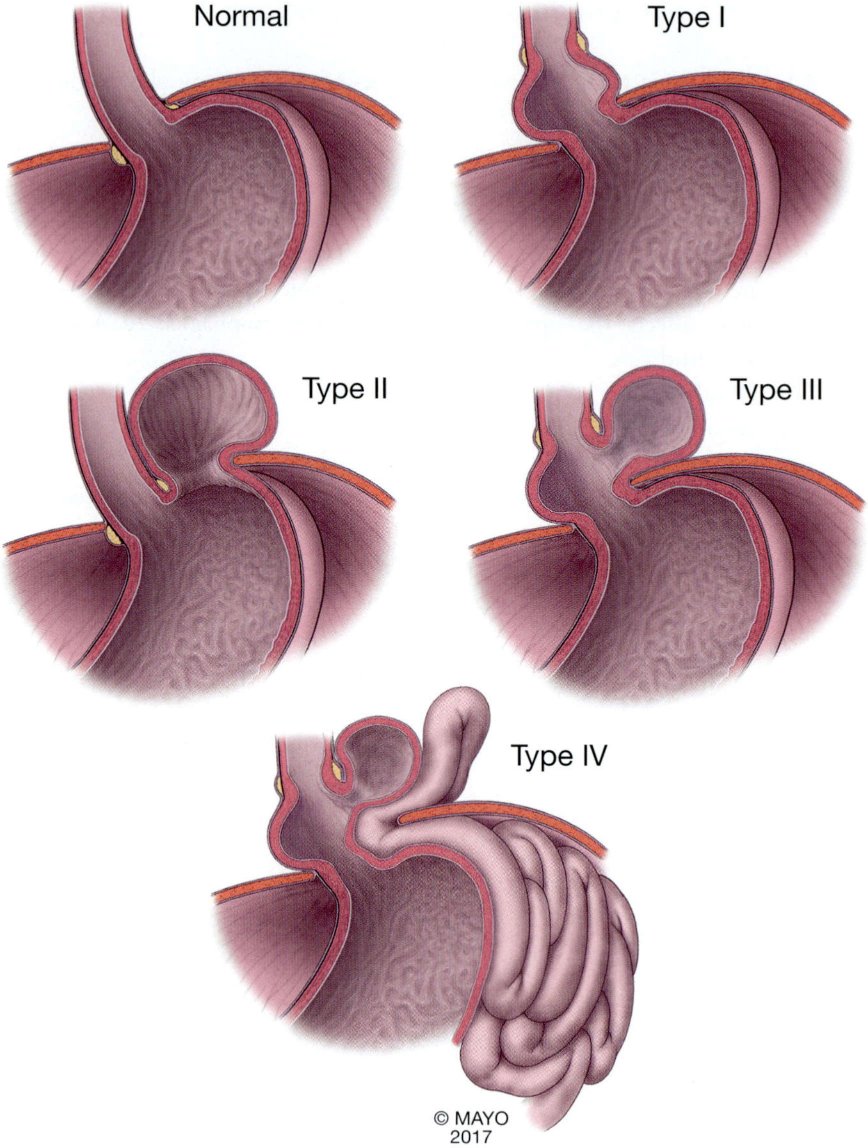

FIGURE 7.7. The Four Types of Hiatal Hernias.

8

Gallbladder

Embryology

The endodermal diverticulum of the caudal foregut develops into the GB.

Anatomy

The GB lies between liver segments 4B and 5 (Video 8.1) and is supplied by the cystic artery (branch of right hepatic artery). Small veins drain from the GB into the liver. The cystic duct lies within the Calot triangle (Video 8.2). The biliary system drains via the CBD into the second portion of the duodenum through the ampulla of Vater.

Physiology

Cholecystokinin and vagal stimulation result in GB contraction, delivering bile (synthesized in the liver) into the duodenum. Bile emulsifies fat, allowing it to be absorbed. The enterohepatic circulation recycles bile salts by active transport through the terminal ileum.

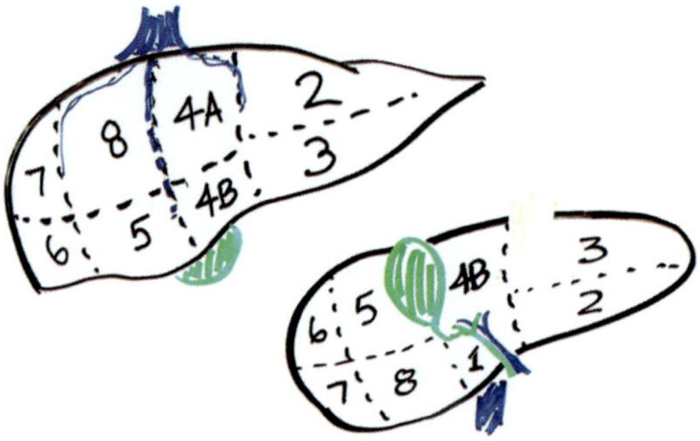

VIDEO 8.1. Liver Segments and Adjacency of Segments 4B and 5 to GB.
Transcript: The gallbladder is intimate with the liver. The liver has basically 8 segments. The right lobe of the liver is 5, 6, 7, and 8; the left lobe is 2, 3, 4A, and 4B. When we try to take out the gallbladder, we think about segment 4B and segment 5 being close behind. If we flip the gallbladder up, looking from the underside when we extend the gallbladder up for a laparoscopic cholecystectomy, 4B, segment 5. The rest as you see, the caudate lobe is down near the vena cava. The vena cava is important for liver anatomy. Cantlie line is where the middle hepatic vein is, dividing right and left, between each other. The left hepatic vein slides in and the right hepatic vein, as well, become the dividing points of the sectors. So, 8 segments of the liver—1, 2, 3, 4B, 5, 6, 7, 8; from the gallbladder standpoint, 4B and segment 5 are adjacent to it.

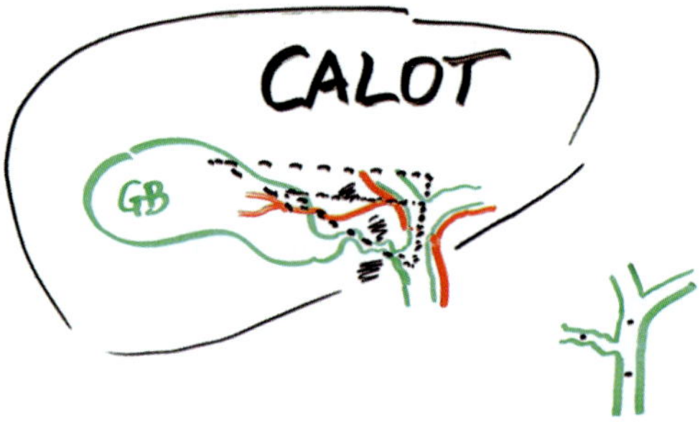

VIDEO 8.2. Calot Triangle.
Transcript: Calot triangle is an imaginary triangle that talks about the hepatic duct, the cystic artery, and the cystic duct. Knowing that, this is a high-rent district to find the duct and the artery. There's also another triangle that people talk about, and that's the cholecystohepatic triangle, and it's basically a bigger triangle that takes the edge of the liver and slides down the common hepatic duct and the cystic duct. The key thing is what we're all talking about is trying to find the cystic duct, the common hepatic duct, and the common bile duct, and when we dissect them, we've got to think about this. Looking for the critical view, we clean off below it, in between the artery, in between the liver and the artery. We're trying to find and dissect Calot triangle to find a duct going into the gallbladder and an artery going into the gallbladder. Calot triangle is important for safe gallbladder surgery.

Clinical Presentation

More than 80% of gallstones (cholelithiasis) (Figure 8.1) are of the cholesterol type. Pigmented stones occur in patients with hemolytic disorders, cirrhosis, or infection; they often lead to primary CBD stones. Most patients with gallstones are asymptomatic; most are female (also fertile, fat, and forty) (Video 8.3). If the cystic duct is obstructed, biliary colic or acute cholecystitis (Video 8.4) may occur. GB cancer is rare and is best treated with resection of surrounding liver, the GB, and lymph nodes along the bile ducts.

Imaging

Porcelain GBs (Video 8.5) can be seen on plain radiographs. Patients with RUQ pain should undergo US (Video 8.6) to look for gallstones (Video 8.7), bile duct dilatation, and signs of inflammation (Video 8.8). At least 10% of gallstones are radiopaque. Cholescintigraphy or hepatobiliary iminodiacetic acid study (Video 8.9) is used to evaluate biliary dyskinesia or define patients who may not benefit from a cholecystectomy.

Operation

Unless GB cancer is suspected preoperatively, or dense adhesions are likely, laparoscopic cholecystectomy (Videos 8.10 and 8.11) is the operation of choice. Obtaining the critical view enhances safety (Figure 8.2). An open approach is associated with greater morbidity and longer hospitalization.

Complications

Injury to the CBD (0.5%), duodenum, and liver parenchyma is uncommon but is a serious complication.

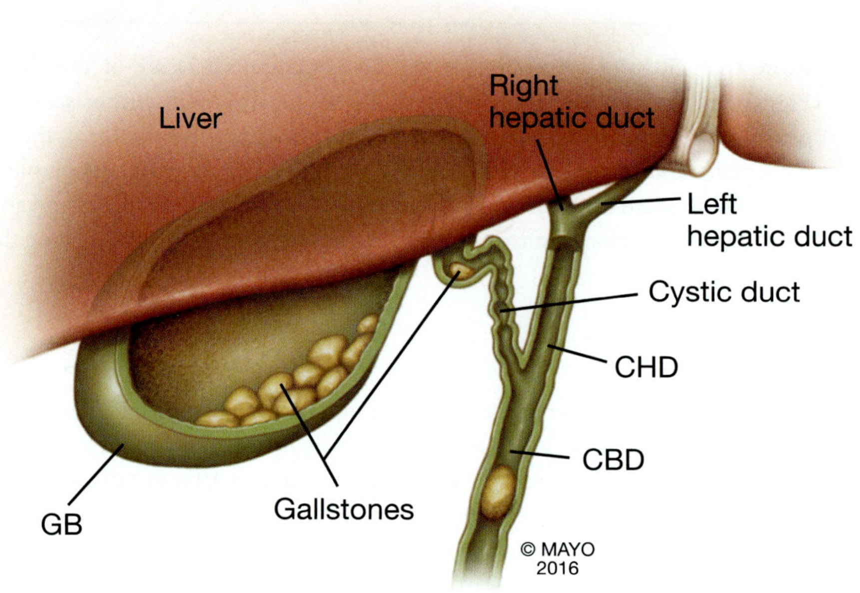

FIGURE 8.1. Anatomy of GB With Gallstones.

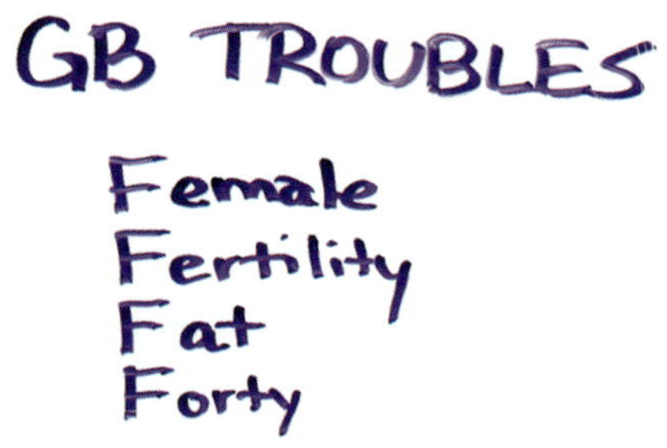

VIDEO 8.3. Causes of GB Problems: Female, Fertile, Fat, Forty.

Transcript: Roughly 700,000 people get their gallbladder taken out every year. Who gets it taken out? Well, there's a 4F mnemonic that people talk about with symptomatic gallbladder problems. It's more common in women, so it's "female." It often happens around child-bearing times, where they get symptomatic. Maybe they're eating more (bigger) or fatty meals. Female, fertile. Oftentimes, the patients are a bit overweight. And then, again, it's usually not in the elderly. It can happen at any time, but a lot of gallbladder troubles occur in females, around fertile periods, they're fat, and they're about the age of 40.

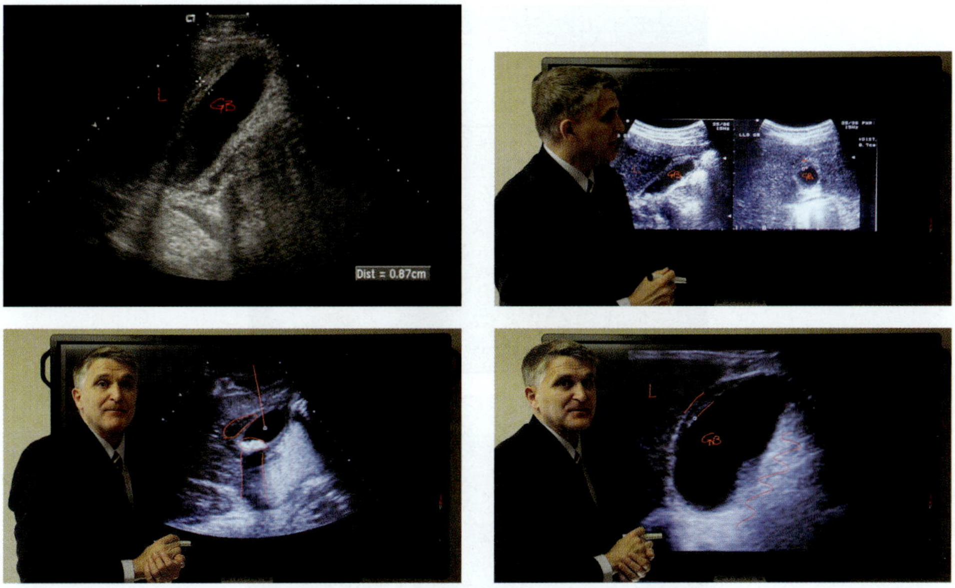

VIDEO 8.4. Acute Cholecystitis.

Transcript: Acute cholecystitis. "Acute" means it's right now, within today or tomorrow. "Cholecysto" means the gallbladder, and "-itis" means inflammation or infection. Putting those all together, it means the gallbladder is swollen, edematous, inflamed, and you're fighting an infection because bacteria are having their way with the gallbladder. That's something that needs to be evaluated and treated rapidly. Probably the best way to do it is with ultrasound, and it also gives us some pearls about acute cholecystitis. Here's an ultrasound of the gallbladder. I've got the liver up here, and this is the gallbladder. What this ultrasound is showing us is the thickness of the gallbladder wall. Down here it says 0.87 cm, or 8.7 mm. If it's bigger than 3, that's a thickened gallbladder. This is inflamed. It could be chronically or acute, but that depends on the patient's presentation.

Let's take a look at a couple other pictures. We've got a gallbladder here, we've got the liver, the gallbladder. We've got an end-on view. Remember, with ultrasound you can change it around; it doesn't always look like a water-filled balloon. Now the question becomes, is this thick or not thick? Without the markers here, I can't tell. I've got some markers here, and now I've got to find out where it is. Ah, it's 7 mm. This is acute cholecystitis.

The gallbladder will also sometimes show us some stones and show some echogenicity. Stones block the sound waves, kick back up, and we'll see some funny patterns. Not every gallbladder looks the same. We can also get a sense of some fluid over here. This is pericholecystic fluid. This is a really hot gallbladder. This patient is in pain. They either need the gallbladder out or need a percutaneous drain to drain that material and bacteria out of there.

Another picture. What do you think? You can find the liver. When we get this funny sort of look over here, sometimes air doesn't show up very well on an ultrasound, but we've clearly got a gallbladder. It's distended, but I'm hopeful that you'll notice over here it's way too thick and there may be some fluid there. Acute cholecystitis—we need to take care of this patient.

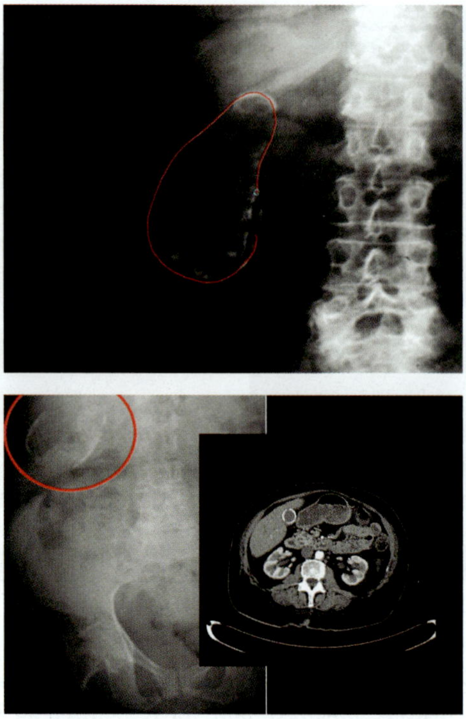

VIDEO 8.5. Porcelain GB.

Transcript: Porcelain gallbladders. Porcelain, that's brittle, it will break; the vase will drop and break. Porcelain gallbladder is nothing more than calcium within the wall of the gallbladder. We can see calcium in the vertebral bodies and calcium in the ribs. This is a plain, old-fashioned, long-ago KUB, a flat plate of the abdomen, seeing a calcified gallbladder. This is sort of something that must happen over time (it doesn't happen over days) and it sort of represents evidence of chronic cholecystitis, usually in elderly men and women, maybe women a bit more than men. The thing that we need to know about porcelain gallbladders is some folks suggest there's maybe a higher risk of having a cancer in there, and so oftentimes people have these removed if the patient is fit enough and healthy enough.

Here's another picture. Porcelain gallbladder we can see on an x-ray. It doesn't guarantee or mandate that there's a cancer there, but it suggests that person has been depositing calcium in the wall of the gallbladder for a long time. We can see similarly in a CT scan that little porcelain gallbladder; it just shows us where that gallbladder is and suggests they probably had some aches and pains over time. If the person was 95 and on death's door, there's nothing that needs to be done, but if somebody was 25 and had a porcelain gallbladder, I would suggest it should be removed.

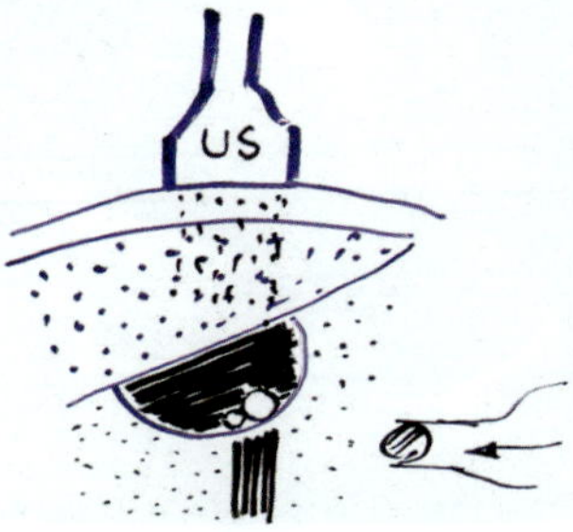

VIDEO 8.6. US of GB.

Transcript: When men and women have symptoms of gallstone or abdominal pain, 1 of the first tests to get is what's called an ultrasound. Basically a probe that sends signals, if you will, underneath that probe through the skin and the liver and sends sound waves down, and they bounce and they hit structures. The transition in structures sends a lot of things back so you'll get an image, and oftentimes it will look something like this. Fluid, or bile, looks black; it's anechoic, no echoes. We talk about echoes when it's ultrasound. There may be gallstones, and they'll be hyperechoic, or whitish, if you will. Because those sound waves come down and hit those stones and bounce back, there'll be no echoes from here, much like there are no echoes with water. There's nothing to bounce it back; it just slides through. So this is what's called acoustic shadowing, and it will have a very representative look. You can take the ultrasound probe and ask your patients to move, and as they move, gravity will take these gallstones and roll them down toward the center of the Earth. They're freely mobile within the gallbladder. There are some times when the ultrasound probe will see a thickened bile duct and sometimes can't see the gallstone that's stuck in it, but we can see a bigger gallbladder or duct being blocked.

So the ultrasound is a fantastic tool. It has no radiation, it's cheap, it's painless, it's quick, and you can look at biliary anatomy, you can look at the wall of the gallbladder, how thick it is, and that gives you a sense about inflammation. You can find out about stones and sludge. It's a wonderful tool. An ultrasound should be the first test that people think about with someone with gallstones.

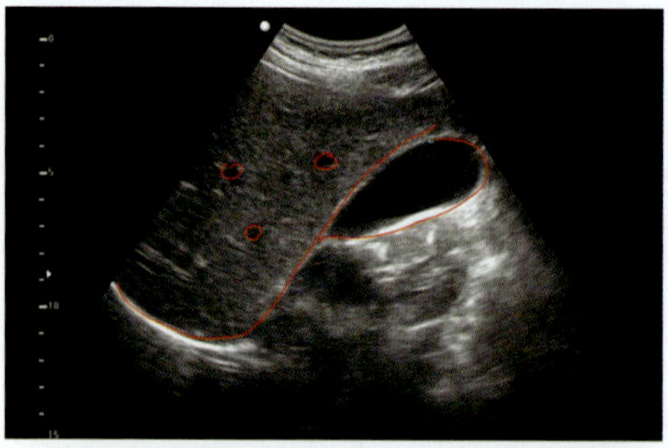

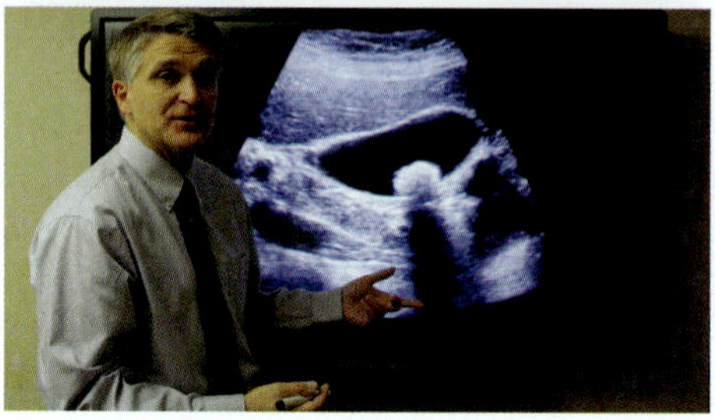

VIDEO 8.7. US Images of GB: Normal GB and GB With Gallstone.

Transcript: Ultrasound. Echogenicity. See a good-looking liver here on the side, likely some hepatic veins. They don't have the whitish outlining of the portal triad stuff. We can see what? I'm hoping you're telling me that's a gallbladder, and it's normal. It's not thick, it's a normal rind, and it's less than 3 mm. I don't see any stones and no acoustic shadowing. Normal gallbladder.

Okay. Again, left lateral sector or the liver up above. See the gallbladder below. I'm hoping you can see a hypoechoic shadow. That means there's obviously a mass there. Is it a polyp? It's pretty doggone dense. A polyp would give us more signal through it. It's likely a stone. We can get the patient to move around, and that stone can roll around. But a normal-appearing gallbladder wall thickness, no pericholecystic fluid; just a gallstone floating in the bile.

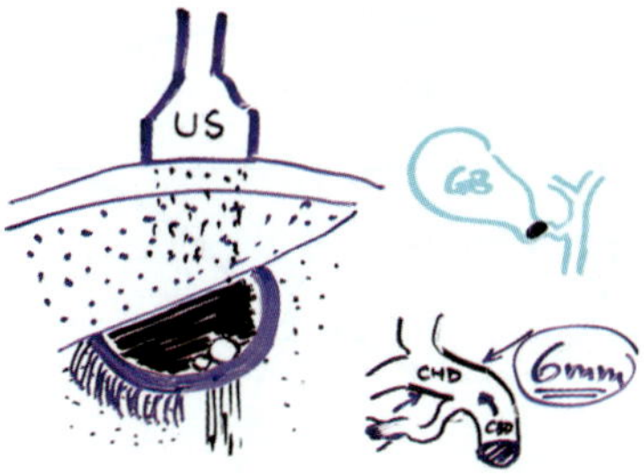

VIDEO 8.8. US Signs of Inflammation of GB.

Transcript: The gallbladder, cystic duct, common bile duct, and common hepatic ducts are in close association. When we get gallstones stuck in the cystic duct, the gallbladder enlarges, and usually the stone will pop back into the gallbladder. Sometimes it slides down and is deposited in our waste. Sometimes it's stuck in the cystic duct or the common bile duct. If it gets stuck in the cystic duct, when we look with ultrasound, we will get a chance to see oftentimes that the wall of the gallbladder is thickened, and with inflammation this will get thicker than 3 mm. So our radiology colleagues and ultrasound doctors, when they see a gallbladder wall that's greater than 3 mm, they think about cholecystitis. "-Itis" means inflammation; that's different from symptomatic cholelithiasis. Gallstone attacks are one thing, they come and go, but "-itis" sticks, and some of these people need emergent operation or urgent operation.

So that's 1 sign, is a thickened gallbladder wall. Other times we'll see on ultrasound fluid around the gallbladder wall, so-called pericholecystic fluid. That means it's more inflammation and further along. If we can get a chance to zoom in on the bile ducts, sometimes we can see a stone stuck down in the duct or we may not see that; we may get a sense that maybe there's a stone in the common bile duct, and if so, this backs up the bile such that the size of the common hepatic duct, which is very consistent (usually less than 4 mm and most people it's 3 mm or so), enlarges. When we see common hepatic ducts that are bigger than 6 mm we really start to ponder there's something here—either a tumor or likely a stone.

So ultrasound looking at inflamed gallbladders can tell us a lot—thickened wall, pericholecystic fluid, and the size of the common hepatic duct or the common bile duct. When these structures start getting bigger, the common bile duct bigger than 7 or 8 mm, the common hepatic duct bigger than 4 and certainly 6 mm, we think about obstructive symptoms.

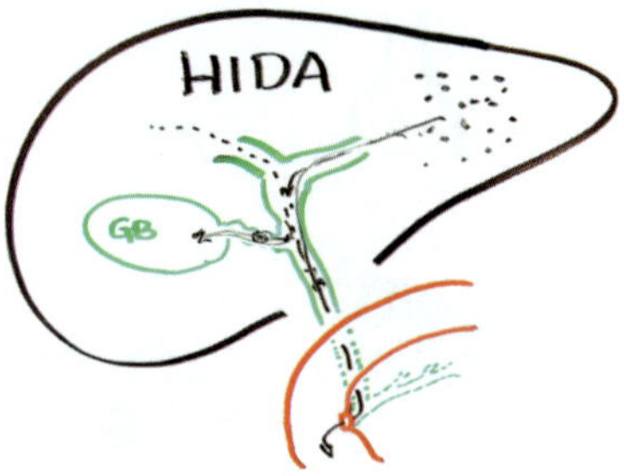

VIDEO 8.9. Hepatobiliary Iminodiacetic Acid (HIDA) Scan.
Transcript: The liver makes bile all day long, and that bile comes down the ducts, and if we're not eating and drinking, it heads back into the gallbladder. There are times that a HIDA scan, so-called hepatic iminodiacetic acid study, is important for a surgeon to make sure a patient doesn't need an operation. Sometimes people have funny aches and pains, and the question is, do they have a stone here or do they have a stone here, is it blocked off?

Sometimes the ultrasound can't help us, when people have lots of air in the duodenum or the stomach, and we have this test. It's a technetium-label study, and the little radiolabeled things are picked up by the liver and slid down into the biliary tree, and if there's a blockage, the dye will stop and it won't slide in. It should go into the gallbladder, but if there's a stone blocking that, it won't. These HIDA scans are helpful from time to time, identifying people that have funny problems. A surgeon is thinking about surgery, but if this dye goes all the way down through and out the duodenum and it goes into the gallbladder, there are no problems here. It's saved a lot of people operations that wouldn't have helped them.

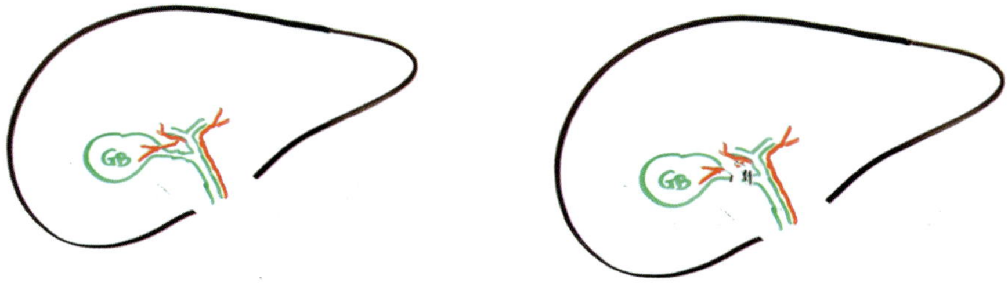

VIDEO 8.10. Laparoscopic Cholecystectomy.
Transcript: Cholecystectomy means removing the gallbladder. Laparoscopically means doing it with a laparoscope. It could be done with a robot or in an open fashion. The key thing about laparoscopic surgery is to safely divide the cystic duct, usually with a couple of clips, and divide it, and carefully divide the cystic artery and clip it, without hurting the common bile duct, the common hepatic duct, or the right hepatic artery. These are the main goals of taking out a gallbladder, and it happens 700,000 or 800,000 times. Unfortunately, they're going to injure the common bile duct, the common hepatic duct, or the right hepatic duct about 1 in 200 cholecystectomies.

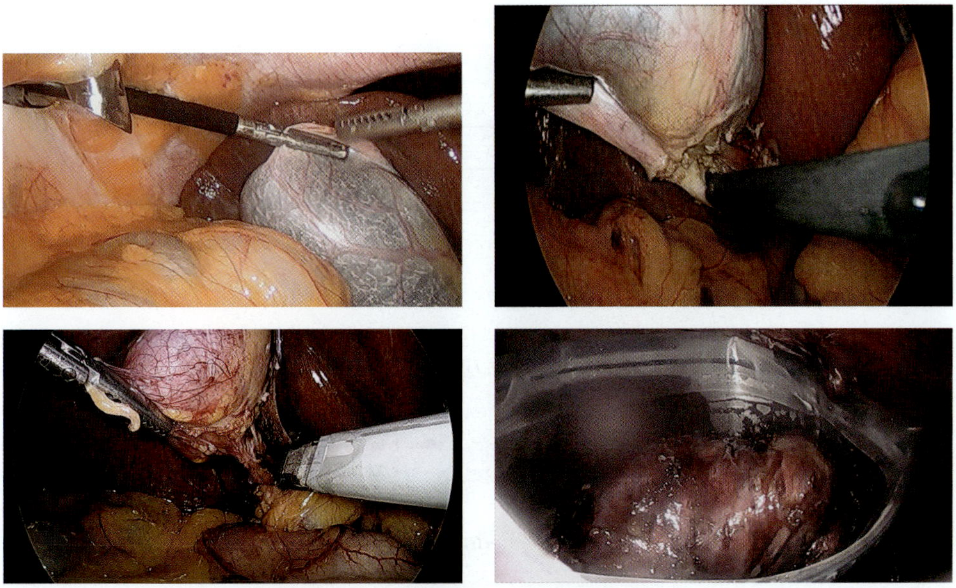

VIDEO 8.11. Laparoscopic Cholecystectomy: Intraoperative.

Transcript: Laparoscopic cholecystectomy, coming in from the belly button, looking at the right upper quadrant. Omentum plastered up beneath there. This looks like a benign gallbladder. It's got some lymphatics filled with fatty tissue. We use the hook cautery, trying to find the cystic duct. It's right there. We use this little gadget to try to find the cystic duct, the cystic artery, and create spaces between them and see the liver behind them. It's what's called the critical view of surgery. We've got a grasper in our left hand, pulling what's called Hartmann pouch, sort of the bottom of the gallbladder.

Now we can see the cystic duct being cleared off, and we've got 2 tubular structures there. One's the cystic duct and one's the cystic artery. We just need to make sure it's not the common hepatic or the common bile duct. We can see gallbladder with a little yellow stone in it. The clip applier has put 2 clips nicely on the cystic artery, 2 clips on the cystic duct. We put a third clip on the specimen side, and then we'll be able to cut between them and take the gallbladder out from the bottom up. You can see the bile duct underneath there, near the duodenum. A lot of close structures here we've got to be careful of. Here's a clip on the specimen side of the gallbladder, on the cystic duct, and after transecting those structures, now we need to take the gallbladder away from the liver. Beautiful demonstration of tension, traction, and counter-traction, light touch, just a little cautery, hit the button, and it falls apart. We can see it little by little. We've just got to be careful that we don't burn a hole in the gallbladder and spill bile.

Gallbladder is out; this is the more difficult gallbladder that I showed you at the start. We've changed a little bit. That's the liver. It tends to bleed a little bit on the raw edge. Patients with a laparoscopic gallbladder operation typically go home later that day. This is that inflamed gallbladder. That person might stay overnight; they might be a little more sick than somebody with an easy gallbladder. It's nice to do it with little bitty operations, little bitty incisions. Here, putting it in an endobag and pull that thing out, usually 1 to 4 little incisions. Patients have some pain but typically go home later that day.

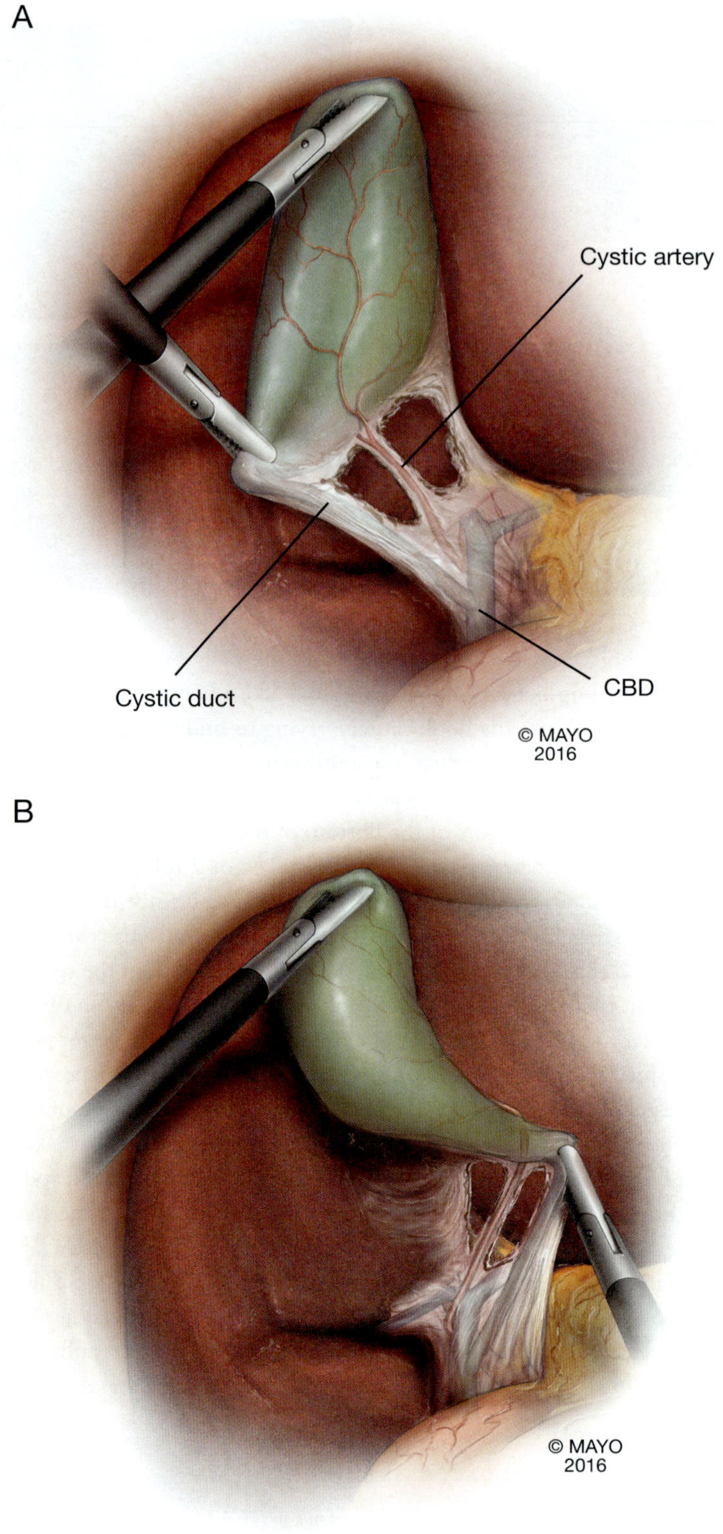

FIGURE 8.2. Views of the GB During Surgery. A, The critical view of safety for cholecystectomy. B, Mobilization of the GB allows visualization of the back side of the GB and vessels.

Gallbladder Challenge Questions

8.1. What is gallstone ileus?
8.2. Who is likely to get acalculous cholecystitis?
8.3. Define Mirizzi syndrome.
8.4. Who was John Benjamin Murphy?
8.5. What is Courvoisier's law?
8.6. What is biliary colic?
8.7. Explain what the critical view involves.
8.8. When is a cholangiogram useful?
8.9. What percentage of people have normal bile duct anatomy?
8.10. Where is the Calot node?

Answers to Gallbladder Challenge Questions

8.1. A large gallstone may erode into the duodenum, pass down the GI tract, and lodge at the ileocecal valve.

8.2. Patients who are ill or compromised, often in the intensive care unit, receiving total parenteral nutrition, and bedridden.

8.3. Impacted gallstone in the cystic duct causes inflammation and often secondarily obstructs the CHD or CBD.

8.4. A prominent surgeon from Chicago who first described inspiratory arrest on deep palpation at the subcostal margin when a patient with cholecystitis takes a deep breath.

8.5. A palpable GB in a jaundiced patient void of pure pain likely has a periampullary malignancy.

8.6. Temporary blockage of the cystic duct from a gallstone causing constant RUQ pain lasting less than 6 hours.

8.7. Dissecting and exposing the cystic duct and cystic artery clearly so that the liver is visible behind and between them and both structures emanate from the GB.

8.8. A cholangiogram is useful to assess for abnormality (eg, stones, debris, tumors) in the CBD, CHD, or right and left hepatic ducts.

8.9. Twenty-five percent to 50%. Variations are normal.

8.10. Anterior to the cystic duct.

9

Inguinal Region and Hernias

Embryology

Failure of fusion of the processus vaginalis (Figure 9.1) in childhood can predispose to indirect inguinal hernias. Communication with the peritoneal cavity may lead to hydroceles.

Anatomy

The inferior portion of the EO muscle runs between the ASIS and the pubic tubercle; as it folds underneath itself, it forms the inguinal ligament (Figure 9.2). Medially, the EO aponeurosis has an opening (external inguinal ring) through which the spermatic cord (Video 9.1) (men) or round ligament (women) passes. The internal inguinal ring (Video 9.2) is a defect within the transversalis abdominus and internal oblique layers. The inguinal canal runs from the internal inguinal ring toward the external ring for approximately 4 cm. The floor of this canal lies within the Hesselbach triangle (Figure 9.3).

Physiology

A hernia is the protrusion of a hollow viscus through a musculoaponeurotic opening. Inguinal hernias result from a patent processus vaginalis, weak abdominal fascia, or increased intra-abdominal pressure (eg, coughing, sneezing, lifting). Hernias can occur at any age.

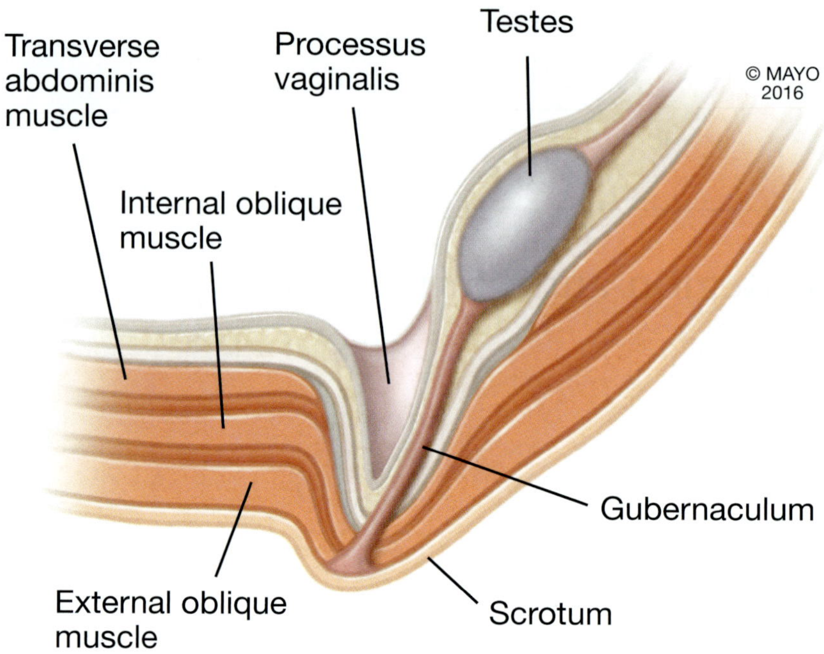

FIGURE 9.1. Embryologic Anatomy of the Male Inguinal Region.

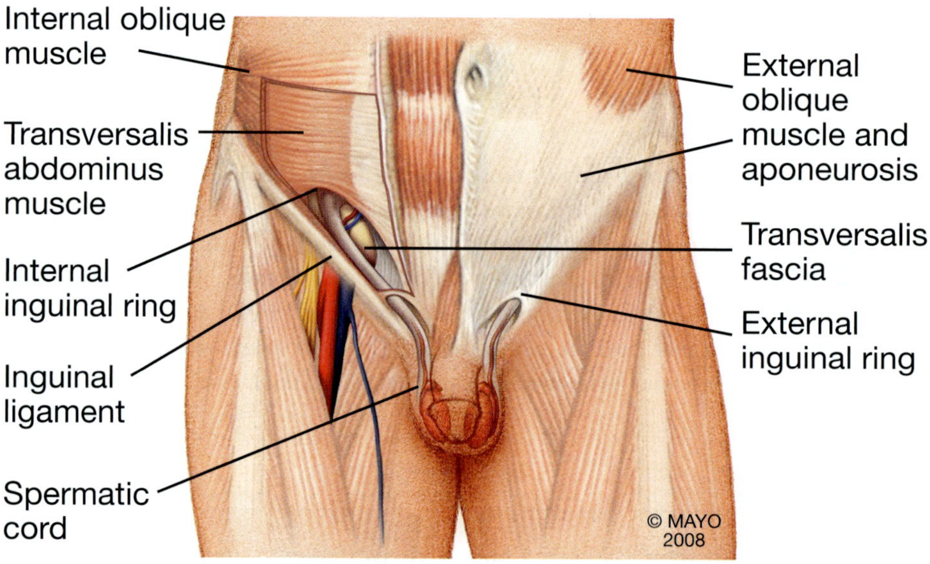

FIGURE 9.2. Muscle Anatomy of the Lower Abdomen.

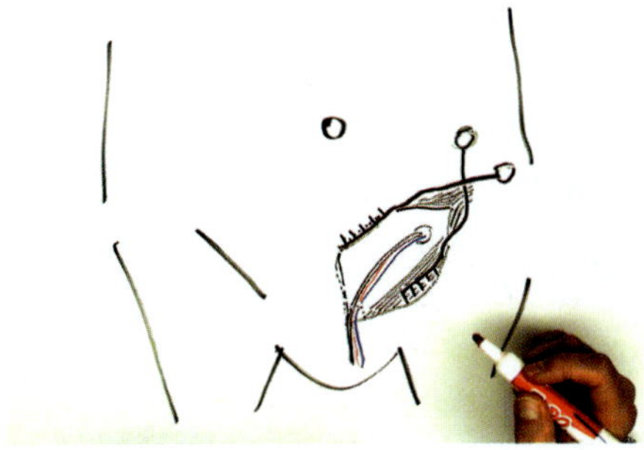

VIDEO 9.1. Spermatic Cord.
Transcript: The spermatic cord exists in a man. The cord here in a woman is the round ligament. The spermatic cord carries the vas deferens where the sperm travel through, the testicular artery, the gonadal vein, and a variety of other structures. There will be a branch at the ilioinguinal nerves, sometimes often with the spermatic cord, and then the genital branch of the genitofemoral nerve. This is the spermatic cord coming through the internal ring, the deep internal ring, and exiting the external or superficial ring. This drawing shows the external oblique fascia being filleted open and the spermatic cord will lie underneath. In a female, that will be the round ligament.

Clinical Presentation

Groin discomfort and a palpable bulge (Video 9.3) are common. The hernia sac is nonreducible in incarcerated hernia (Figure 9.4); it may or may not be painful, and surgery is often necessary in the near future. Strangulation (Video 9.4) means the blood supply of the hernia contents are compromised; an emergency operation is indicated. Incarcerated hernias may progress to strangulation.

Imaging

Hernias should be diagnosed on the basis of signs and symptoms. CT (Video 9.5), MRI, and US are reserved for patients with unusual symptoms of a hernia or vague physical findings.

Operation

Symptomatic hernias are repaired with open mesh (Lichtenstein repair [Videos 9.6 and 9.7]) or laparoscopic (totally extraperitoneal [Video 9.8]; transabdominal preperitoneal [Video 9.9]) approaches. Open tissue-based repairs (McVay, Bassini [Video 9.10], Shouldice [Video 9.11]) are less commonly used.

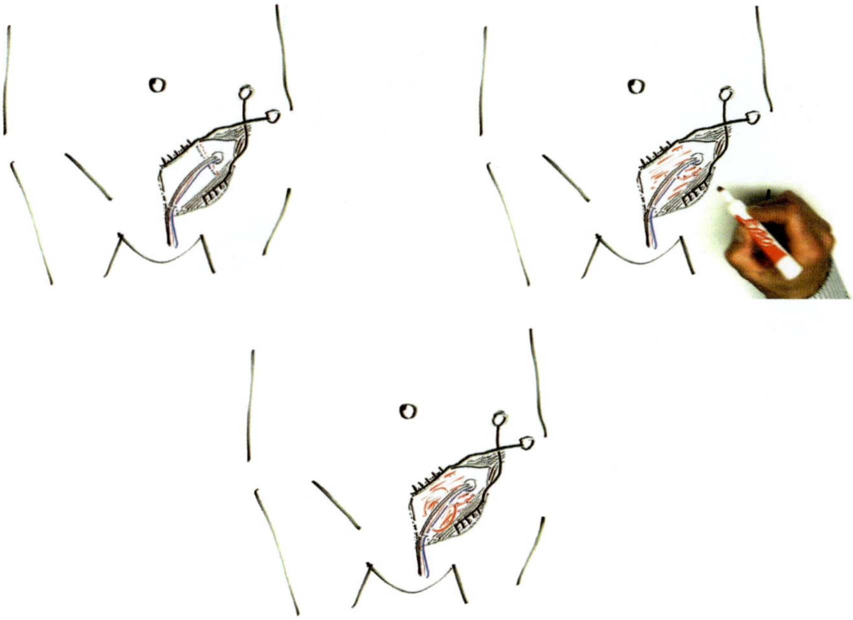

VIDEO 9.2. Internal Inguinal Ring.
Transcript: The internal inguinal ring allows the spermatic cord contents, or the round ligament in a female, to slide down caudally toward the pubic bone and into the scrotum in a man. The internal ring is marked by deep inferior epigastrics that run just medial to the internal ring. You don't see them because these vessels are deep, they are coming off the external iliac artery and vein, lying posterior to the transversalis muscle and internal oblique musculature—they are hidden underneath there. So, hernia surgeons need to be careful and know that those vessels are there. The internal ring is a landmark. Indirect hernias, when the peritoneum sneaks through the internal ring, are called indirect defects. A direct hernia through Hesselbach triangle is more medially placed. The internal ring is crucial for fixing and identifying inguinal hernias in both men and women.

Complications

Early postoperative complications include urinary retention (1%-10%), hematoma (1%-2%), and superficial skin infection (about 1%). Long-term complications include hernia recurrence (1%-10%), chronic pain (2%-10%), and ischemic orchitis (<1%).

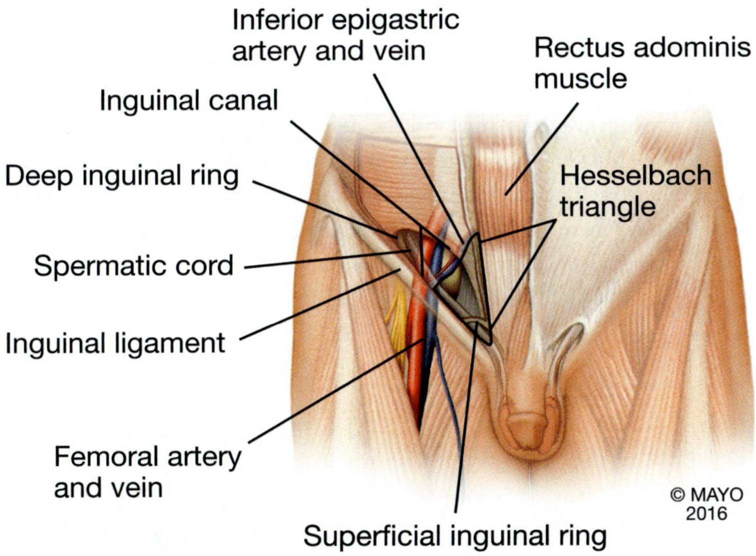

FIGURE 9.3. Anatomy of the Inguinal Canal and the Hesselbach Triangle.

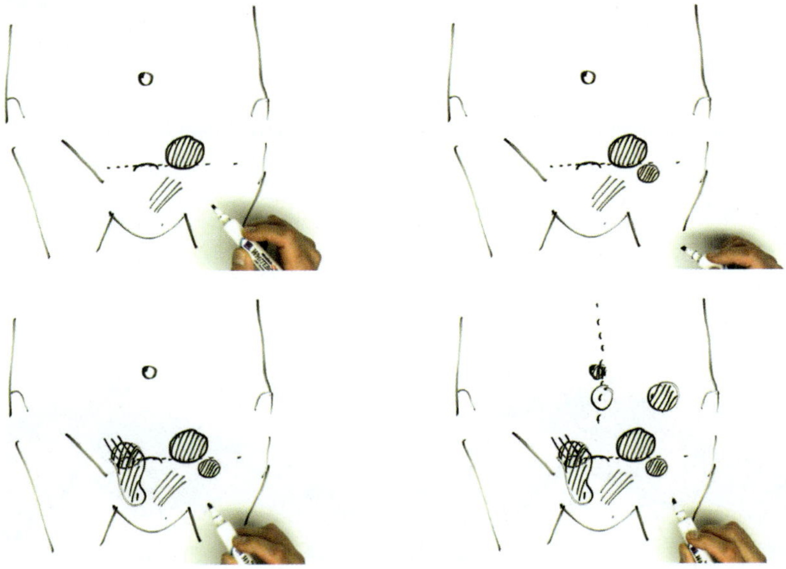

VIDEO 9.3. Palpable Hernia Bulge.

Transcript: Hernias oftentimes will show a palpable bulge. You need to find the pubic bone, scrotum, and genitalia below; palpate that pubic bone, and slide to the side. In a man, with a scrotum, finger slides up toward the pubic bone and slides laterally up into the external ring. The bulge that you will feel or the patient will show you, or see, is important where it is located. If that bulge, that hernia, is cephalad to that edge of the pubic bone, it is likely an inguinal hernia. If it is below that line, it is likely a femoral hernia. So it is important when you examine patients—where is the bulge?

VIDEO 9.3. Continued

Most bulges will be inguinal hernias; they will be cephalad to the pubic bone and lateral to it, coming out in men, the external ring, that sits down here. That bulge will typically be here. The larger it gets, it can slide down into the scrotum. But the hole and the defect is typically above the pubic bone.

If somebody has a palpable bulge on the abdomen, it may be up higher, that could be a spigelian hernia. It could be a belly button hernia. It could be an incisional hernia. This section is on inguinal hernias. Find the pubic bone; take a look at where the bulge is. Ideally, inguinal hernias are above that line of the pubic bone. In the groin or the crease, it is likely a femoral hernia.

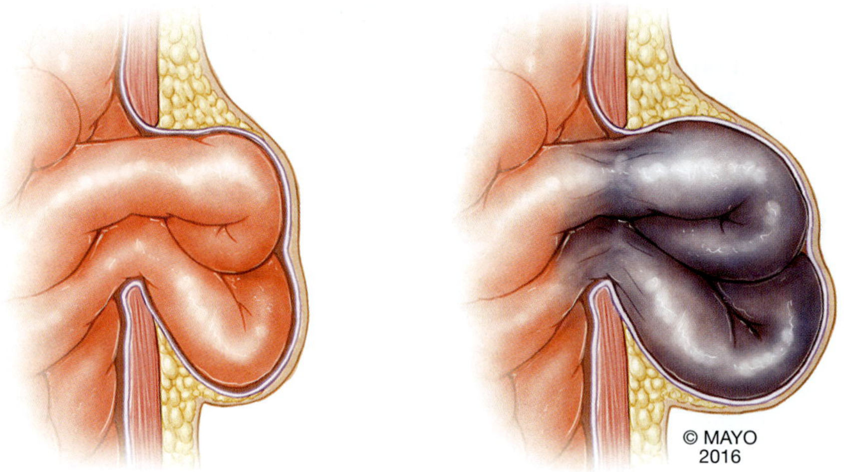

FIGURE 9.4. Hernias: Incarcerated Bowel (left) and Strangulated Bowel (right).

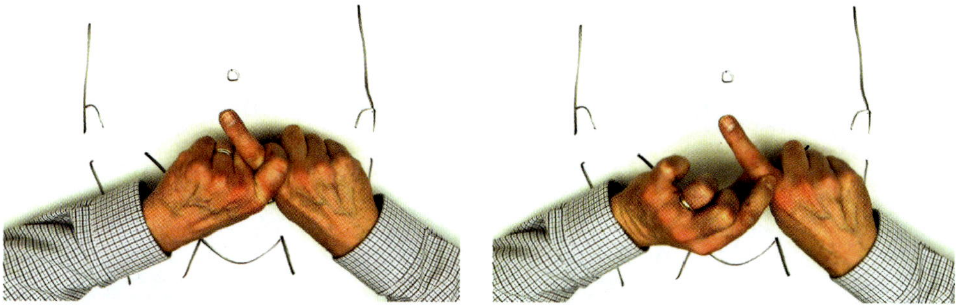

VIDEO 9.4. Strangulated and Incarcerated Hernias.

Transcript: We are often asked to see a bulge in the groin and patients are worried about strangulation or incarceration. Let me give you a brief demonstration. Strangulation means you are losing blood supply, it's becoming ischemic. My finger is just fine, I am going to cutoff the blood flow—that finger will be dead in 6 hours because there is no blood flow. Incarceration means that it is stuck, it's not going anywhere. It's not hurt and it's not a problem. The difference between strangulation and incarceration—prisoners are incarcerated, 3 meals a day, air conditioning and heat, a roof over their head—incarceration, not a bad

VIDEO 9.4. Continued

problem. Strangulation that is a noose around the prisoner's head; that is going to be a lethal problem. If we don't release this tourniquet, we are going to have a dead finger in 6 hours.

When you see somebody in the emergency room with pain, a palpable mass, think about strangulation. If you see somebody, your grandma, your grandpa, your uncle, with a mass that is stuck, they are eating and drinking and are happy and healthy. Are they nervous and scared? No. That is incarceration, the mass is stuck. Maybe it should be fixed.

But a strangulated hernia, that is an emergency. That person needs treatment right now.

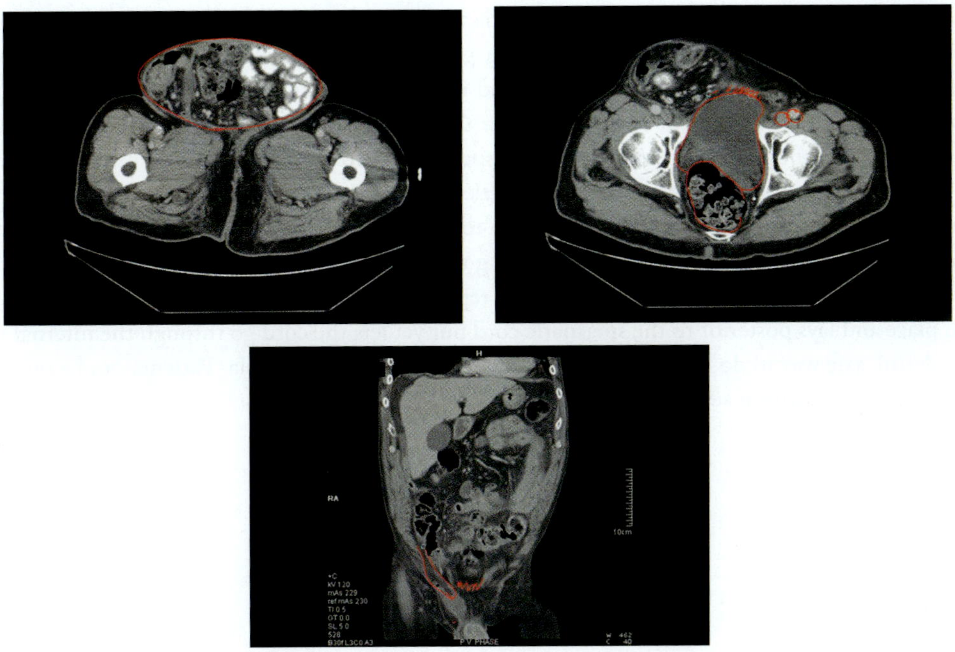

VIDEO 9.5. CT of Hernia.

Transcript: CT scan is not common to take a look at inguinal hernias; but, here is a nice CT scan, actually at midthigh. The graphic thing here to understand is that this is all hernia sac. This is an elderly farmer that has bowel and colon; this is a classic picture for colon with stool in it, small bowel with contrast. This is an amazingly large hernia.

As we go back upstream, this is the same patient, pelvic bones on the side, rectum down below, this is his bladder, the skin on the outside, the muscles on the left side, there is the femoral artery and femoral vein, and now we see this big bulge on the right side. This is a right inguinal hernia, likely an internal hernia, it slides down through the internal ring, through the external ring, down into the scrotum, and far beyond. Skin, fat, and muscle layer—this is the rectus abdominis here. It is tough to see anything on this side. He has had this hernia for 30-some years.

We take a look at a different section, a coronal section, in a different patient. Here we see the rectus abdominis coming down nice, the musculature coming down nice, and the genitalia down below here. Interestingly enough, this person has an appendix that is sitting through the internal ring. This is an Amyand appendix or hernia. Sometimes people can get pain and problems down there, but the key thing for a surgeon is to make sure we don't hurt that appendix as we fix the inguinal hernia.

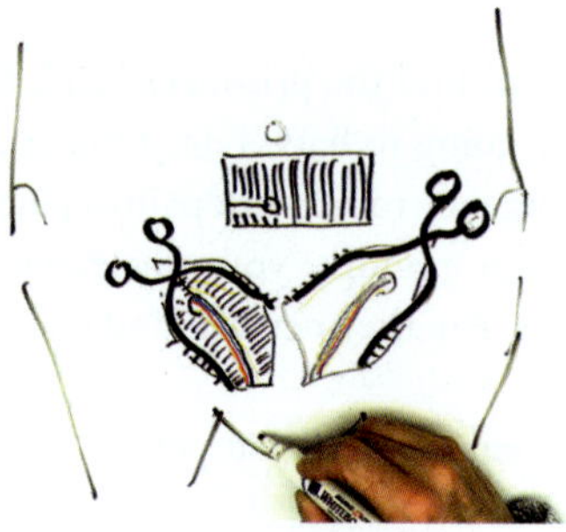

VIDEO 9.6. Lichtenstein Repair.

Transcript: Dr Lichtenstein did a lot of work on fixing hernias. By the 1980s, his plan for fixing a hernia was the best way possible and probably still remains that way, although folks will argue. A Lichtenstein hernia repair—left groin with spermatic cord, right groin with spermatic cord—we have got it exposed and we take a piece of mesh, something like so, and it is prolene, it is nylon, it is something simple; we make a couple little cuts in it, a cut with a hole. If you could turn that mesh and put it in here, now that mesh is going to sit underneath or posterior to the spermatic cord and be sewn in place. With a cut here, we are going to sew this together so that the spermatic cord comes through the hole, through the internal ring through the hole in the mesh and slides down to the scrotum. The mesh is sewn in place inferiorly and tacked elsewhere trying to avoid the underlying nerves—we don't want to damage any of those organs. So this is what is called a Lichtenstein hernia repair, that is a panel of usually nylon, prolene mesh, sewn in place and lays posterior to the spermatic cord but yet lets the cord go through the internal ring. It is a wonderful, safe way to do hernia surgery, under attended local anesthesia. Patients can be outpatients and be back to work within several days.

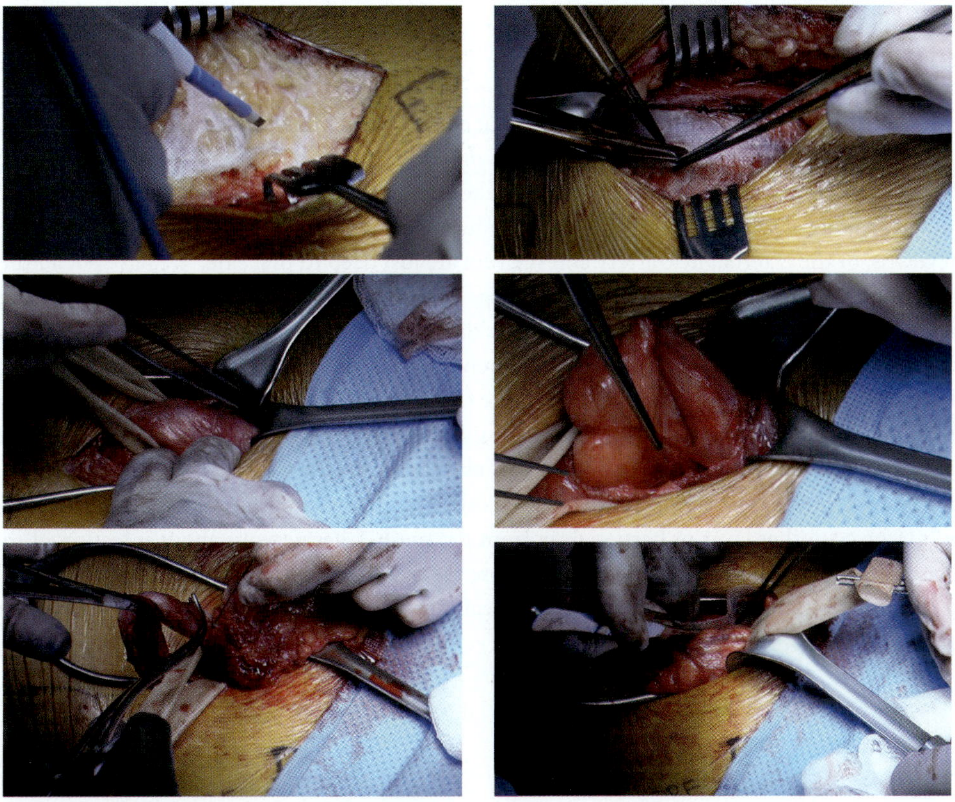

VIDEO 9.7. Inguinal Hernia With Lichtenstein Repair: Intraoperative.
Transcript: This is an open right-sided inguinal hernia. The pubic bone is to the right, the anterior superior iliac spine is to the left, and the genitalia are inferiorly. Add some pick ups with electrocautery dividing the fatty tissue. Traction and counter traction creates tension, and we use the tip of the cautery and the tissue lightly falls apart, beautiful work. Before you get to Scarpa fascia, there is usually a superficial epigastric artery and vein; I like to tie those off to minimize bleeding, especially in patients on Coumadin or Plavix. Postoperatively, a hematoma of the groin can happen.

There are lots of different pickups here, traction and counter traction trying to get a sense of where to go. We have got Murphy rakes exposing and we now find the external oblique fascia. We want to put a nick in the fascia, we have done that, we want to take our scissors and spread that layer open knowing that the spermatic cord is just deep to us. The ilioinguinal nerve, the iliohypogastric, will be just below us, so you can't cut deep to it. We are cutting towards the pubic bone towards the external ring. We have created that space and now we have got the external oblique cut. We have our Weitlaner, or self-retaining retractor, and we are going to push that fascia open and get those other clamps out of there. We find the spermatic cord and the surgeon gets their finger around the cord. The cord has a testicular artery and vein, the vas deferens, and in this person, a big indirect inguinal hernia.

So again, we are going to try to find the peritoneum, light touch with the tip of the cautery—the surgeon, medical student, and resident. There is a big bulge and we are going to pull this thing and pull it out of the scrotum and up into the wound. It is a big bag of water or a big bag of omentum. The structure on the right is the sac, the peritoneum, the fatty tissue and the vessels within the spermatic cord are to the right. We are going to clamp that sac as long as there is no bowel or nothing evil in there. We tie it off,

VIDEO 9.7. Continued

and we are going to transect and get rid of that sac. Hopefully that sac then will slide into the abdomen once we are done with it.

Now with the sack in the belly, we are going to put a piece of mesh on top, which is called a Lichenstein hernia repair. What we want to do is put that mesh on the internal oblique and transversalis, but put the mesh deep to where the spermatic cord is. This is a tough picture to look at but we are sewing from the pubic tubercle along the ilioinguinal ligament. We have got to be careful sewing that mesh because the femoral vessels, or the external iliac artery and the vein are just deep to that side. We have got a little gauze in there and we are now creating a new internal ring. We put a cut in that mesh and it is sewn inferiorly, a couple of stitches and we have got a hole where the spermatic cord goes through. These are prolene stitches tacking the mesh to the internal oblique, careful not to hurt the nerve (ilioinguinal or iliohypogastric). We are now going to close the external oblique fascia over the top of the mesh and the cord; and we want to do this in a tension-free manner and make sure we don't cut or injure the spermatic cord below.

We are just about finished up closing the external oblique, a running suture. Young surgeon at the helm and a little slower, but no problem, does that very nicely, that is a running suture. Now Scarpa fascia, I like to close it to give another layer or barrier away from the mesh. I get nervous about infection of the skin. Scarpa fascia is closed and then we will want to close the skin with a running, absorbable suture. Ideally making this cosmetic and tension-free and it will heal nicely. Nice job! Need to close up the skin and we are all done.

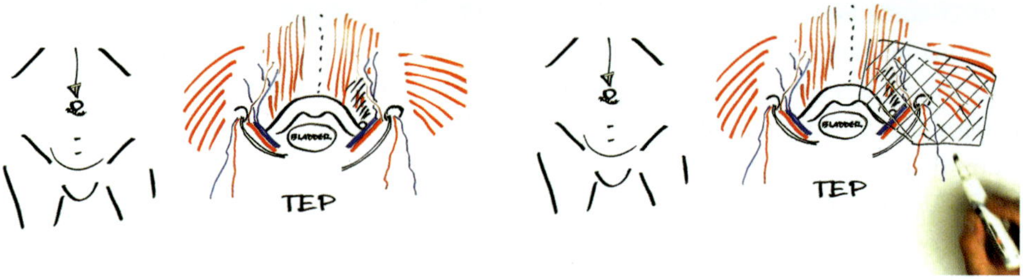

VIDEO 9.8. Totally Extraperitoneal Laparoscopic Repair.

Transcript: Similar to a TAPP, a TEP incision initially starts out underneath the belly button. Two other little incisions that allow us access into the preperitoneal space. But TEP stands for totally extraperitoneal. Unlike when we put the camera in on a TAPP, on a TEP, we never get into the abdomen. We don't see the gallbladder, we don't see the appendix, and we don't see the bowel. The tricky thing is we slide in just anterior to the peritoneum and blow up a balloon and we get to see this space with the bowel and contents behind us. It is a wonderful opportunity to see the internal ring, the deep inferior epigastric arteries and veins, femoral hernia, Hesselbach's triangle; and the nice thing about the operation is that we are not going to hurt the bowel or create adhesions within the abdomen. The downside is that it is a smaller space and it is not as easy to get at and it is a little bit more confusion than a TAPP. It is my own bias on how to fix a hernia, because I think it is a good way to do it. Once we find out where the hernia is, we cut a piece of mesh and cover the defect. Another advantage of both TAPP and TEP, it will fix 3 hernias at the same time: an indirect, a direct, and a femoral defect. It is a good option for inguinal hernia repairs.

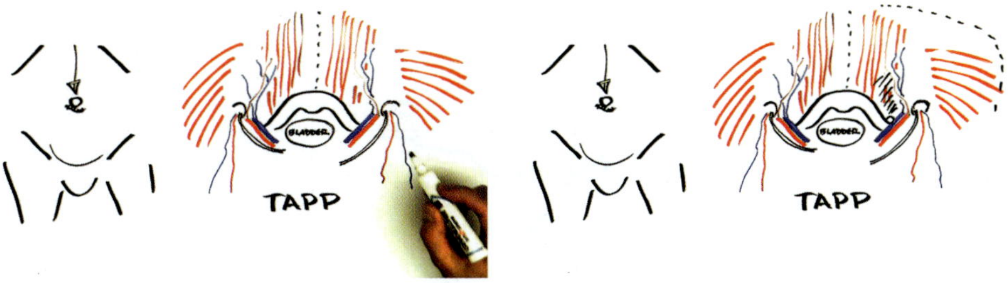

VIDEO 9.9. Transabdominal Preperitoneal Laparoscopic Repair.

Transcript: Inguinal hernias can be fixed laparoscopically. We typically get into the abdomen through the infraumbilical region. Into the abdomen, allows us to do a transabdominal preperitoneal inguinal hernia repair (TAPP in video). When we slide into the abdomen, we look down toward the pelvis. So the camera is looking down this way into this pelvis and we will see linea alba, the rectus abdominis muscle, the pubic bone with the pubic symphysis, the bladder, we might be lucky enough to see the external iliac vein and artery. And as we dissect and take a look at things, we might find an indirect hernia, in the internal ring, a direct hernia, a Hesselbach triangle, or a femoral hernia right near the external iliac vein.

Transabdominally into the abdomen, we can also see bowel, colon, and a variety of things. The peritoneum covers this area. What hernia surgeons will do is incise the peritoneum, sneak that peritoneum down, and then dissects out the hernia sac, place a piece of mesh, and put that peritoneum back up. The nice thing about this is that you can look at the gallbladder, appendix, and see around the rest of the abdomen. It gives a big space to slide into. The upside is that you have put a hole through the belly and you may have caused some problems with adhesions doing this or you could injure the intra-abdominal contents. It is a very safe operation and most surgeons that do laparoscopic inguinal hernia repair use a TAPP procedure.

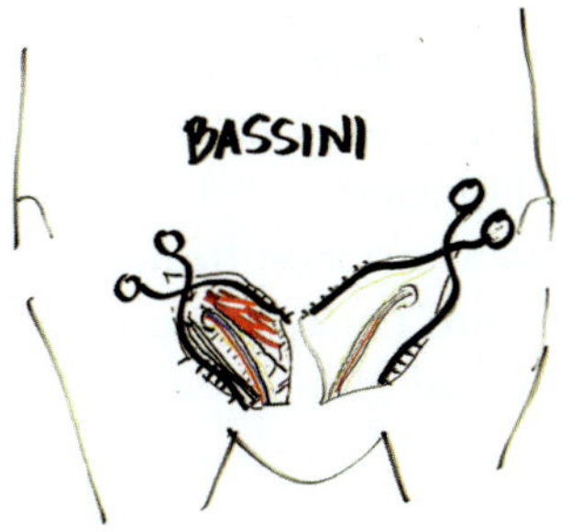

VIDEO 9.10. Bassini Repair.

Transcript: A Bassini hernia repair is historically the most effective of long ago. Dr Bassini, in Padua, Italy, he fixed hernias in the 1880s and what he did was whether the hernia was around the internal ring or in Hesselbach triangle, he decided to cut from the internal ring all the way down to the pubic tubercle. That tissue would open up and the spermatic cord was there. He would get the spermatic cord and mobilize it and then he would stitch from what is so called the conjoined tendon; the transversalis fascia, and the internal oblique and sew that to the shelving edge of the inguinal ligament, so-called the Poupart ligament. So if you could imagine taking a bite of tissue, sneak it underneath the cord and taking a bite of tissue and passing it back to move this ligament underneath and move the muscle underneath, such that at the end of the cord is in place. But the defect that Bassini cut and moved is moving the conjoined tendon to the inguinal ligament, sewing that up posterior to the spermatic cord. So, the cord stays intact, but using permanent suture—no mesh—sewing it in place. This is a wonderful technique, higher recurrence rate, but you don't need to use mesh.

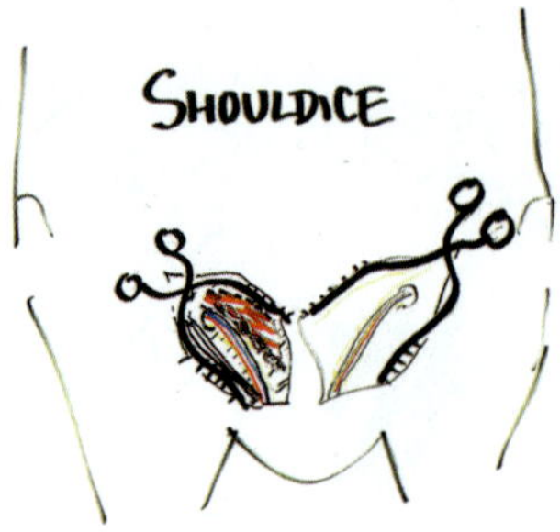

VIDEO 9.11. Shouldice Repair.

Transcript: The Shouldice repair is a hernia repair popularized by the Shouldice Clinic, outside of Toronto, Ontario. Wonderful operation, no mesh, tension free, but instead of Bassini or McVay's technique, trying to get the shelving edge of the inguinal ligament sewn together with a conjoined tendon, not with interrupted sutures, but with running sutures down and back and down again. Basically, 3 layers of tissue, trying to create more scar tissue and strength to hold it together. The downside, perhaps, it is sometimes hard to get that tissue together. The upside, it has gotten wonderful results, low recurrence rates, done as an outpatient. It is a wonderful operation in the hands of experts; the Shouldice repair.

Inguinal Region Challenge Questions

9.1. What are Bassini, McVay, and Shouldice repairs?
9.2. What is the absolute contraindication to laparoscopic repair?
9.3. When is laparoscopic repair indicated?
9.4. What is the triangle of doom? What is the triangle of pain?
9.5. When is an open repair better than a laparoscopic repair?
9.6. What does NAVEL stand for?
9.7. What are 4 important sensory nerves in the inguinal region?
9.8. What is the round ligament?
9.9. Which type of groin hernia most frequently leads to emergency surgery?
9.10. What are the chances of a man having an inguinal hernia in his lifetime?

(Answers appear on page 138)

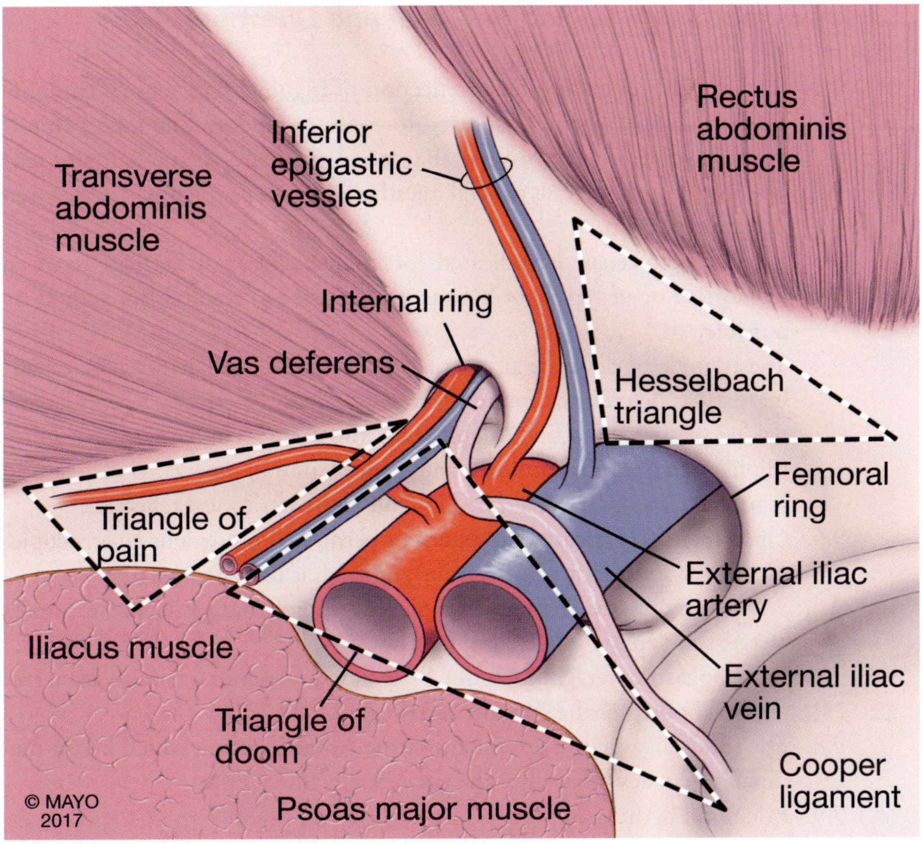

FIGURE 9.5. Triangles of Doom and Pain in the Left Inguinal Region.

Answers to Inguinal Region Challenge Questions

9.1. Bassini: Sutures approximate reflection of inguinal ligament to conjoint tendon; McVay: Cooper ligament sutured to conjoint tendon; Shouldice: Imbrication of the transverse fascia, transverse abdominal aponeurosis, and conjoint tendon.

9.2. The inability to tolerate general anesthesia (eg, hypovolemic shock, severe cardiac decompensation).

9.3. Laparoscopic repair is indicated for bilateral inguinal hernias, recurrent hernia from prior open repair, or a patient's necessity to resume full activity as soon as possible.

9.4. The triangle of doom is an area to avoid injuring in laparoscopic repair of groin hernia (vas deferens or round ligament medially, spermatic vessels laterally, external iliac vessels inferiorly) (Figure 9.5). The triangles of pain involve sensory nerves (iliohypogastric, ilioinguinal, and genitofemoral) lateral to iliacs, posterior to inguinal ligament, medial to ASIS, and above peritoneal reflection.

9.5. Open repair is indicated for recurrent hernias with previous laparoscopic repair, if mesh is contraindicated (infection), or mesh is to be removed.

9.6. NAVEL represents the contents of the femoral triangle lateral to medial: *n*erve, *a*rtery, *v*ein, *e*mpty space, *l*ymphatics.

9.7. Iliohypogastric nerve, ilioinguinal nerve, lateral femoral cutaneous nerve, and the femoral branch of the genitofemoral nerve.

9.8. The round ligament is a remnant of the gubernaculum, which lies in the inguinal canal in females (instead of the vas deferens in males).

9.9. A femoral hernia.

9.10. Twenty-five percent of men have an inguinal hernia in their lifetime.

10

Jejunum and Ileum

Embryology

During development, there is physiologic herniation of the midgut into the umbilical cord, and it then slips back in with a counterclockwise rotation. Malrotation of the midgut can lead to a volvulus.

Anatomy

Jejunum (about 1.5 m) and ileum (about 3.5 m) occupy the mid abdomen and pelvis (Figure 10.1). The jejunum has a thicker wall, larger lumen, and less mesenteric fat than the ileum. Plicae circulares (circular mucosal folds) (Figure 10.2 left) increase surface area for nutrient absorption and are characteristic of the jejunum; these folds are smaller in the ileum. Jejunal and ileal arterial branches arise from the SMA and form loops, arcades, and vasa recta (Figure 10.3). The jejunum has fewer arcades and longer vasa recta than those of the ileum. Venous drainage is by the valveless portal venous system.

Physiology

The jejunum is involved in calcium and magnesium absorption. The ileum contains lymphoid tissue (Peyer patches) (Figure 10.2 right) at the antimesenteric border. Bile salts, fatty acids, vitamin B_{12}, and fat-soluble vitamins are absorbed in the terminal ileum.

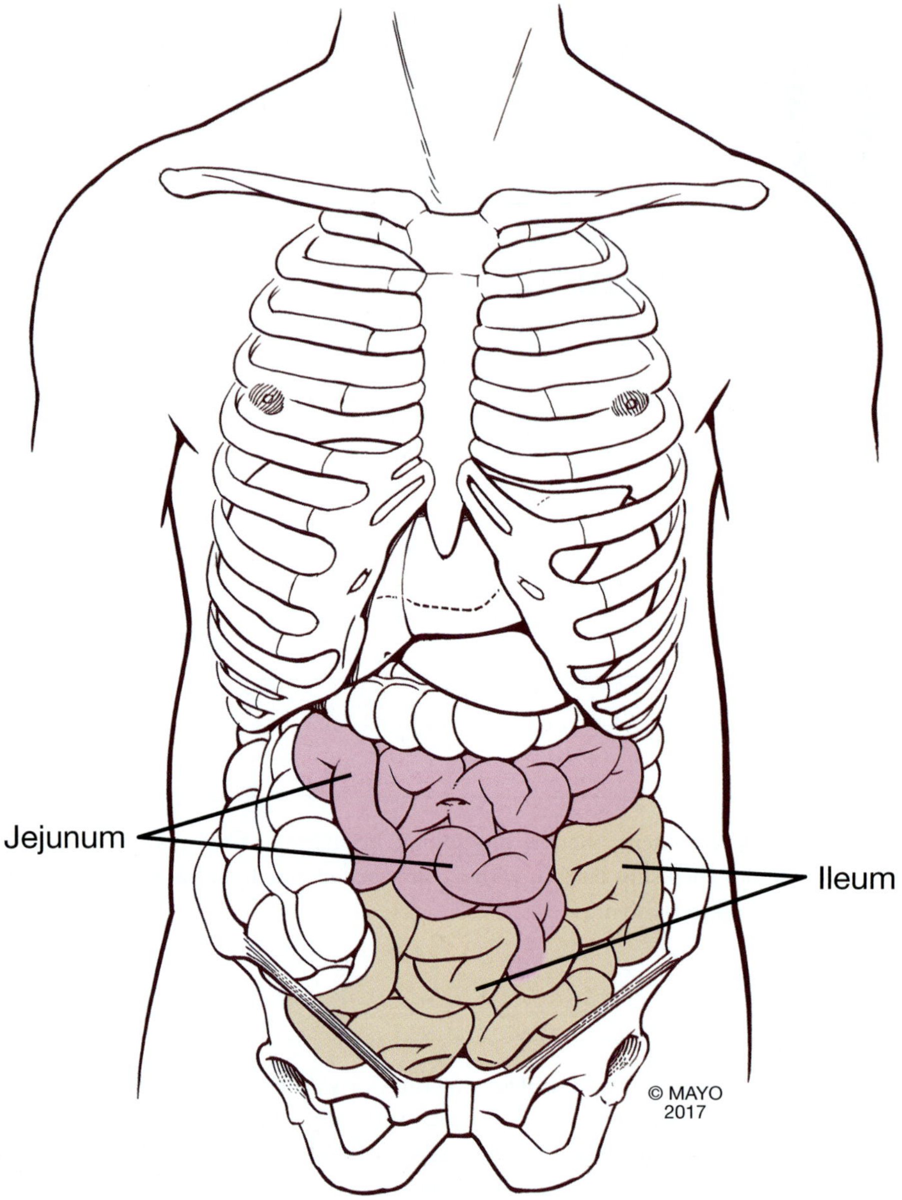

FIGURE 10.1. Anatomy of the Jejunum and Ileum.

Clinical Presentation

Small bowel infections present with a range of symptoms from diarrhea to severe dehydration to sepsis. Other common diseases of the small bowel are inflammatory bowel disease (Video 10.1), lactose intolerance, celiac disease (Video 10.2), and SBO (Video 10.3). Signs of SBO are emesis, distention, fever, acidosis, tachycardia, and leukocytosis. The main cause of SBOs worldwide is hernias; in developed countries it is postoperative adhesions.

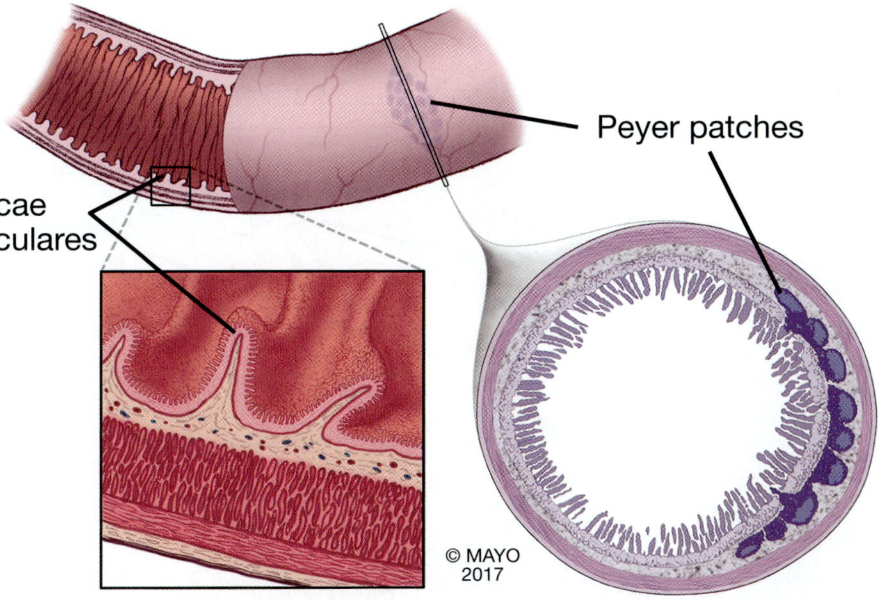

FIGURE 10.2. Plicae Circulares (left) and Peyer Patches (right).

Imaging

Suspected SBO can be evaluated with plain radiography (Video 10.4), upper GI studies (meglumine diatrizoate vs barium), or CT. Dilated loops or air-fluid levels are prominent. Dilated small bowel may look like a stack of coins (caused by thin mucosal folds, termed *plicae circulares* or *valvulae conniventes*) (Video 10.5). Capsule endoscopy, conventional endoscopy (Video 10.6), UGI (Video 10.7), and CT may be useful for evaluating small intestine disorders.

Operation

The treatment of SBO is initially nonoperative (IV hydration, nasogastric suction, nothing by mouth); most obstructions (90%) resolve within a few days. Patients with peritonitis, free air, or unsuccessful medical management require laparoscopy or laparotomy. Adhesiolysis or formal small bowel resection may be required for SBO, cancer, ischemia, and other disorders. A pancreatojejunal anastomosis (for a Whipple procedure) is often indicated to treat tumors of the pancreas, intestine, and bile duct (Video 10.8).

Complications

Paralytic ileus (Video 10.9) occurs in many patients after abdominal surgery and is treated with IV fluids, nothing by mouth, and electrolyte replacement. Anastomotic leak, bleeding, and adhesive SBO can occur.

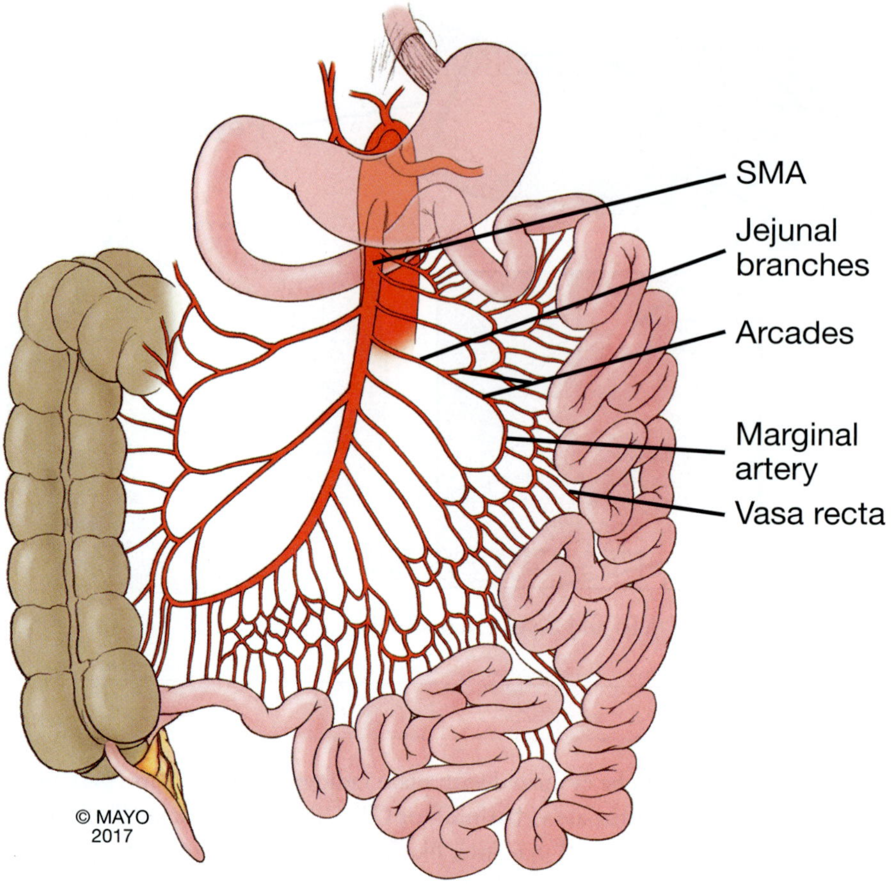

FIGURE 10.3. Jejunal and Ileal Arterial Branches.

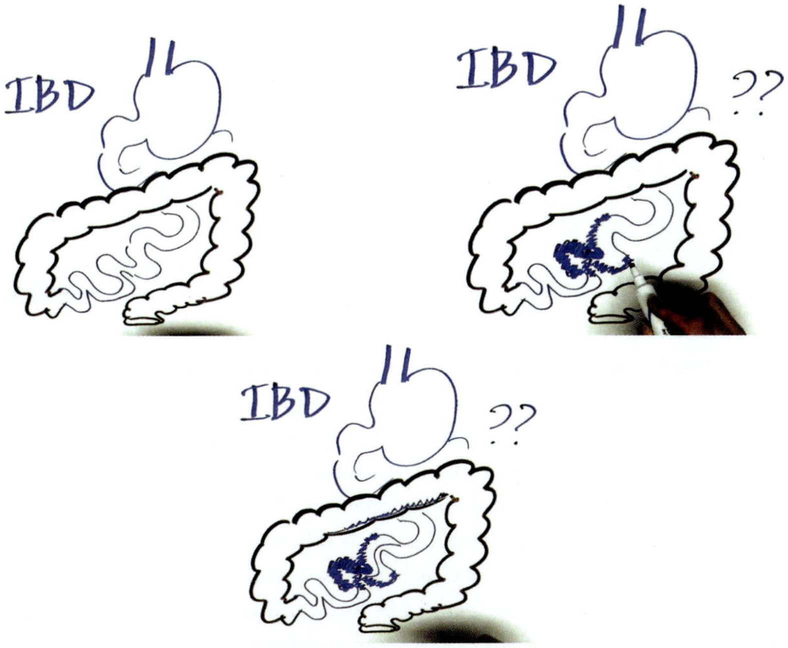

VIDEO 10.1. Inflammatory Bowel Disease (IBD).
Transcript: Inflammatory bowel disease is a group of disorders that are problematic, painful, irritable, and sometimes lethal to our patients. When I think about irritable bowel disease I think about Crohn disease, which can happen from the mouth to the anus. I think about ulcerative colitis, or colitis in general, which is typically just the colon but sometimes the rectum. There are other disorders, sprue, and a variety of things that cause problems. Most of these things consistently have environmental and genetic factors, but we honestly don't know what causes some of these things—Crohn disease especially, we are waiting for the cure. Patients with Crohn disease will oftentimes have thickening of the entire intestinal wall and that often leads to obstruction. It sometimes can lead to bleeding. It can have obstructive symptoms with nausea, vomiting, and weight loss. People will have significant pain.

Folks with ulcerative colitis, it's typically the lining of the colon that gets inflamed and red and may lead to bloody diarrhea. But it is a constellation of symptoms and folks with IBD may have other problems besides the colon and the small bowel. There may be things wrong with the liver, the joints, ankylosing spondylitis, arthritis, skin manifestations, and eye problems. There must be something going on globally with these things. Inflammatory bowel disease, Crohn, ulcerative colitis, and a host of other struggles.

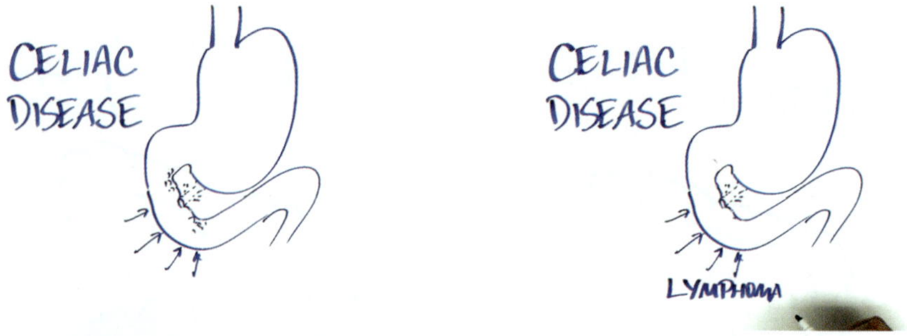

VIDEO 10.2. Celiac Disease.

Transcript: Celiac disease is not uncommon. People can have it and have real difficulties. Oftentimes you will see it on an upper GI study; little ulcerations, outpouchings, aphthous ulcers of the duodenum especially. Young folks that are eating gluten and have sensitivity to it and create antibodies; basically, the body is fighting itself. The nice thing about this is that if we could avoid gluten protein, or gliadin, basically the body will settle out and these ulcers will heal and people can do just fine.

Now the thing about celiac disease, or what I used to call sprue, is there is an increased risk of other problems, including lymphoma. So patients that have sprue need to be followed up consistently. They don't just get to go home and take care of themselves forever. But they need to avoid gluten; otherwise, they will run into serious trouble. Celiac disease is more common than you think.

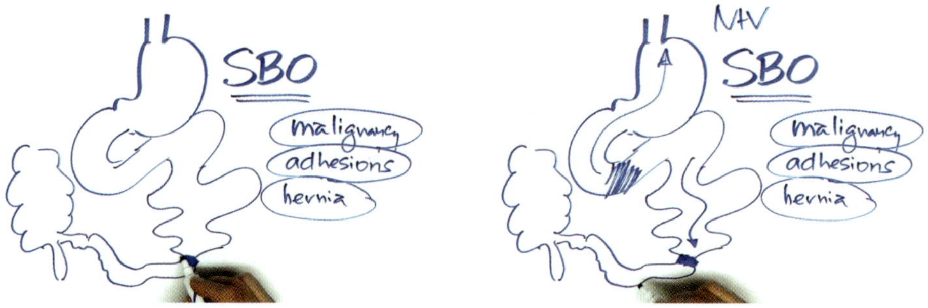

VIDEO 10.3. SBO.

Transcript: Small bowel obstruction happens for a variety of reasons. Most times after surgery it settles out. Some people need surgery for this.

If we are in a developed country with a good health care system, small bowel obstruction is typically related to a malignancy, or hernia, or adhesions. If we are in an undeveloped country, the number 1 reason to have a small bowel obstruction is a hernia. In a developed country with lots of surgery, adhesions would be the choice. But there can be underlying cancers for this. Looking at a small bowel obstruction, what does that mean? An obstruction, something is narrowed out and the material can't get through—it is backed up. When things get backed up, that causes problems. If the blockage is early on in the small bowel, in the duodenum, people will block up quickly and will have nausea and vomiting. If they have the blockage down here in the ileum, this will swell up later. They will eventually get nausea and vomiting, but first they will get obstruction, dilatation, tympany, and a big belly. If they have the obstruction in the colon, then this will happen far, far later and people will have different symptoms. So, the more proximal obstruction, the more likely it is that you will have nausea and vomiting. The more distal of obstruction, look for somebody with a big belly that has tympany.

VIDEO 10.3. Continued

Small bowel obstruction can be a lethal problem. It can be due to cancer, if there are adhesions that are related to ischemia and a segment of bowel dies that can be a lethal problem in hours. Even a hernia, incarcerated or strangulated bowel can be a problem. Fortuitously, most people with a small bowel obstruction, adhesions, the twist settles out and people are better. If it is a malignancy, we usually can resect it and take it out. If it is a hernia, we can definitely fix that.

But a small bowel obstruction, one should never let the sun set if somebody has a small bowel obstruction. You need to find out right now why that is happening.

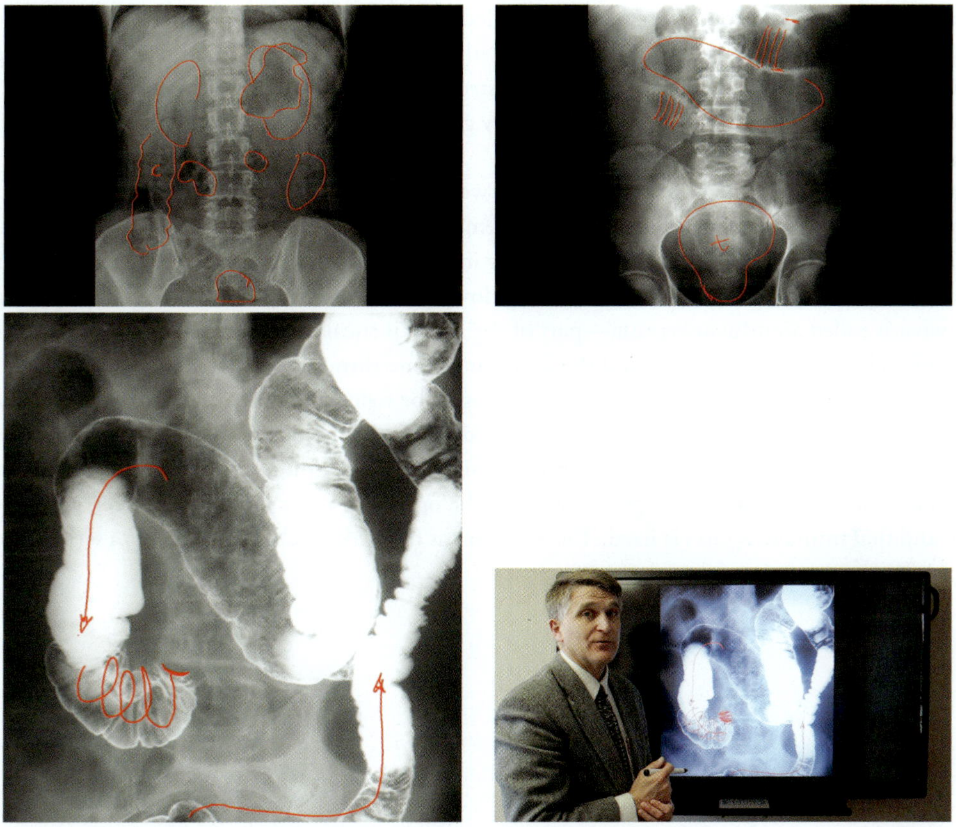

VIDEO 10.4. Plain Radiograph of the Abdomen. CAT (in narration), computed axial tomography.
Transcript: A plain x-ray of the abdomen. Historically called a KUB—kidneys, ureter, and bladder. But this is a KUB, a plain x-ray of the abdomen—and it is a normal one. There are lots of different things to look at. We can see the spine and the ribs, but most general surgeons and most surgery trainees are thinking about something else; they are looking at the cecum. We can see the stool in the colon, cecum, descending, and ascending colon. We see air in the stomach; it is a gastric air bubble. If we look closely, we actually can see the kidneys sitting back there, tougher to see over here, but they are there.

Oftentimes when you are looking at a KUB, or a flat plate of the abdomen, we are looking for gas. We can see some gas here and some air in the intestine and stool in the colon. Then ideally, look down at the bottom to see if there is gas in the rectum.

VIDEO 10.4. Continued

Let's take a look at a couple of pictures that are not normal, and their KUBs, if you will. So here is a picture of a young man that comes to the emergency room that has got abdominal pain and he has got tenderness and he has got a bigger belly. Lying flat on his back, a flat plate if you will; this is what his abdomen looks like. I hope that you can see that there is dilated bowel and they have these thin little lines, the so-called valvulae conniventes. This is small bowel that has got lots of air in it. So we have to think about why does the body have a lot of air in it? Most people do not have a lot of air in their small bowel; they quickly get into the colon. But this person must have a blockage point at some point. Lying flat on the table, we are not sure where it is. Is there any gas or stool down here? I don't see any. I don't see much over here, but I do see big loops of small bowel intestine. I am thinking that he might have a small bowel obstruction or maybe the colon is blocked someplace.

Let's change it, instead of being a flat plate, let's stand him upright. When you stand upright, gravity is your friend because know you can see what are called air fluid levels, lots of them. These typically occur in the small bowel. So we have lots of gas in here with some air, and liquid mixing around. Until proven otherwise, this person does have a small bowel obstruction or very proximal colonic obstruction. These tests don't tell you exactly what is going on, but they give you a sense that this person is not making it up, he needs some help.

So a couple of different ways to think about it, we could get a CAT scan or another study, or this is a study you might have seen before—a barium enema. Barium is placed through the rectum and under pressure, sneaks all the way around and if you allow it enough time, it gets into the ascending colon, into the cecum, and then we see a funny sort of thing down here, it stops and something is happening here. This is what is called an intussusception—part of the ileum is sneaking through but it is so tight that it is kinked off and the contrast can't go and the food can't come through from below. So this person has an emergency and either needs an operation or this thing to be reduced. Sometimes the barium can actually push the bowel back and intussusception can be cured—frequent in kids. Oftentimes happens when they are 2, 3, and 4 years old. But in adults, oftentimes this intussusception occurs because there is a tumor, a cancer, a carcinoid, a polyp. So this person went to the operating room and had a cancer, a carcinoid removed, and that intussusception is fixed. The KUB led us to thinking about that this is a serious problem.

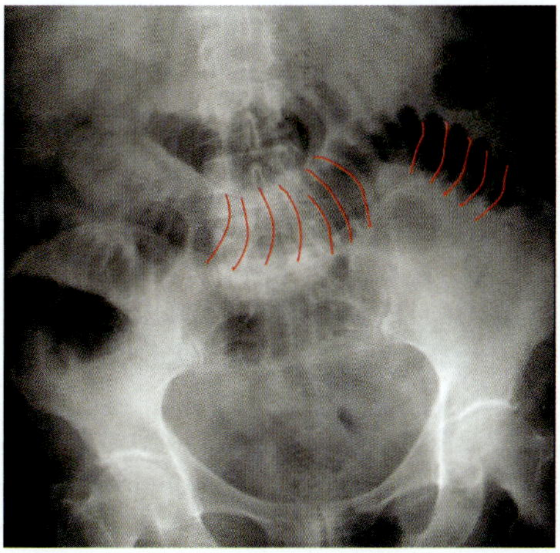

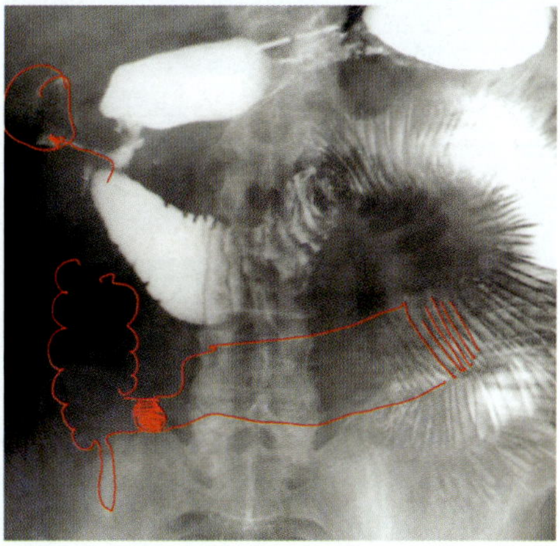

VIDEO 10.5. Valvulae Conniventes (Plicae Circulares).

Transcript: The ileum and the jejunum are amazing organs for absorption. They have lots of surface, they have valvulae conniventes, they have plicae circulares; basically lines that help this fluid move through and help absorb it. But we shouldn't see these lines on a flat plate of the abdomen. There is way too much gas here. This is a KUB showing someone with a small bowel obstruction. These lines depending on whether they are oriented or not, sometimes look like stacked coins.

This is a wonderful barium study that shows exactly what I think people are talking about stacked coins with a line. All of that material should be moving through, it shouldn't stay there. This is a wonderful picture showing us some stacked coins; ileum and jejunum that is lightly obstructed, with the colon or something downstream. Interestingly enough, we have got a problem up here with the gallbladder as well. There is some dye leaking out. This might be someone with a problem of what is called gallstone ileus, an inflamed gallbladder. The stone erodes through and sneaks all the way through; but because the ileocecal valve down here near the appendix and the ascending colon isn't very big, the stone gets stuck down here and everything behind it becomes massively dilated. This is a great picture showing a barium contrast study of somebody with a gallstone ileus.

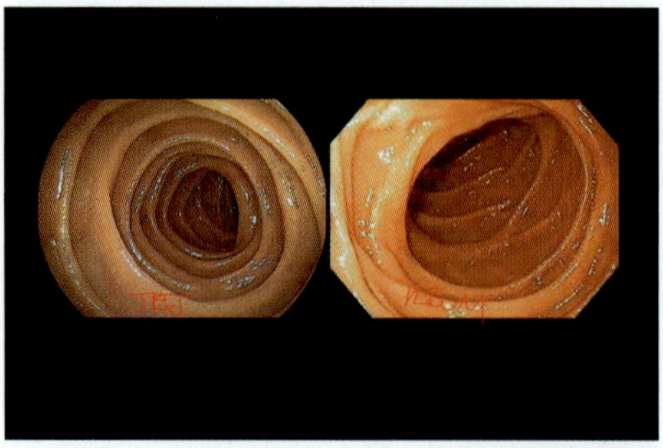

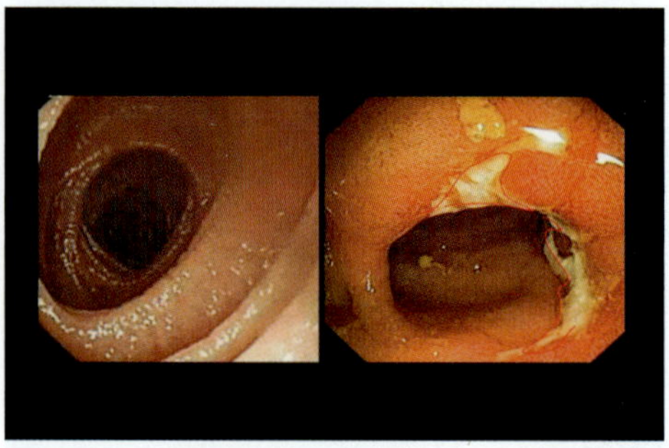

VIDEO 10.6. Endoscopy.

Transcript: Modern medicine, short of surgery, the best way of looking at the ileum or the jejunum is usually with an endoscope. This is the jejunum on this side. It is thicker; it is a little more robust. The ileum tends to be a little thinner. Having said that, these are normal pictures of the jejunum and ileum, wide open, they're glossy, they're nice, and they are healthy—that is not always the case.

Take a couple other pictures, the jejunum here on the left is sort of a little beaded, it is not as smooth and it is not as healthy looking. This is likely celiac sprue disease, it's got nodularity to it, maybe not the best blood supply. Maybe they are eating gluten. If they stop eating the gluten, they will be much, much better. Over here the ileum, often seen through the colonoscope, as opposed to the jejunum, it's the endoscope from above. This is not normal. This is scar tissue; this is material that shouldn't be here. This is likely Crohn disease. This is a granulomatous disease; full thickness, its woody, it's boggy, and it is not any fun for patients to have. But what a beautiful way to diagnose without making a big incision on somebody—somebody with Crohn's or sprue. The treatment for each of these things is oftentimes medical; avoid gluten, here there are medications, steroids and others that alleviate this temporary or long-term. So endoscopy is a wonderful way to get to the small bowel: the jejunum from above through the esophagus, stomach, and duodenum, and then the ileum from below through the colon. The problem with endoscopy for the small bowel is in the middle of the small bowel—the more distal jejunum and the more proximal ileum.

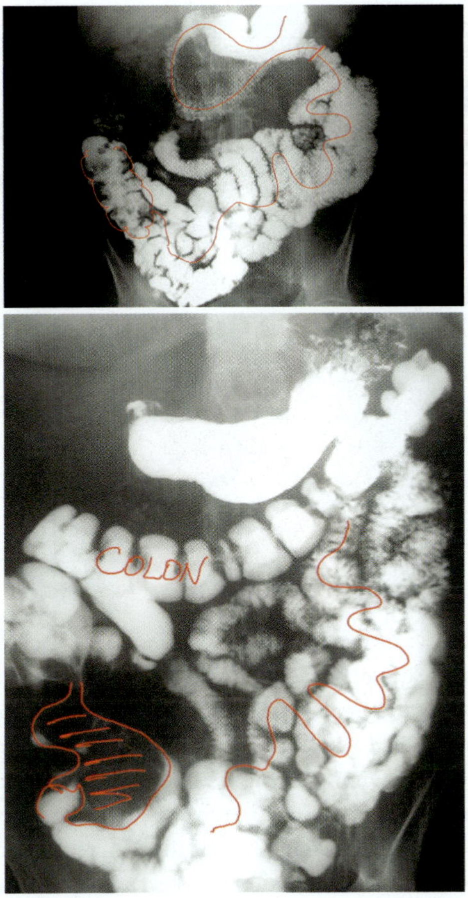

VIDEO 10.7. UGI Radiograph.

Transcript: This picture depicts an upper GI study. What I would say is upper GI small bowel follow-through. Meaning you have waited long enough to see the dye come through. So we are up in the body of the stomach, the antrum, the pylorus, duodenum, and now from here on is jejunum and ileum. And it weaves its way through, eventually to the ileocecal valve where we see the cecum and ascending colon. This is a normal upper GI small bowel follow-through. It may take 1 or 2 hours for this test and if somebody has an obstruction or slow motility, it may take 6 to 8 hours to get pictures like this. But you don't just immediately drink it and get a photo like this. You have to watch this, and so every few minutes or 30 minutes another picture is taken to see how it percolates through.

Let's take a look at something that may not be perfectly normal. Well, we see stomach here, our dye is here, and we are sneaking it through and actually we can get a sense that it is percolating all the way through. We haven't waited long enough to find out about the rest of the colon. So far, so good.

In a patient like this, what do we see? We have waited a long time because we can see that there is contrast in the colon and the good news is that the contrast gets through the colon. So, the person is not completely obstructed. But, lots of dye, lots of barium sneaking down and we get over to here and something funny happens. There is this area that doesn't have any contrast to it. So, is this inflammation, is this cancer, is this Crohn's disease, and is this an abscess from the appendix? This is clearly abnormal and it's somebody that is having chronic pain, right lower quadrant pain, or eating or drinking problems. This is going to let know that there is an abnormality here. Nowadays, CT scan or endoscopy might give us more information. But this is a good screening test to let us know where the trouble is—this is abnormal.

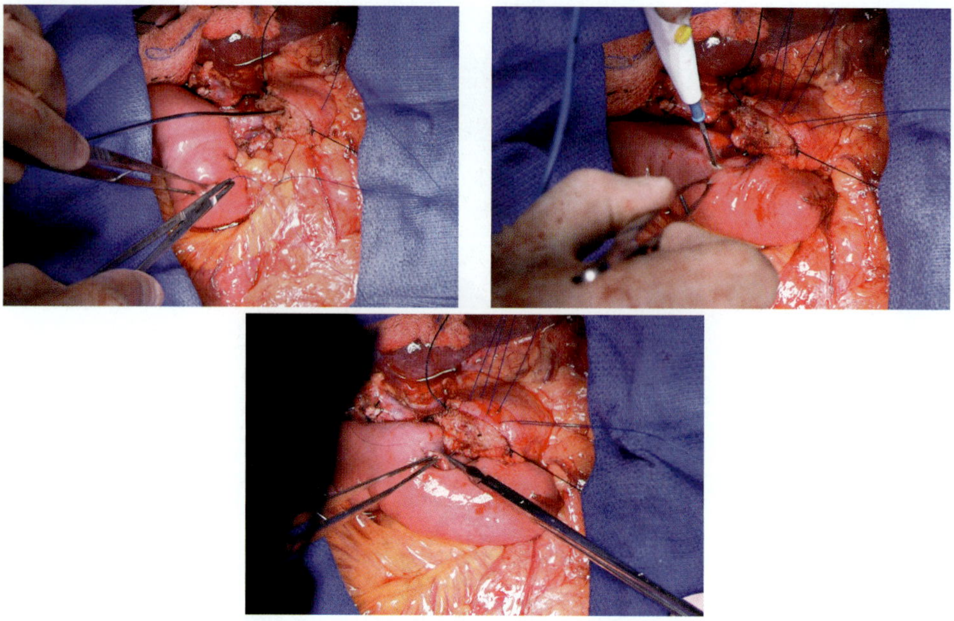

VIDEO 10.8. Pancreatojejunostomy: Intraoperative.

Transcript: This is an open pancreatic operation—it's a Whipple operation—the jejunum and the pancreas are there. We are going to try to match it up. It looks like the pancreatic duct inside the pancreas is maybe 2 or 3 mm. This is what is called a Bakes dilator, sliding in to just make sure the pancreatic duct is okay, and it may be 3 or 4 mm in size, not very big, so it's easy to stenose or have a stricture. So we have got a couple of silk sutures marking the pancreas and now we are going to use some suture, probably PDS, probably 4 or 5-O and we are going to take a big bite of the pancreas, pronate our wrist, supinate it out, take a big bite of the small bowel, that is the jejunum. And eventually we are going to pull pretty hard and pull this neck of the pancreas, or the cut edge of the pancreas, abut up into the jejunum.

We have got some bites in there. You can see both the pancreas and the small bowel are well perfused. This is a healthy person—relatively fit. Another bite that is going to sort of dunk this pancreas toward the small bowel. But eventually what we want to do is do a mucosa-to-mucosa anastomosis. Right now this is sort of a back wall setting things up and we are going to be able to pull that bowel up against the pancreas snug. Little bit of bleeding here. Anytime the needle goes through a well vascularized structure like the pancreas, or the small bowel, you get a little bit of bleeding. But most of that will stop on its own. The surgeon is backhanding this. Going from pronation to supination and supination to pronation, whatever angle is best and going to spin that needle out.

So, the back is all done. Now we need to make a little hole in the jejunum, pop into that lumen, and we have got to sew the pancreas duct to this tiny little opening. Oftentimes we will put a little stent in here to help us with it, but here the surgeon is taking a bite of the small bowel, may pull that back and set ourselves up to open it up, tying some 1-handed knots. And every surgeon has a little bit different strategy. That mucosa is now sewn to the serosa on that small bowel. Here comes a bite, a careful one through the pancreatic duct. Going to catch the bottom or the posterior aspect of that duct, little bitty sutures; this is all magnified. Nice bite of the pancreas, we have got mucosa, the pancreatic duct, now we are going to take a little bit of a bite to catch the outside of the serosa, a little bit of the mucosa, and sew these together. That is the back part, probably going to take several other sutures to do this well; 4, 5, or 6 stitches. Pancreatojejunostomy, mucosa-to-mucosa repair.

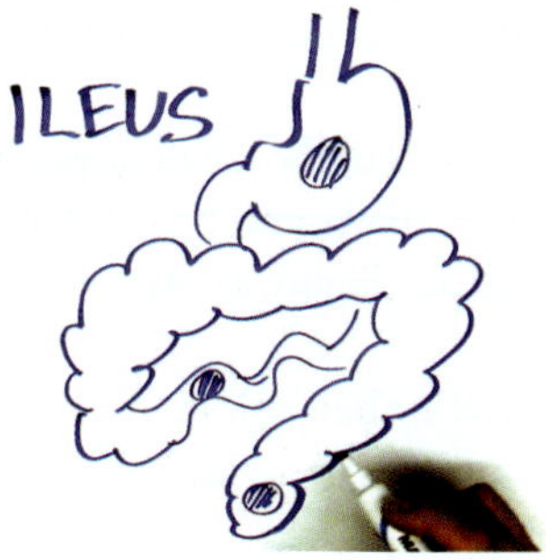

VIDEO 10.9. Paralytic Ileus.

Transcript: Ileus is a problem for surgeons and patients alike. The bowel doesn't work—temporarily it's out of order. That can be from handling it, that can be from surgery, that can be from metabolic problems, electrolytes out of abnormality, or kidney function is bad. But when you think of ileus, you have to be thinking of a couple different things. Ileus means that the whole bowel is sort of shut down, but there should be air in the rectum. There should be air in the small bowel, and there should be air in the stomach. If there is air throughout the small bowel, but nothing in the colon or rectum, then you need to think about an obstruction. So the key thing in my mind is that if somebody has an ileus, correct the metabolic electrolyte abnormalities, but make sure they don't have a small bowel or large bowel obstruction. The best way to tell that initially early on is with a flat plate of the abdomen and see gas throughout the intestinal tract. If you have got somebody downstream that doesn't have any air in the rectum or the distal colon, and they haven't been passing gas or stool, you need to think about an obstruction. An ileus, that will just take time. Back off the narcotics and get your patient up and out of bed moving around, IV fluids, make sure the electrolytes are a-okay, and avoid narcotic medications is really helpful.

Ileus is a temporary irritation, usually not a significant, lethal problem.

Jejunum and Ileum Challenge Questions

10.1. What is the "rule of 3's" for the small bowel?
10.2. What marks the start of the jejunum?
10.3. What malignancy is associated with metastasis to the small intestine?
10.4. What is the order of return of motility from paralytic ileus?
10.5. What is the most common location of lymphoma in the small bowel?
10.6. What is the most frequent site of anticoagulant-induced SBO?
10.7. What is the most common cause of enteric infection by drinking water from a stream?
10.8. What is blind-loop syndrome?
10.9. What is a likely cause of B_{12} deficiency of the small intestine?

Answers to Jejunum and Ileum Challenge Questions

10.1. The normal dimensions of the small bowel: bowel wall less than 3 mm thick, bowel folds less than 3 mm thick, and bowel diameter less than 3 cm wide.
10.2. The ligament of Treitz (Figure 10.4).
10.3. Melanoma.
10.4. Small bowel, stomach, then colon.
10.5. The ileum (Peyer patches are lymphatic tissue).
10.6. The proximal jejunum.
10.7. *Giardia* species.
10.8. Bacterial overgrowth in the small intestine.
10.9. Resection of the terminal ileum.

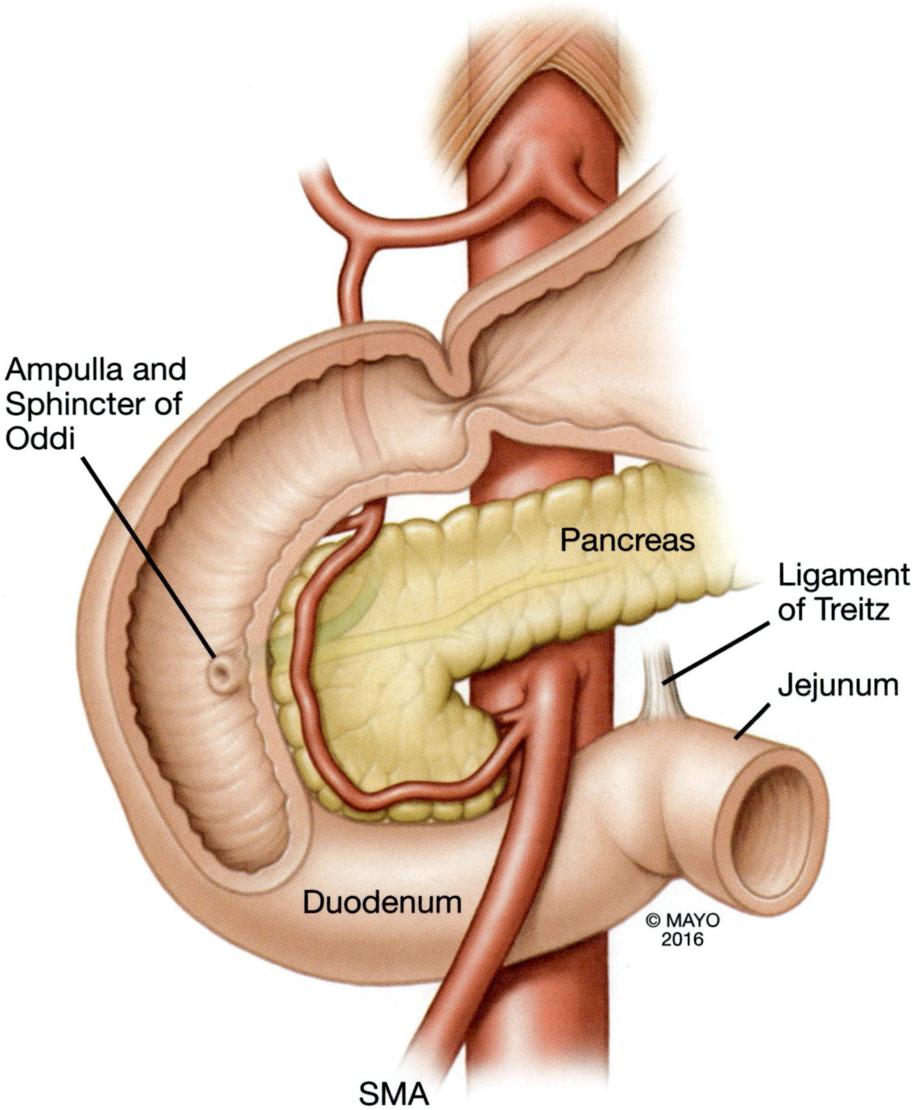

FIGURE 10.4. Ligament of Treitz and the Start of the Jejunum.

11

Liver

Embryology

The liver arises from the foregut-midgut junction. The endoderm differentiates into hepatocytes (liver and parenchyma) and cholangiocytes (epithelial cells of bile ducts).

Anatomy

The liver is contained in the Glisson capsule, and the falciform ligament attaches the liver to the anterior abdominal wall (Figure 11.1). The Cantlie line (Figure 11.1) is an imaginary line from the IVC and GB fossa dividing the liver into left and right lobes. The Couinaud segments (Figure 11.2) divide the liver into 8 segments. The center of each segment has a branch from the porta hepatis (liver hilum) (Figure 11.3) where the hepatic ducts, arteries, and portal veins enter and leave the liver. Blood supply is from the portal vein (75%) and proper hepatic artery (25%) (Figure 11.3). The components of the portal triad (Figure 11.3) are the proper hepatic artery, portal vein, and CBD.

Physiology

Hepatocytes perform approximately 500 functions. The liver has roles in, for example, metabolism, detoxification, hormone production, protein synthesis, hematopoiesis, lipid and steroid turnover, and storage of glycogen. Bile is produced in hepatocytes and secreted into bile canaliculi to travel through bile ducts.

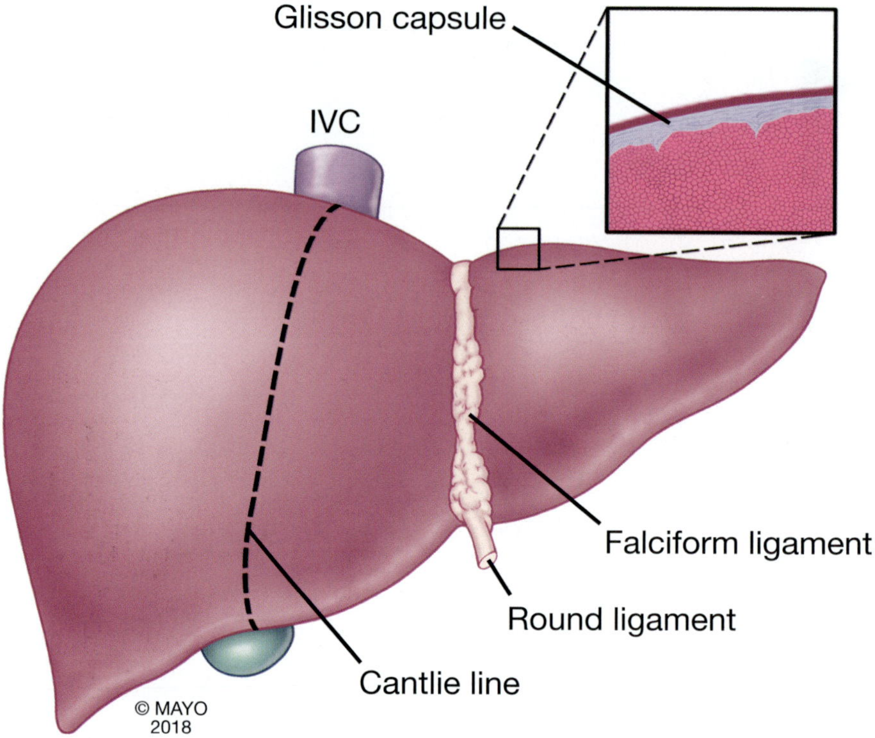

FIGURE 11.1. Anatomy of the Liver.

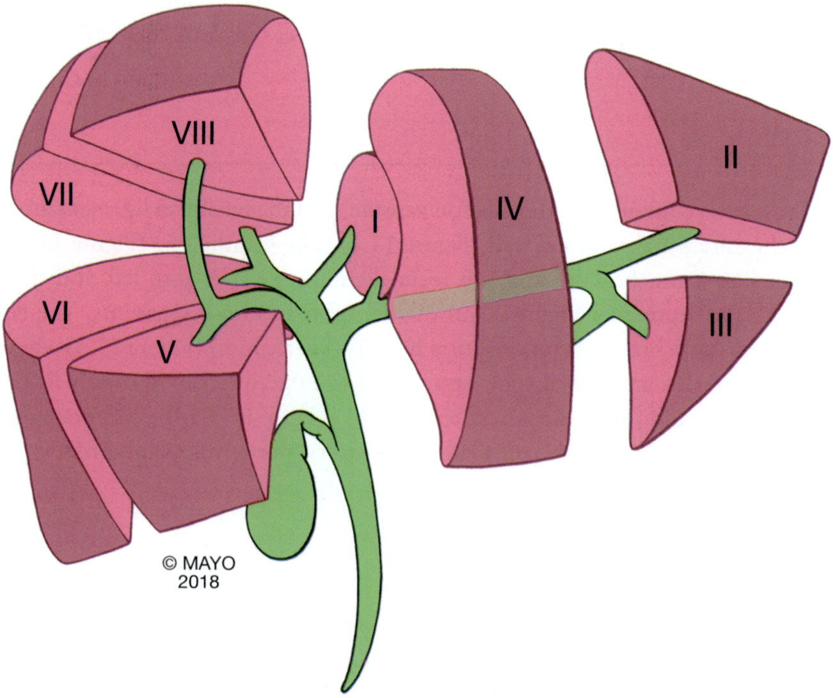

FIGURE 11.2. The Couinaud Segments of the Liver.

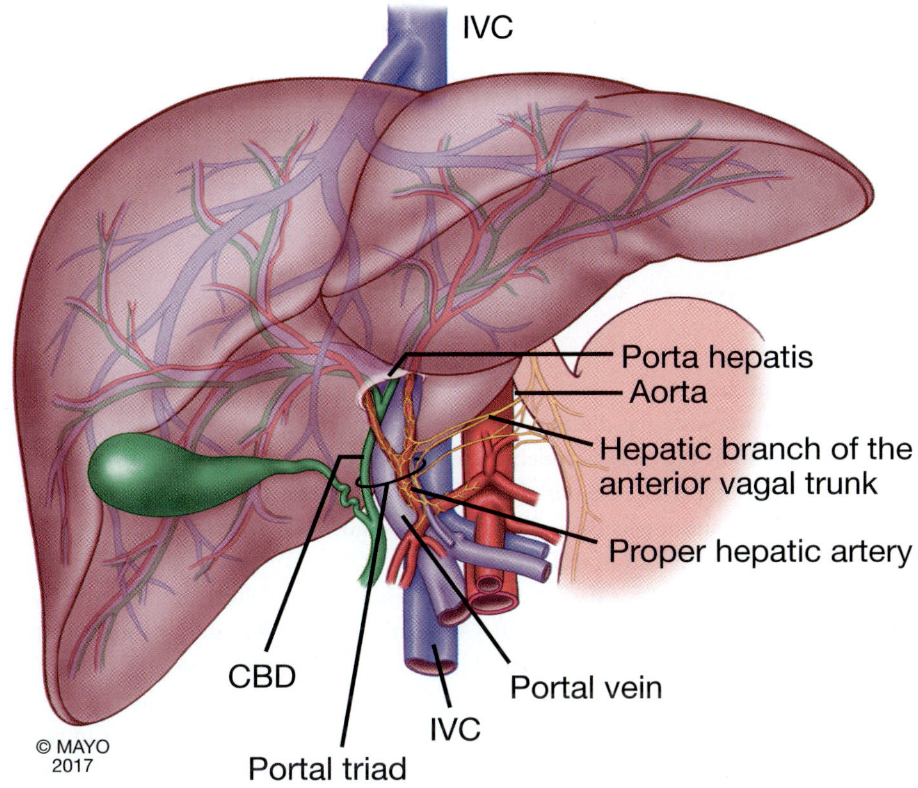

FIGURE 11.3. Blood Supply for the Liver.

Clinical Presentation

Chronic hepatitis C, alcoholic liver disease (number 1 cause in the United States), and nonalcoholic steatohepatitis may cause cirrhosis (Video 11.1) and give rise to liver failure and potentially HCC (number 1 type of first-degree liver cancer) (Video 11.2). Some symptoms of cirrhosis are fatigue, anorexia, nausea, abdominal pain, edema, ascites, jaundice, palmar erythema, and bleeding. Complications from cirrhosis include ascites, esophageal varices, spontaneous bacterial peritonitis, HCC, and hepatorenal syndrome (Video 11.3).

Imaging

MRI, CT (Video 11.4), and US (Video 11.5) are helpful for determining the extent of cirrhosis and detecting ascites, tumors (HCC), and blood flow.

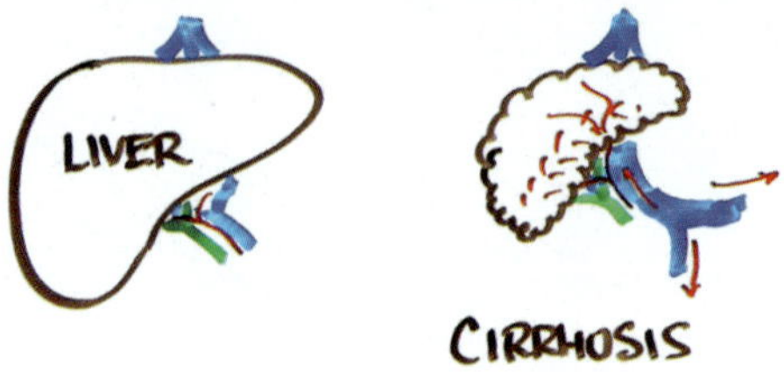

VIDEO 11.1. Cirrhosis of the Liver.
Transcript: Cirrhosis is a devastating disease. We have a normal liver with normal anatomy here. A cirrhotic liver sometimes can be big and distended and edematous, but usually over time it will shrink down and scar; and what really happens is, the portal vessels, the blood that is coming into the liver has a tough time getting into the liver, and it gets backed up. The blood goes backwards and tries to find a different way back to the heart—this can lead to real problems.

The liver does 500-some things for the human body. People with cirrhosis get a lot of problems: they have abdominal pain, they might have nausea, they have anorexia, edema, ascites, they become jaundice, and they can have bleeding episodes. And when things go really bad, they run into real problems; they can have ascites, they can have bleeding, they can die. Cirrhosis is a difficult problem; it's a fibrotic reaction within the liver narrowing things down. The artery with enough blood pressure can get blood into the liver, but the portal vein is a low pressure system. Seventy-five percent of all patients' blood gets to the liver through the portal vein; but not when it's cirrhotic. It becomes a fibrotic backup and the blood can't get there and it goes someplace else; and when it goes someplace else, it causes ascites and bleeding and it defunctionalizes the liver. All sorts of problems are had with liver cirrhosis.

Operation

Fifty percent to 80% of the liver can be resected if the remainder functions well (Video 11.6). Liver transplant is considered in acute liver failure or when cirrhosis progresses to end-stage liver disease. The model for end-stage liver disease (MELD score) (Video 11.7) is used to prioritize organ allocation.

Complications

Liver resections may bleed, leak bile, or lead to infection (cholangitis, hepatitis, abscess). Coagulopathy, ischemia, and obstruction are dangerous problems.

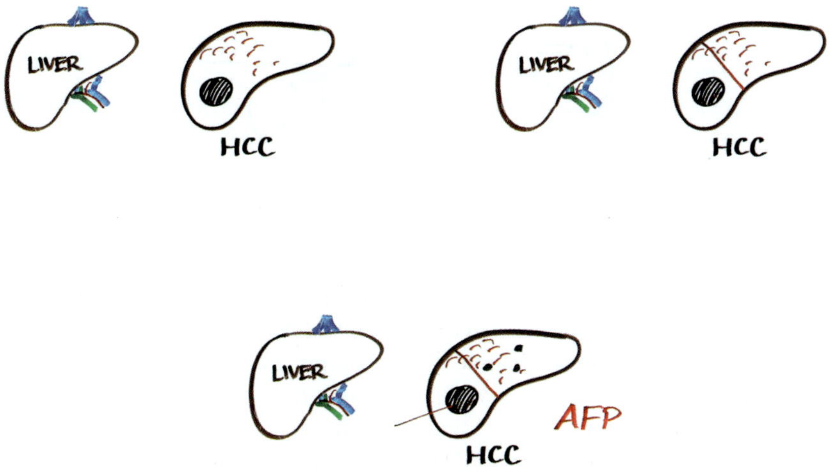

VIDEO 11.2. HCC of the Liver. Mets (in narration) indicates metastases.

Transcript: Hepatocellular carcinoma that is a cancer deriving from the hepatocytes. It's the most common primary type of liver cancer. Metastatic disease to liver is probably the most common cancer in the liver, but HCC is a deadly problem. It is an aggressive tumor and it usually develops from chronic liver disease and cirrhosis; particularly in patients with chronic active hepatitis B and C. So over the course of time the cirrhosis, the fibrotic, the lumps and bumps, change the way these liver hepatocytes grow and replicate. At some point in time, tumors develop, and a larger tumor that can be resected and removed, 50% of those patients do extraordinarily well. The problem is HCC sometimes becomes more than 1 tumor. Maybe it becomes tumors with satellite lesions or other problems. This becomes less likely to cure with an operation. If there is an operation, it is potentially a liver transplant operation.

When we are looking for masses in the liver, one of the things to check for is what is called an alpha-fetoprotein level. It is a marker of hepatocellular cancer. It is not a perfect marker, but if it is elevated it gives us concern.

Oftentimes we can biopsy, CT guidance or ultrasound guidance and get tissue out and diagnosis a hepatocellular cancer. But if given a choice if there is no bony mets or brain mets or lung mets, the number 1 treatment would be surgical resection. The great thing about the liver is you can remove half of it or more if the rest of the liver is normal and patients can do just fine. If you can't remove that liver, then chemotherapy and other agents are possible or consideration for liver transplantation is reasonable.

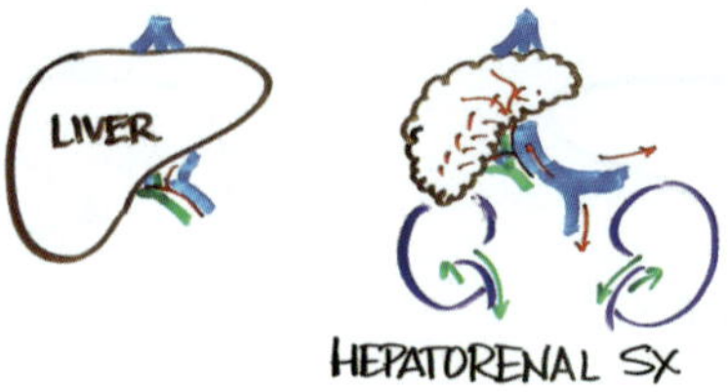

VIDEO 11.3. Hepatorenal Syndrome.
Transcript: Hepatorenal syndrome is a function of bad liver function and it gets so bad that it goes from normal liver to bad/normal liver. At some point in time, the 500 different factors that the liver can do are going to affect your kidneys and decrease the volume of urine output and decrease the function of the kidney.

There are a couple different kinds of hepatorenal syndrome. Type 1 progress rapidly; the kidneys basically shut down and no longer function. Type 2 is not quite so dramatic, but people develop ascites. This is backup of fluid from the liver and then the kidneys don't work, and there is a backup of fluid here as well. So what happens is the liver is the problem. There is nothing wrong with the kidneys, but because the liver is so bad, whether that is from hepatitis, alcoholic hepatitis, cirrhosis, malignancy, or whatever problem, the kidneys begin to fail and when that happens it is called hepatorenal syndrome and it can be a devastating complication.

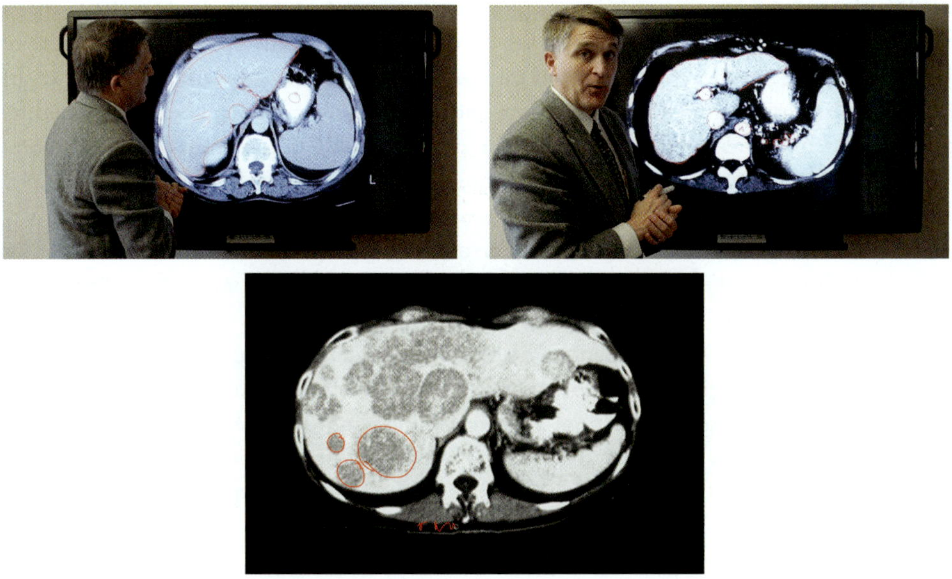

VIDEO 11.4. CT of the Liver.
Transcript: Computed tomography (CT) of the abdomen, especially of the liver, is very accurate and very telling. This is a normal CT scan in a normal patient. It's got some contrast in the stomach and it's maybe got a little bit of dye in the aorta, in the IVC, but this is our liver. It is a good looking liver. It occupies about half of the abdomen here. If there isn't any dye, then the spleen and the liver should be the same density; everything is density here and when you see funny little things like this that is fat density that is a falciform ligament. We are starting to see some blood vessels here as well. This is normal. Let's take a look at something that is not so normal.

VIDEO 11.4. Continued

This is a CT scan and it has a lot of dye in the aorta and the vena cava so it will be bright, and it definitely is, but we can get a sense here that this liver is a little bit bumpy, it's got a little bit of roughness to it. We can see down here, especially. This is a cirrhotic liver, maybe not the worst cirrhotic liver you have seen, but this is a fibrotic liver that sometimes you can get big but eventually is going to get small and it's going to block off the ability to get blood to go through it. The big vessel that goes through the liver is the portal vein—and here it is right here. It is almost the size of the aorta; that is uncommon. This is a big structure and it's getting blocked; and in fact, it is blocked back up so that there are blood vessels back here that are heading back towards the spleen. This is what is called portal hypertension.

Let's take a peek at another CT scan—a different person. Big liver, we can see it, but I am guessing and hoping that you can see bumps on the top. This is a cirrhotic liver as well—very advanced. It is an ugly looking thing and you can see that there is this cut out sort of features, it's not consistent, and it's not homogeneous. This is a liver that is functioning poorly.

Let's take a picture of a different patient with a different liver. You can see some lumps and bumps; unfortunately, these lumps and bumps are inside the liver. These are tumors that are growing. This is potentially a lethal problem. This is metastatic cancer disease. Fortunately for this patient, its carcinoid, it's a neuroendocrine tumor, and some of these people can have these tumors for decades and tolerate that and get along, others can't.

This looks like metastatic disease. Might this be a colorectal cancer or a melanoma? This is an advanced metastatic process that is likely going to kill this person. In fact, you can get a sense they're skinny on the outside, there is not much fat. They are probably losing weight because these tumors are using up all the patient's nutrition.

Another picture—a beautiful CT scan, again with dye in the aorta and the IVC, and here is our portal vein, left branch and right branch. But, the problem is that this should be a homogeneous density and we have got all these tumors here. This is likely somebody that has metastatic disease.

Same sort of thing here, maybe harder to see, but almost the entire right lobe is replaced with tumor. Surgeons can take that out, but the problem for this young person is that there are additional tumor burden and you can't live without a liver.

CT scan is a very effective way to look at the liver.

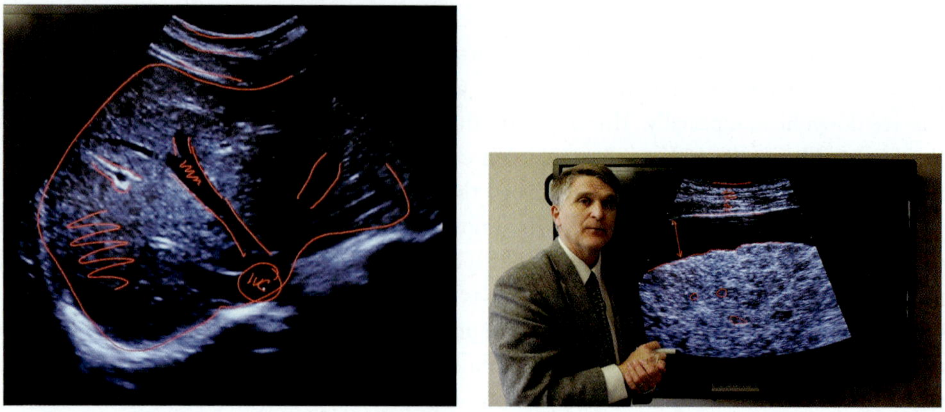

VIDEO 11.5. US of the Liver.

Transcript: Ultrasound is a very effective way of looking at the liver. When I think of the ultrasound, I think of echoes, echogenicity. It's hypoechoic, anechoic, hyperechoic, or isoechoic—the level of echoes. So the probe is sitting up on the skin and we have got abdominal wall, muscle, and now we are into the liver. This is all liver here. What are we looking at? This is sort of normal texture of liver on the side. We are going to see some blood vessels that have basically anechoic, no echoes, they are black—that is this stuff here. If it doesn't have a white barrier around the outside or a border, it's likely the hepatic vein. The hepatic veins run by themselves as opposed to those things that are what is called the portal triad: that is the bile duct, hepatic artery, and the portal vein. You see this whitish business here, this is going to be the portal triad, there are going to be 3 things there. Unlike the hepatic veins that don't have that whitish structure to them. The hepatic veins empty into the inferior vena cava. This is a normal ultrasound of the upper liver; let's take a peek.

Something else, closer down, no echoes here, that is the IVC, a nice differentiation between the liver, maybe the kidney, or the retroperitoneum below, and in the middle here we see lots of normal echoes and then we've got a white border. What does that mean? It is part of the portal triad. So that could be the portal vein, and not likely the hepatic artery or the bile duct, but it's likely the portal vein with other structures next to it. There is that fibrotic rind around it. Anything that doesn't have dense echoes would be the hepatic vein. So, if you are looking to find something that doesn't have any borders that is likely a branch of the hepatic vein.

What does it look like on ultrasound when you have a cirrhotic liver? Let me show you 1 picture. Couple of different things, probe on the skin, fatty muscle, peritoneum. This is the liver and it's a little lumpy, bumpy, it's cirrhotic, it's fibrotic. And, you can see it, it is not isoechoic. It's got some areas with more echoes and some with less. But, importantly for this person, they have a lot of fluid that is called ascites. Basically, the blood cannot get into the liver and a lot of fluid weeps out. So this is what ascites looks like with using an ultrasound.

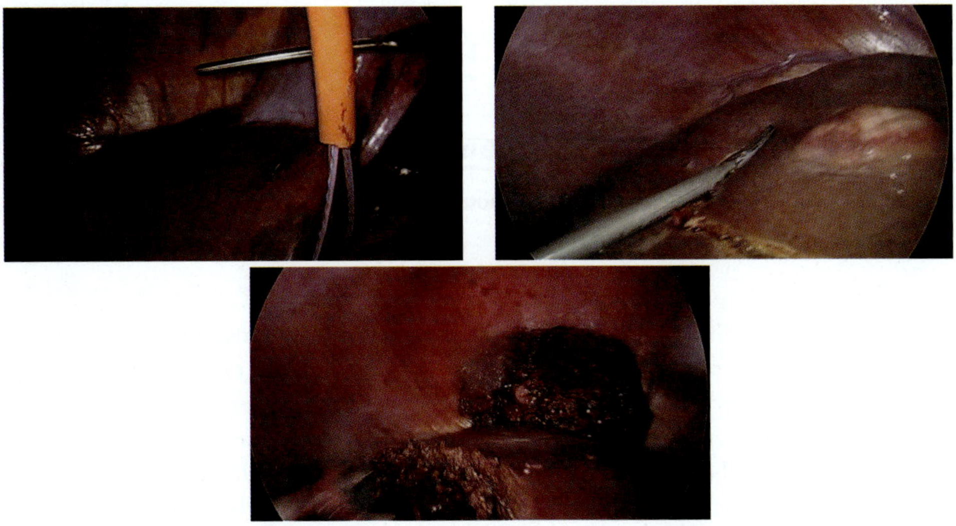

VIDEO 11.6. Laparoscopic Wedge Resection: Intraoperative.
Transcript: We are going to do some laparoscopic liver surgery here. We put the laparoscope in and we are blowing up the abdomen with carbon dioxide and we are putting some 5 mm ports in. We are looking for the patient's right upper quadrant from the belly button. So that is the liver and the gallbladder being dissected. We can see a little bit of stomach and duodenum. What the surgeon is trying to do off the get-go is safely get control of the blood flow into the liver. He is down around what is called the hepatoduodenal ligament. This is basically what is called a Pringle maneuver. We are going into the foramen of Winslow and are just going to pass this vessel loop, a Rummel tourniquet around the portal vein, the hepatic artery, the bile duct, wrapping it up and then have better control because the liver has an amazing blood supply from the portal vein and hepatic artery and you want to control that.

So, now we have got this Rummel tourniquet around that structure and if there is trouble, we can cinch that down and stop bleeding and whether that is done laparoscopically or in an open fashion, at least we have got control. So this is the top of the liver, sort of where the right liver meets the left liver, and the ultrasound is looking to see are there any other metastases or is this a hepatocellular cancer? Ideally, it is just 1 lesion and that is what it is.

The surgical team here now is using a heating element, it is a ligature, it's a harmonic scalpel, it can be the cautery, and it can be the CUSA, a variety of different strategies. The ideal thing is to get at least a centimeter around this bump, because until proven otherwise, this is a cancer. And this is the CUSA device that basically vibrates and spits water in and breaks up the liver and makes it easier to see blood vessels as you divide through. You run into big blood vessels and you need to take a little stapler or some other gadget that takes care of it. But, this little suction device can suck up part of the liver and make it very easy to see and relatively bloodless.

So now we have taken out sort of a tennis-ball–sized mass around this metastasis or primary tumor. Now we are back into the cavity and drying things up. We have got to be nervous about bile leaks and hemostasis. Surgeons take a lot of time with this and it is important that they do. The other thing to be cautious about is that there is a big hole in the liver and with carbon dioxide and pressure you can get what is called an air embolus. Having said that, it is all cleaned up and looks good. And we can put it in a little plastic bag and if the incision is enlarged just a little bit we can usually sneak it out within a 2 or 3 cm incision and out it comes. And the patient can potentially go home perhaps later that day or more likely the next.

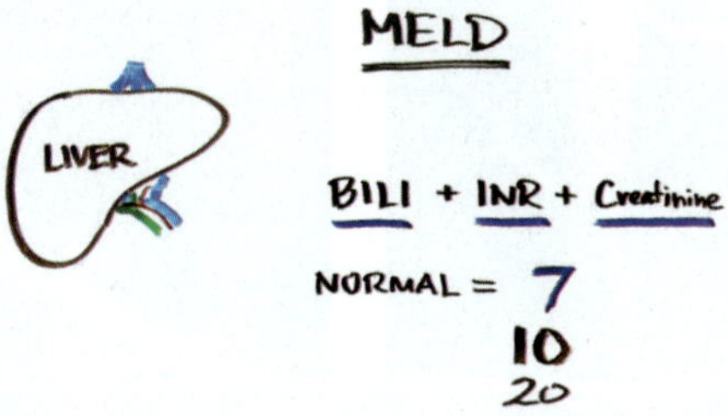

VIDEO 11.7. Model for End-Stage Liver Disease Score. INR indicates international normalized ratio.
Transcript: The MELD score it's what is called the model for end-stage liver disease. Basically, we look at patients with cirrhosis or liver disease and we get a sense from 3 simple numbers; it's a calculation, there is log function and multiplication; but the bottom line is it is the bilirubin level, the patient's INR, and the creatinine level put together. Most patients on the planet that are healthy have a MELD score that is about 7. Patients with chronic liver disease can have a normal score as well, but as they progress over time that number will rise, and it's an important number, such that if it rises to 10, it's somebody that is going to go under an operation and may have a 6% or 10% chance of mortality postoperatively. If the number is 20, the chance of death may be 20% or higher within 3 months of that operation. A MELD score of 30 or 40 has a significant mortality without any surgery. So surgeons especially need to consider the MELD score on patients with chronic liver disease whether they are going to have a hernia fixed, a spleen taken out, or something done to their heart. If the MELD score is above 7, it's abnormal and it puts them at increased risk.

A model for end-stage liver disease, it is a wonderfully simplistic calculation. Find out what your MELD score is and know the risk after surgery.

Liver Challenge Questions

11.1. What is Kasabach-Merritt syndrome?
11.2. What complications are associated with Denver and LeVeen shunts?
11.3. Describe the Pringle maneuver.
11.4. What is the most common cause of a bacterial liver abscess?
11.5. What is vanishing bile duct syndrome?
11.6. What organism is likely to form a liver abscess with "anchovy paste"?
11.7. What type of liver mass can form in females taking over-the-counter prescriptions?
11.8. What medications are used to treat hepatic encephalopathy?
11.9. What laboratory value is thought to correlate (not cause) with the degree of encephalopathy?
11.10. Which clotting factors does the liver create?

Answers to Liver Challenge Questions

11.1. Hemolytic anemia + platelet trapping + loss of fibrinogen in liver hemangiomas.
11.2. Diffuse intravascular coagulation, infection, and catheter malfunction.
11.3. Compression of the hepatoduodenal ligament, including the hepatic artery and portal vein.
11.4. Biliary tract obstruction.
11.5. Chronic liver rejection.
11.6. Amebic.
11.7. Hepatic adenoma.
11.8. Lactulose with or without neomycin.
11.9. Serum ammonia.
11.10. Clotting factors 2, 7, 9, and 10.

12

Pancreas

Embryology

The pancreas forms from the dorsal and ventral endodermal buds, which develop at the foregut-midgut junction. Abnormal development of the pancreas includes pancreatic divisum (Figure 12.1) and annular pancreas (Figure 12.2).

Anatomy

The head of the pancreas (Figure 12.3) lies in the duodenal C-loop, anterior to the IVC and left renal vein. The pancreatic neck is anterior to the SMA (to left) and superior mesenteric vein (to right) (Video 12.1). The uncinate process lies posterior to these vessels. The pancreatic body lies posterior to the stomach; the tail lies in the splenic hilum. Blood is supplied through branches of the celiac artery and SMA (Video 12.2).

Physiology

Islets of Langerhans (Figure 12.4) carry out the endocrine function of the pancreas. Alpha cells secrete glucagon; beta cells, insulin; and delta cells, somatostatin. Pancreatic exocrine secretion (Video 12.3), including cholecystokinin and secretin, is under control of the vagus nerve.

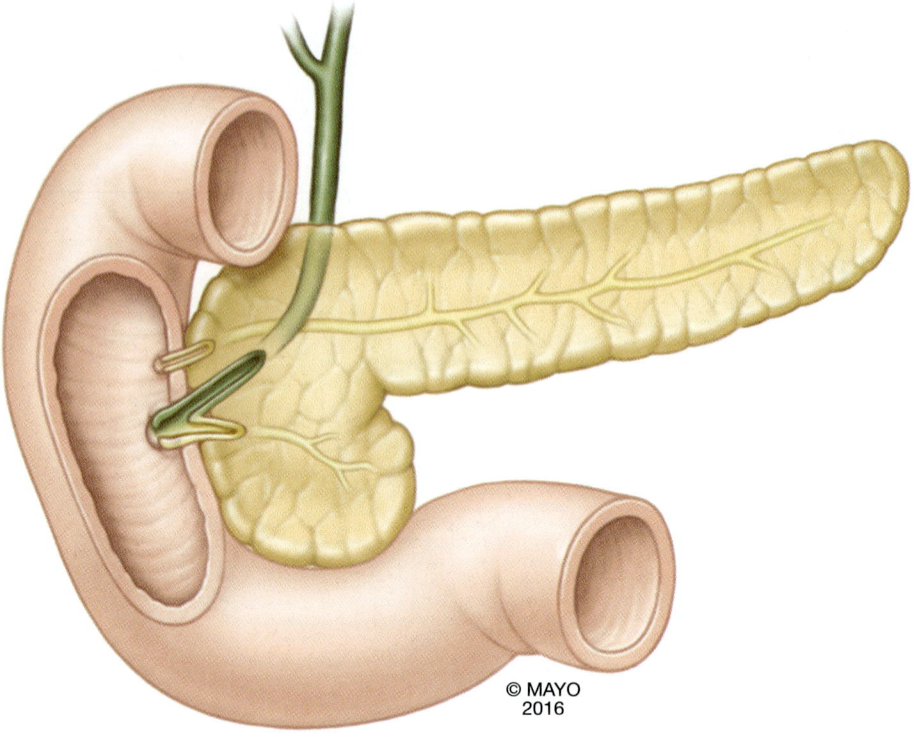

FIGURE 12.1. Pancreatic Divisum.

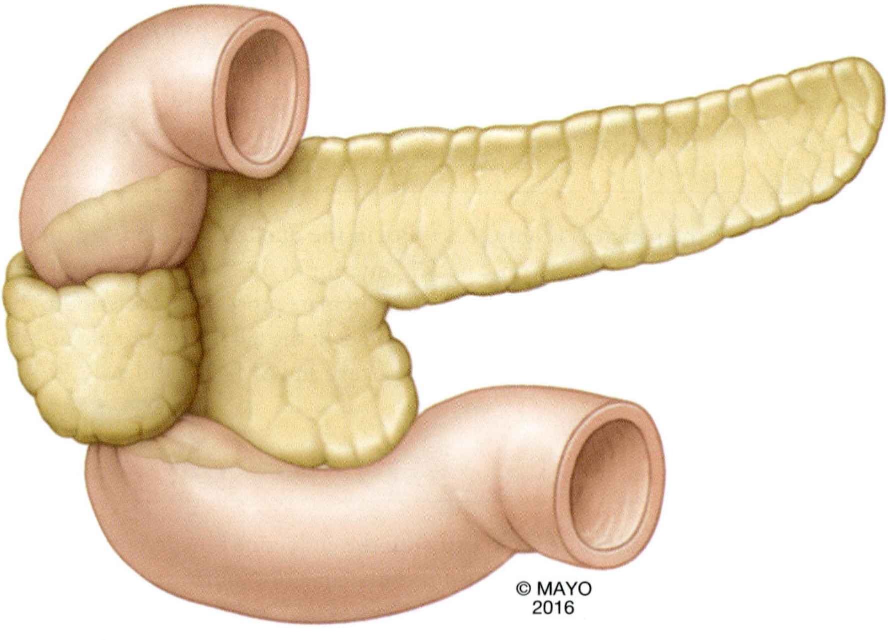

FIGURE 12.2. Annular Pancreas.

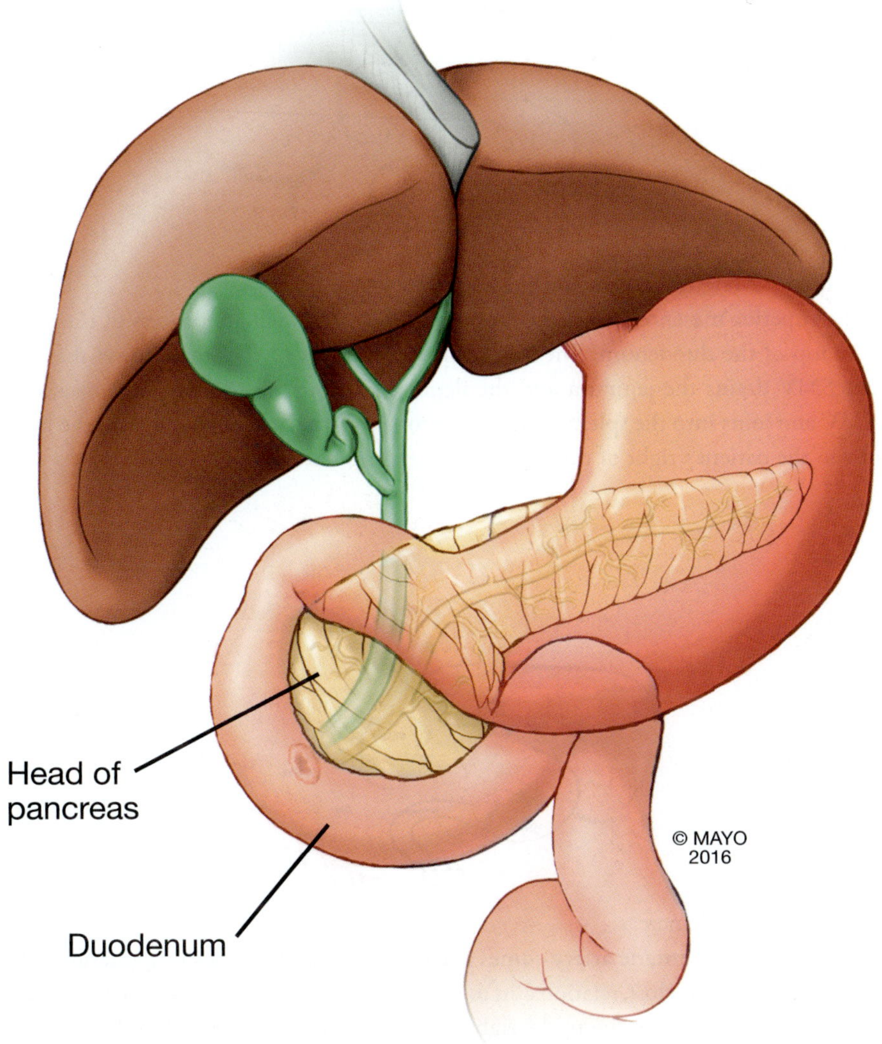

FIGURE 12.3. Anatomy of Pancreas in Duodenal C-Loop.

Clinical Presentation

Acute pancreatitis is caused by gallstones (40%), alcohol (40%), and trauma (15%). Epigastric pain radiating to the back is common; most patients improve with supportive care, but some may become critically ill. Ranson criteria (Video 12.4) are often used by physicians to estimate the risk of mortality in patients with acute pancreatitis. Chronic pancreatitis leads to fibrous replacement of pancreatic parenchyma with endocrine/exocrine dysfunction and pain. Pancreatic cancer (Video 12.5) may be indicated by painless jaundice or Courvoisier sign (Video 12.6).

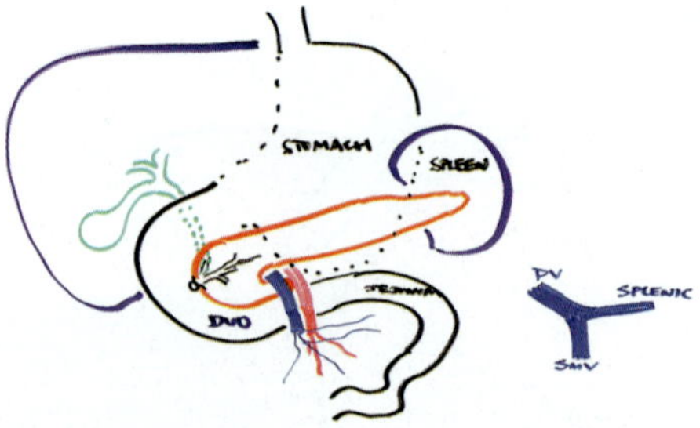

VIDEO 12.1. Superior Mesenteric Vein and the Pancreas.

Transcript: The superior mesenteric vein sits just anterior to the uncinate process of the pancreas. It extends over the top of the duodenum. The duodenum is this part of the small bowel that joins into the jejunum. The SMV drains the jejunum and the ileum and brings all the nutrients back to the liver. It drains the SMV and joins into the splenic vein and becomes the portal vein going into the liver. The SMV is located just to the patient's right of the superior mesenteric artery.

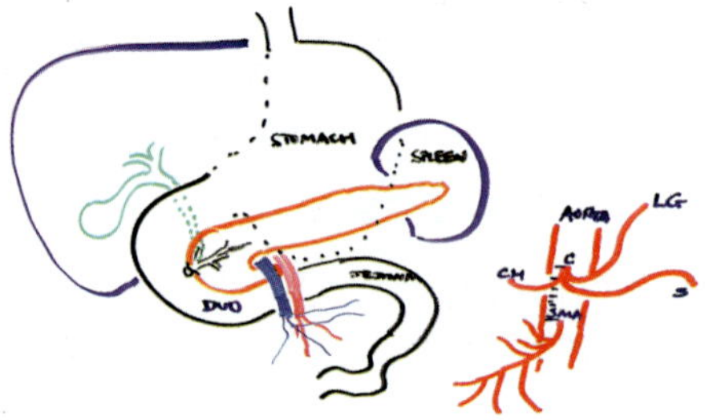

VIDEO 12.2. SMA and the Pancreas.

Transcript: The superior mesenteric artery comes from the aorta and it slides just anterior to the uncinate process of the pancreas. It's in close relationship to the superior mesenteric vein. The blood coming out of the SMA goes to the jejunum, the ileum, the right colon, and the transverse colon. It will also have blood vessels that supply the duodenum and parts of the pancreas.

We look more closely at the aorta. The first branch off the aorta in the abdomen is the celiac artery; it gives off the common hepatic and left gastric and splenic. About 1 cm to 1.5 cm, this distance blown up here, is really no more than 1.5 cm. It is a small space and is tightly all packed in here in the retroperitoneum. The SMA, the first branch comes back to the duodenum and the pancreas; and others come to the middle colic, the right colic, all the way down to the ileocecal valve to the appendicle artery and then the blood supply to the entire small bowel. The SMA is a crucial artery to blood flow within the abdomen.

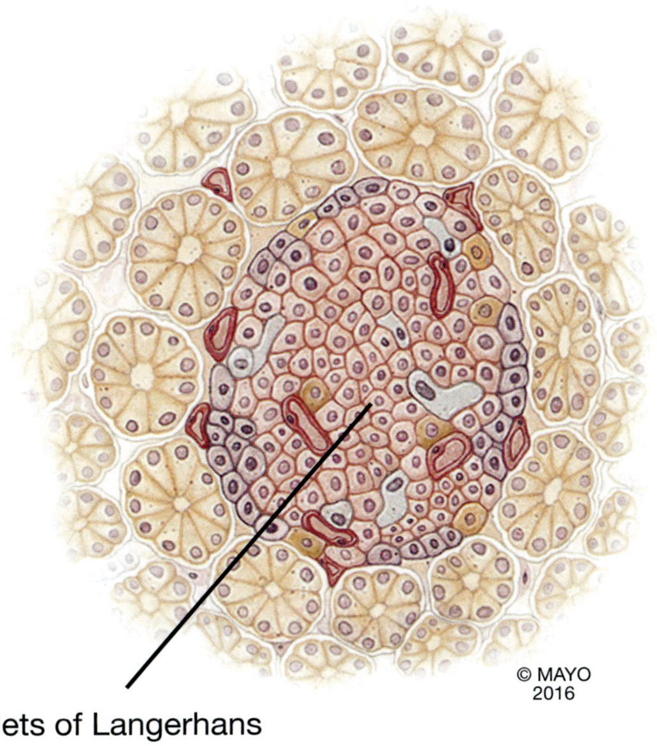

FIGURE 12.4. Islets of Langerhans.

Imaging

CT (Video 12.7) with an IV contrast agent may be used to diagnose pancreatitis (Video 12.8), pancreatic cancer (Video 12.9), or complications (Video 12.10) after pancreatic surgery. ERCP (Video 12.11) and MRI may also be of use.

Operation

Most patients with acute pancreatitis are managed conservatively (Video 12.12). Surgical débridement is indicated for infected pancreatic necrosis and abscesses. A Whipple procedure (Video 12.13) may be indicated for adenocarcinoma of the pancreatic head. Puestow (Video 12.14), Beger (Video 12.15), Partington-Rochelle, Child, or Frey (Video 12.16) procedures are options to treat severe chronic pancreatitis pain. Distal pancreatectomy is shown in Video 12.17.

Complications

Pancreatic leaks occur in approximately 20% of operations on the pancreas. Bleeding, delayed gastric emptying, and infection do occur. Need for long-term total parenteral nutrition is rare.

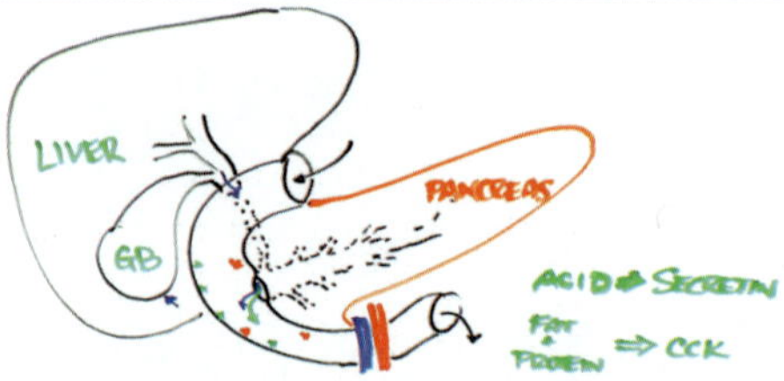

VIDEO 12.3. Pancreatic Exocrine Secretion. CCK indicates cholecystokinin.
Transcript: The pancreas secretes as much as 1 or 2 liters of fluid a day. That fluid will come out of the pancreas into the duodenum to help break down food products. This simplistic drawing of the stomach enters into the duodenum and the duodenum enters into the jejunum.

The pancreas is regulated by the wall of the duodenum. The duodenal wall allows us to make enterokinase which will activate lipase and amylase coming out of the pancreas. The duodenum itself will secrete secretin, which also stimulates the pancreas when there is acid around. So the secretin senses the acid from a stomach, kicks up, and the pancreas puts out secretin which is alkaline. It is a basic solution which helps neutralize the contents of the lumen. When we see fat and protein into the duodenum, CCK will emanate from the wall as well and that will stimulate the gallbladder to secrete and put bile down into the lumen, which will help break down food. It's a complex process—the pancreas is crucially important for digestive break down of foods. If you are missing your pancreas, meaning you have lost the entire thing because of pancreatitis or surgery, you can still take enzymes and break down food products. But, it is a heck of a lot handier to do it this way!

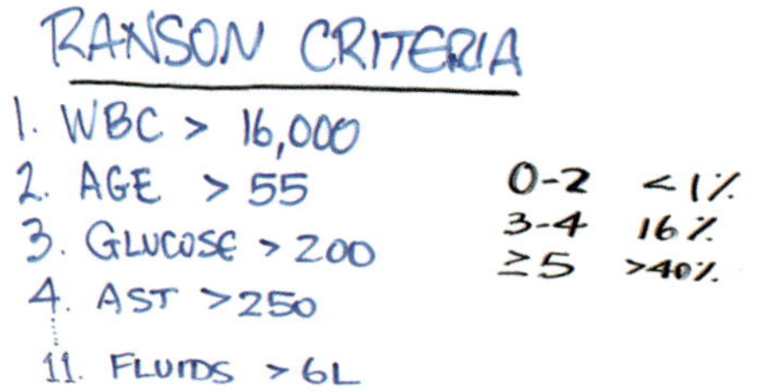

VIDEO 12.4. Ranson Criteria. AST indicates aspartate aminotransferase; WBC, white blood cells.
Transcript: The Ranson criteria were developed some 30 years ago trying to treat and care for patients with acute pancreatitis. And it started out with a few criteria and is now blossomed to 11 such criteria. When a patient comes in through the emergency room with severe acute pancreatitis, they are in great disarray. If their white count is above 16,000, then that is a bad sign. If they are older than 55, that is a problem. If their glucose is >200, their AST is >250, and a variety of other criteria including you need >6 L within 48 hours to make their blood pressure better, they have a serious mortality.

If there are 0 to 2 Ranson criteria, those patients will mostly do well. Less than 1% will die, but again we are talking about mortality here. Three or 4 criteria—16% mortality; ≥5, >40% mortality. So heaven forbid somebody comes in with a white blood count of 20,000, they are 60 years old, and their glucose is 220, and they have got some liver function tests that are abnormal, that patient, that family, and the surgical and medical team taking care of that patient need to understand that this is a serious problem with nearly 50% mortality. The Ranson criteria are very predictive.

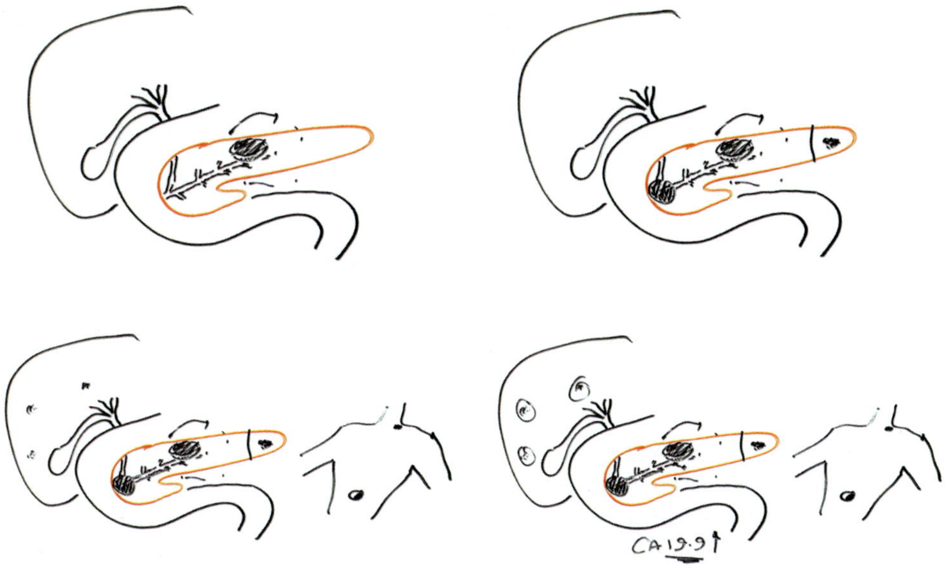

VIDEO 12.5. Pancreatic Cancer.

Transcript: Pancreas cancer is the fifth leading cause of death from cancer in the United States. It usually presents at an advanced stage. If the tumor is located someplace in the body or neck of the pancreas, it rarely causes symptoms until it is extended into nerves and blood vessels and at that point, people have symptoms of weight loss, back pain, they are miserable. They are obviously ill.

Fortunately, some cancers start near the ampulla or near the proximal portion of the head of the gland. If that is the case, then the pancreas backs up and the bile duct backs up and people will have what is called painless jaundice. They become yellow, they become icteric. Liver function tests will be abnormal. If this is caught early a Whipple operation can remove that tumor. Or by serendipity, or luck, or symptoms, small tumors in the tail, they can also be removed. It depends where the tumor starts and how fast it moves along. Most pancreas cancers are adenocarcinomas, they are ductal adenocarcinomas. The lining of the ducts, they bring us the pancreatic juice and they are a lethal problem. Most patients die of their disease. Having said that, if it is caught early and resected, surgical cures are possible. Some folks will come to their doctor losing weight, back pain, they are miserable. They will have liver metastasis. They may have in their abdomen at the umbilicus, a firm little nodule; it's called Sister Mary Joseph sign. That is a metastasis of a lymph node near the umbilicus. They may also have in the neck what is called a Virchow node that means the tumor has gone from the abdomen all the way to the neck. Not likely a curable problem.

Blood tests—can we find pancreas cancer before we can tell it is there? Typically not. One of the markers used is CA19.9; it's a marker that when it is elevated, it's a very bad prognostic factor. Typically there are metastatic deposits. It doesn't show up early with tumors in the pancreas. It is typically something that after you have taken out a tumor, we check patients with their 19.9 levels and follow up to see how well they are doing. If it stays low that is encouraging. If it is rising that means there are likely tumors spreading throughout.

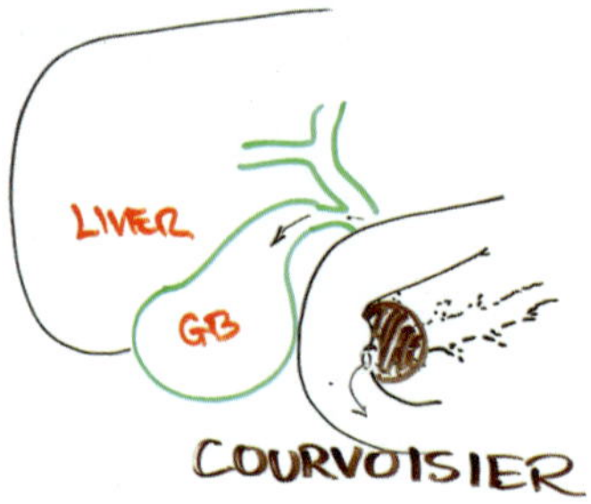

VIDEO 12.6. Courvoisier Sign.
Transcript: Courvoisier sign is an ominous sign. It basically relates to a tumor that blocks the bile duct. And that could be a tumor of the duodenum, it could be a tumor of the pancreas, it could be a tumor of the ampulla, or it could be a tumor of the bile duct itself. So 4 different things can do this and once you block the bile duct, the bile that is normally flowing through now is backing up and it fills up the gallbladder. And Courvoisier sign is no more than a palpable gallbladder on physical exam in someone that is jaundice. So if your grandma or grandpa looks yellow and you feel their abdomen, their upper abdomen and you feel this tight ball that is no longer hidden behind the liver because it is big like a grapefruit, this is Courvoisier sign and it is likely a distended gallbladder due to a mass in the head of the pancreas, the bile duct, ampulla, or duodenum.

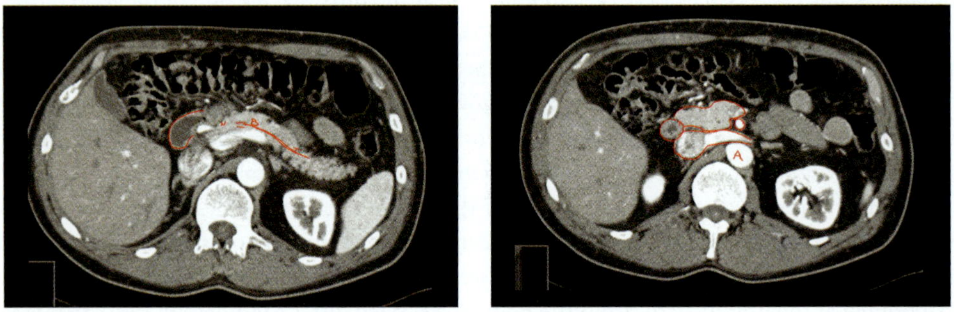

VIDEO 12.7. CT of Normal Pancreas.
Transcript: We have got an axial CT with contrast. The aorta is lit and so is the vena cava so it is mixed up. We see the left kidney and the spleen. The tail of the pancreas comes to the hilum of the spleen. This is a normal looking pancreas. Healthy tissue, maybe a little fatty tissue within it, it's a healthy pancreas all the way through. This little structure right here in the middle would be the pancreatic duct caught on 1 section. If we follow this up and down, we might see this sneak all the way out. Vena cava, this would be the duodenum and this is the neck of the pancreas, body of the pancreas, and the tail of the pancreas. This structure is likely going to be the portal vein. This is a normal CT scan of a pancreas.

This cut of the CT scan is closer toward the feet. We have the duodenum right there. We have the vena cava and the left renal vein. We have the SMA and the aorta. This is normal head of the pancreas with a little part of the pancreatic duct identified. This is a normal bit of pancreas. This is small bowel and this is pancreas. Let's take a look again without all those markers on there, normal pancreas, duodenum with some fluid, IVC with dye, left renal vein, put that in your brain. If you can understand that concept, aorta, left renal vein, SMA, head of the pancreas.

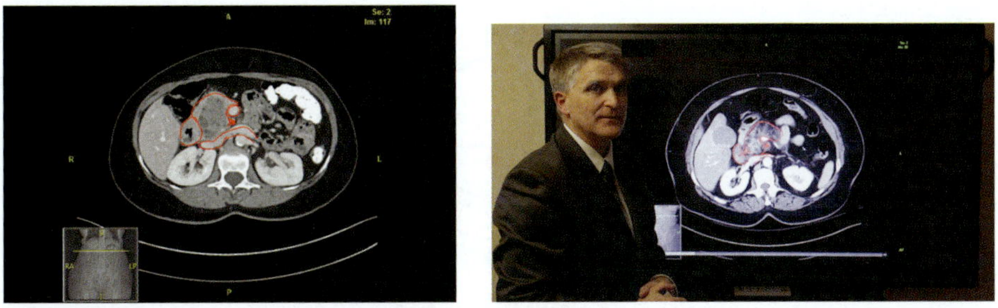

VIDEO 12.8. CTs of Pancreatitis. IPMN, intraductal papillary mucinous neoplasm.
Transcript: So CT scan is probably the best way to find a pancreatic mass. We see a couple of normal kidneys and the liver. The pancreas, the head of the pancreas, sits next to the superior mesenteric vein and the superior mesenteric artery—vein and artery. We have the vena cava underneath, and this is the renal vein going over the top to the left kidney. This structure right here in the middle is a pancreatic mass. This looks like it is kind of a cystic mass and it's important to note that you have the duodenum here and this is pancreas, all pancreas here.

Pancreatic mass, when we think about that, we think about 80% of the time they are cancers, ductal adenocarcinoma that block the bile duct and make people jaundice. A CT scan will show a dense mass. This one is kind of a cystic mass; hopefully, this is benign or what is called IPMN that is resectable for cure.

Another cut: we see the liver and the gallbladder sitting here and this is all pancreas here. It's markedly inflamed and it's probably twice as big as it should be and it's filled with water. This is more normal color down here and this is basically water. It could be a dilated pancreatic duct, but this is a real problem. This gland is inflamed either from gallstone pancreatitis, or from alcohol, or sometimes we get trauma accidents, or other choices are in the hospital we cause problems with drugs or interventions here.

Further toward the feet more caudally or inferior, we can see the superior mesenteric vein, the superior mesenteric artery, and the renal vein. That is a great marker. The left renal vein coming out across the SMA, the artery, and the SMV, and what we should see is a normal gland sort of this density. This is the duodenum here and the ampulla is going to draw in and slide in. The rest of this gland is all inflamed. This person is going to have abdominal pain, swelling, an elevated white count, and this is edema. This is classic pancreatitis.

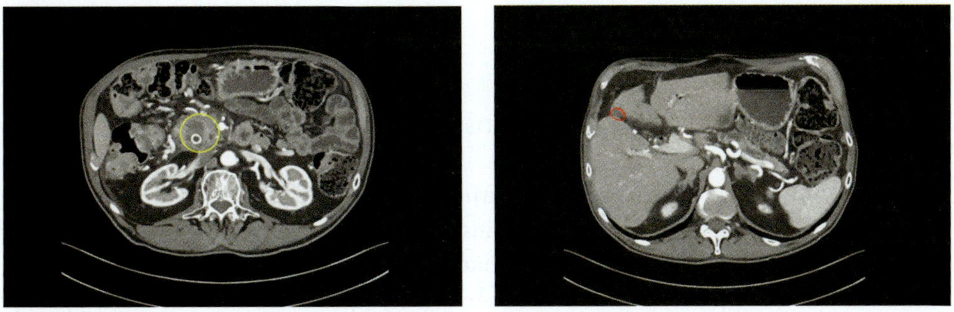

VIDEO 12.9. CT of Pancreatic Cancer.
Transcript: Here is a CT scan of a patient with cancer and an elevated CA19.9 level. Hopefully you are looking in the center and see that biliary stent. The patient is jaundice with a big mass in the head of the pancreas. This is the head of the pancreas with lots of little blood vessels around it being trapped by the cancer. If we go a little bit more cephalad, we see the liver, we don't see any obvious metastases, but perhaps we see a little bit of potential metastatic deposit in the liver. If we look at the pancreas, can you find that there next to the splenic vessels? This pancreatic duct is dilated underneath and that is the entire pancreas body and tail. It's obstructed from that cancer below. This is a CT scan of a bad pancreas cancer.

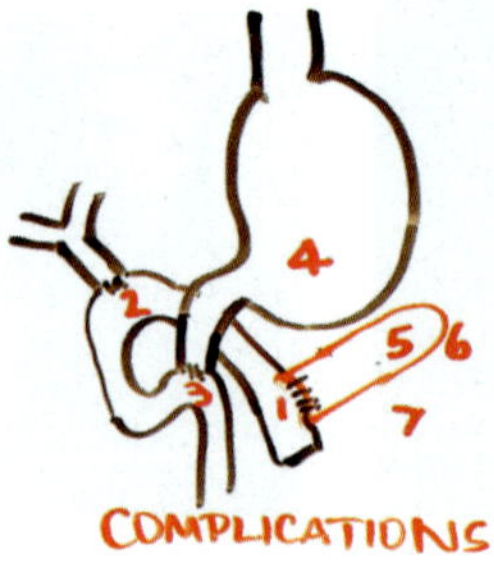

VIDEO 12.10. Complications of Pancreatic Surgery.
Transcript: Following any pancreatic surgery complications do happen. At least 10% to 20% of the time there will be things that go awry. When we think of a Whipple operation, sewing the pancreas to the bowel, the bile duct to the bowel, and the stomach or the duodenum to the bowel, the first thing we should think about is leak, leak, and leak. Those are the first 3 complications of each of those. The most common is the pancreaticojejunostomy. When that material leaks out, again that is amylase and lipase and that can be a digestive problem causing abscess bleeding and whatnot. So our first concern is a leak from the pancreaticojejunostomy. Easier for the hepaticojejunostomy and the small bowel anastomosis because the tissue are stronger, better blood supply, and less likely to leak. But that can happen.

Delayed gastric emptying, the stomach sometimes just doesn't want to work very well after it has been cut up and sewn to. And that can lead to nausea and vomiting and a long NG tube placement. Fortunately, that is relatively uncommon but 2 to 5 people out of a 100 will have that problem after their cure.

When you take part of the pancreas out most people will do just fine but some people have endocrine and some people have exocrine problems. Meaning that some people can be diabetic and their sugars can be out of whack because they have lost the pancreas. Others with exocrine problems won't digest their food materials properly and have terrible steatorrhea or diarrhea. Enzyme pills will help stop that problem. Sepsis or abscess or wound infection among many other things; heart attacks, strokes, pneumonias, can be problematic. So, pancreatic surgery, at least 10% to 20% of people will have complications after the procedure.

Pancreas Challenge Questions

12.1. What are Cullen and Grey Turner signs?
12.2. State causes of acute pancreatitis.
12.3. Why is morphine contraindicated for analgesia in acute pancreatitis?
12.4. What operation is indicated after biliary pancreatitis resolves and why?
12.5. What CT findings are common with chronic pancreatitis?
12.6. How are pancreatic abscesses, infected necrosis, and pseudocysts managed?
12.7. Who was Allen Oldfather Whipple?
12.8. How is a pylorus-preserving pancreatoduodenectomy performed?
12.9. What other organ may be removed with a distal pancreatectomy?

(Answers appear on page 184)

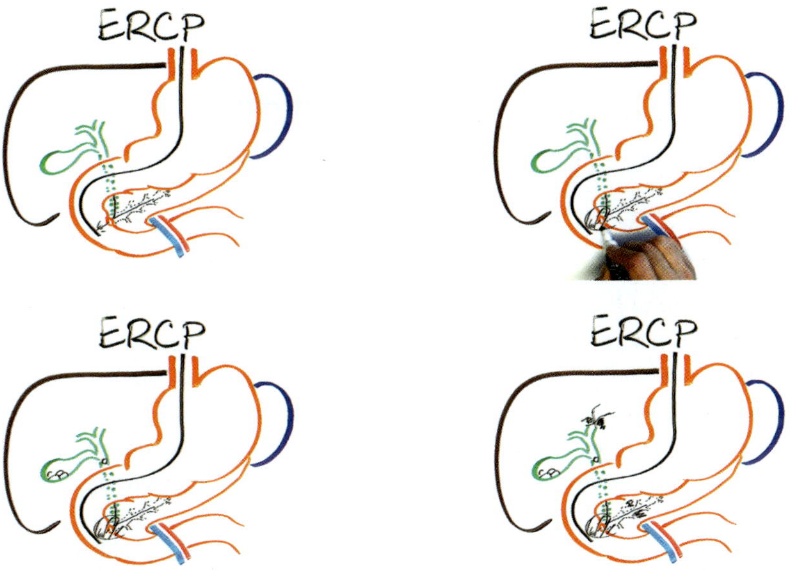

VIDEO 12.11. ERCP.
Transcript: Endoscopic retrograde cholangiopancreatography is basically a tool that uses an endoscope, it sneaks into the stomach and duodenum and it has a side viewing scope to look at the ampulla of Vater and can then take an instrument and either cut that ampulla, put a wire into the pancreatic duct, put a wire or bulb into the common bile duct. And this is done for a variety of reasons. It is a fantastic test. It can cause problems, any time you instrument the ampulla of Vater, an instrument the pancreatic duct, or the bile duct, you can cause pancreatitis which can be severe. Having said that, it is a wonderful tool to assess a variety of different things: 1) it looks for tumors around the periampullary region. You can actually look at it or you can biopsy it. 2) Besides tumors around that region, you can go up the biliary tree. Perhaps somebody has gallstones and maybe a gallstone within the common duct and that can be removed with basket and tools. You can also take a look at the pancreatic duct or the bile duct and inject it with dye and get an image and find out, there is a stricture up high and maybe there is a cholangiocarcinoma or a pancreas cancer downstream. A variety of tools to do this and it is typically done by a gastroenterologist or a surgeon using an endoscope; usually between 1 cm and 1 cm and 4 mm in thickness to slide through the stomach and into the duodenum. People with obstructive jaundice, with gallstones, with trauma, with tumors of the biliary tree and the peripancreatic region, benefit greatly from this.

Complications causing pancreatitis or possible perforation of the bile duct can occur, but are uncommon.

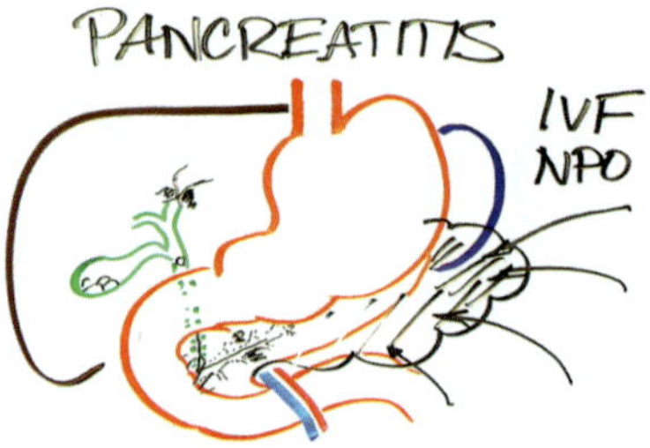

VIDEO 12.12. Management of Pancreatitis.

Transcript: Pancreatitis is exactly that, "-itis" means inflammation, "pancreas" is the gland itself. So for some reason somebody gets pancreatitis: 40% of the time it is related to alcohol, 40% of the time to gallstones that get stuck down here, 15% of the time maybe to trauma or some sort of iatrogenic injury, and then 5% of the time we don't really understand why it happens. But suffice it to say, this pancreas gets big and swollen. Sitting behind the stomach, it becomes massive, edema happens and water is shuttled in. Patients can get deadly sick.

So first things first, if the pancreas gets amazingly inflamed, it's a deadly problem and they need to be in the hospital and invariably need to be in an intensive care unit. Historically, surgeons took people to the operating room; we try to avoid that now. So first and foremost, IV fluid is necessary. Secondly, stop eating; the pancreas likes to secrete hormones, exocrine, and that is problematic. We want to quiet the pancreas down. We would like to put in, usually an NG tube in the stomach to get rid of any sort of fluid in the stomach and then it becomes any sort of things that can help us care for a patient. With fluid into the pancreas and lots of edema, electrolytes can be out of control. Calcium levels can be high and they need to be dropped. Potassium and sodium can be out of whack. So we have got to think about replacing some of these things and we have got to know whether they are high or low. So invariably, people that have pancreatitis need an IV, need blood draws, and sometimes they can be terribly sick and need to be intubated. It's rare that they need a surgical procedure. Now if indeed we find out the cause of the problem is gallstones, then eventually cholecystectomy would be indicated. But if it is related to alcohol consumption, then we need to stop the alcohol intake forever, ideally.

Management for pancreatitis: fortuitously, most people get sick, abdominal pain, and wonder what happened. Some people get really bad sick and show up in the emergency room, a CAT scan shows an inflamed pancreas and these people need IV fluid, they need to be NPO, they need to get their electrolytes taken care of, an NG tube to decompress, quiet down the pancreas. Most people within a few days are better. If not, it can be a long hospitalization.

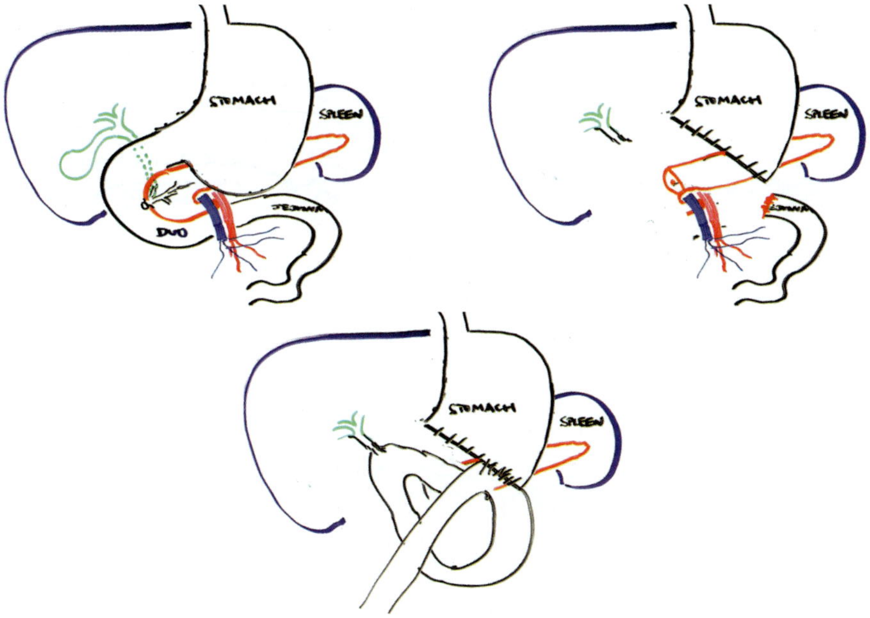

VIDEO 12.13. Whipple Procedure.

Transcript: The Whipple operation is named after Dr Allen Oldfather Whipple, a surgeon in Rochester, New York, that in the 1920s and 1930s developed an operation that dealt with masses in the head of the pancreas or the duodenum. It is a difficult spot to take out. Because if you take out the head of the pancreas, the duodenum, the gallbladder, and part of the bile duct, you have some serious reconstruction ahead of you. And back then when Whipple did this he would take out at least half of the stomach and part of the jejunum. So what happens is you end up with half of the stomach, a little bit of bile duct, and you have a pancreas that has been cut, and we can see a little hole in the pancreas. So now what we do is we have to sew the jejunum, and the stomach, and the bile duct, and the neck of the pancreas back together again. And how do we do that? Artistically it can happen in about a minute, in real life it is going to take about 4 hours to do this operation.

So the first thing is the bowel is sewn to the pancreas, sewn to the bile duct, and then it is sewn to the stomach. Now the problem here is the artwork, this is all going to be hidden then underneath here and this last anastomosis, something like this. So a Whipple operation takes out the head of the pancreas, the duodenum, and a little part of jejunum, part of the bile duct and the gallbladder, and oftentimes part of the stomach. And now to put that back together again you need a pancreaticojejunostomy, a hepaticojejunostomy, and a gastrojejunostomy—that is a Whipple operation.

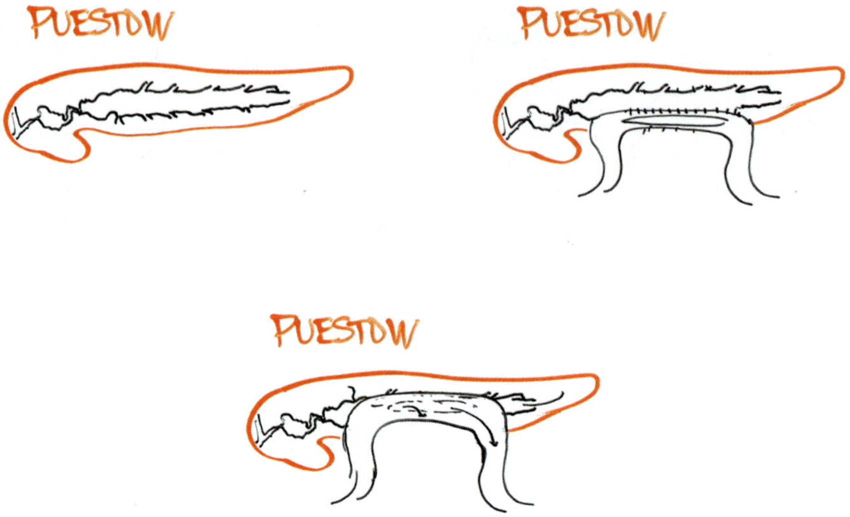

VIDEO 12.14. Puestow Procedure.

Transcript: When patients have chronic pancreatitis, they oftentimes will get a large duct. Sometimes there can be calcifications with it. They can also get stricture and narrowing and you can imagine that this pancreas either from torment of alcoholism over the years or gallstone problems gets blocked and the pancreas can't secrete its juice through here. One way to open that up would be to cut out the head of the pancreas and do what is called a Whipple operation. It tends to be a bit more dangerous.

So surgeons, French surgeons especially, started out and saying let's maybe sew the bowel to this spot of the pancreas. And so what theoretically they do is bring up a loop of bowel and allow this pancreas to be drained so the loop of bowel comes up and now they are going to open this up, and we will see if my drawing can do it justice, they cut a hole in the bowel and they cut a hole in the pancreatic duct and they are going to sew this together and these stitches here will eventually be on this side so it looks like, when we are all done, the bowel will come up and cover this and the pancreas juice from the pancreas here gets to sneak in, come through the hole, there is a hole in this, the connection is so-called anastomosis and we will get it to slide down into the intestine and be useful for digestion. This is what is called a Puestow procedure. Simplistically called a side of the bowel to the side of the pancreas—pancreaticojejunostomy. So a side-to-side pancreaticojejunostomy is the Puestow procedure.

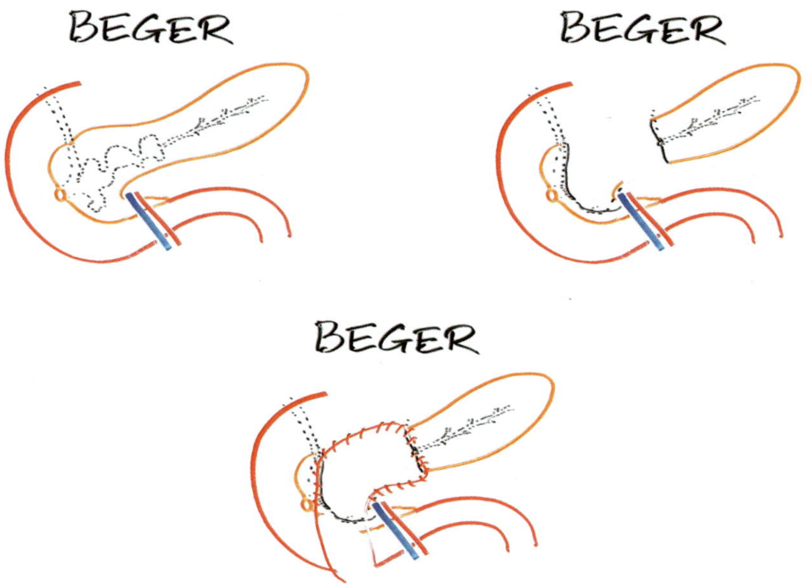

VIDEO 12.15. Beger Procedure.

Transcript: Dr Beger is a German surgeon who gained great fame by coming up with a Beger procedure. It is related to people that have bad pancreatitis, mostly in the head of the pancreas, maybe in the neck as well. Patients with pancreatitis with horrendous pain sometimes get relief if you can break down the obstruction. This fibrotic reaction invariably due to alcoholism, but sometimes to gallbladder disease, one can think about doing an operation short of a Whipple operation which removes the head, the duodenum, and the bile duct. Dr Beger suggested leaving the duodenum in place so people can still eat properly, but thinks about getting rid of virtually the whole head of the gland, but keeps the duodenum intact. So what he opted to do is basically take the neck and the head of the pancreas and core that out, if you will, leave the bile duct behind, and maybe just a thin rim of pancreas and then leave an opening here and bring up a loop of bowel to cover this. So if we went downstream, a loop of bowel over the top is sewn in place.

So the advantages of this operation are it preserves the distal pancreas which is relatively normal, pancreatic juice can come into the intestine and break down the fluid, the food, you keep the ampulla and the bile duct intact, a normal little remnant, a tiny little bit of pancreas is left behind, and that region that causes pain is removed. It is concerning because it can have a leak from any of these spots, but the advantage is you don't destroy the duodenum and people can eat better. And in his study, perhaps 75% of the time, patients felt much better after this and actually got better nutrition and it was a very positive procedure for them.

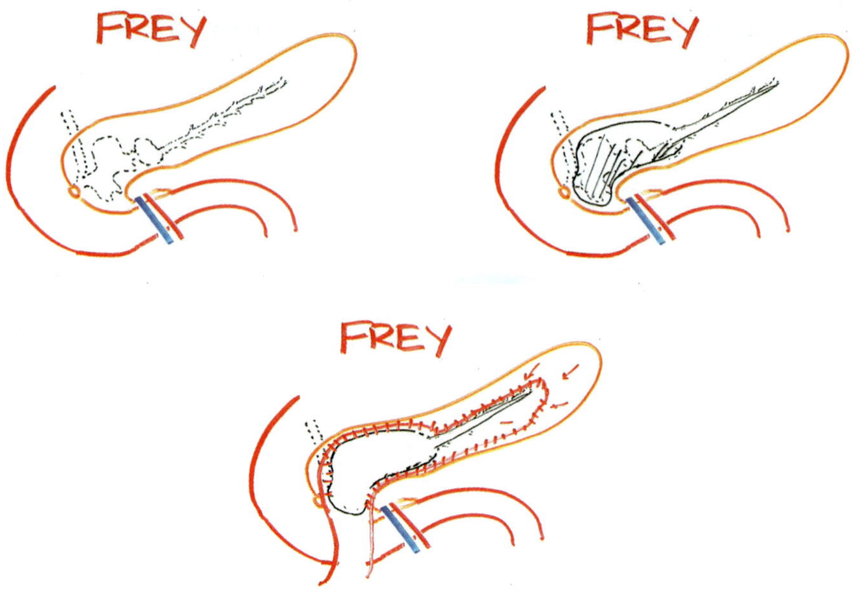

VIDEO 12.16. Frey Procedure.

Transcript: Dr Frey is an American surgeon, and unlike Beger, he decided he didn't like to make an anastomosis to the distal pancreas and then make sure that it doesn't leak from the backside. He decided that that region that was in trouble here, this dilated pancreatic duct with calcifying spots and deposits, he was just going to remove this. Then also open up this duct to make it wide open, which is kind of a Puestow-type procedure, and then because this part of the pancreas is gone and creates a divot, he decided that he would take a piece of bowel just like Dr Beger did and place it on top and sew it to that raw edge. So, this is called the Frey procedure, which is not a whole lot different than the Beger procedure, except that it extends the pancreatic duct opening, and so all this pancreatic juice theoretically shouldn't have any problem getting into this open duct. This is a big cavity where all of the painful obstructions occur with a duct, and he sewed it to the outer rim of this pancreas. And, the nice thing about sewing to the pancreas for pancreatitis is that it's firm and it holds suture well. Again, like Dr Beger, patients typically with alcoholic pancreatitis feel better after this operation, but it too is a big operation. There can be a leak—pancreaticojejunostomy—there can be complications from a big procedure like bleeding. But, all things considered, this is helpful and useful to patients with severe and chronic pancreatitis.

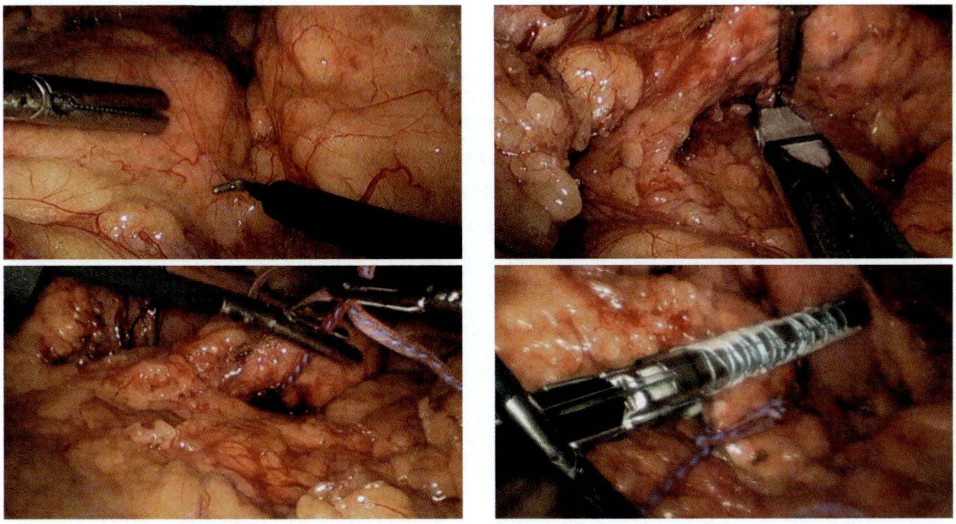

VIDEO 12.17. Distal Pancreatectomy: Intraoperative.

Transcript: This is a laparoscopic distal pancreatectomy. Harmonic scalpel cutting through the fatty tissue, grasper in the left hand. There is the stomach. The surgeon is going to use some tools to retract and get the stomach out of the way, allow it to be held up. A lot of crafty different strategies. Actually tied it up temporarily, when they are done with the operation they will untie that. The stomach can tolerate a stitch without any problem. So the stomach is up toward the diaphragm. You can see the beating heart up there.

We have a variety of different gadgets and can say to ourselves, alright we have got to find the pancreas. This is kind of a fatty person, so we are in the lesser sack, and believe it or not, the pancreas is sitting right there to the left in that fat. It is a little bit of a salmon color. The left hand is grabbing right on top of the pancreas, but doesn't want to grab the whole thing. That is an L-hooked cautery working on the bottom side of the pancreas. This surgeon is pretty gifted, they are quick. They are blasting ahead and there is some fibrofatty tissue on the backside of the pancreas, little bitty blood vessels along the splenic vein. The splenic vein comes out of the spleen. The splenic artery will be back there as well. They are trying to save those blood vessels so the spleen doesn't get divided. It's easier and faster to take the spleen out probably, but it is good to save it for the patient. They will appreciate having the splenic function. So the pancreas is draped over the top, and now we are trying to get underneath all the way around it, and there it is; stomach above and pancreas there. A little string to sneak underneath and it is going to allow us to retract that pancreas anterior toward the abdominal wall. This again is another handle. You don't really want to grab the pancreas. It tends to be crushed easily, you could develop some pancreatitis, and you can crack it, and cause a problem. So it is kind of nice to have one of these things called a Rummel tourniquet and these little strings, if you will, to allow us to hold it up with some traction without hurting it.

So this person likely has a tumor, a lump, and I think you can sense that there is a lump to the right side. Now we are going to use a stapling device and we are going to transect the pancreas and cut it with this stapling device. It has some whitish tissue around it and usually that helps decrease the fistula rate and the bleeding rate; it seals it off. The splenic artery is underneath there, carefully preserve that. The specimen is to the right. The splenic vein is just deep to the splenic artery. The surgeon is trying to aspirate, trying to keep it clean. They are using the harmonic scalpel to divide fibrofatty tissue without dividing that splenic vein. Now we have got to decide, all right, are they actually going to take the splenic vein or are they going to take an artery? And it looks like they decided, this is too difficult, too dangerous; we can't preserve it so therefore we are going to divide the splenic vessels. This is a vascular stapler and it transects the blood vessels. It is important that it does so in a bloodless fashion.

VIDEO 12.17. Continued

Now we can be a little more bold in taking out the pancreas and the spleen, because the blood supply has been taken and it won't be quite so dangerous. You can see as the heater goes in, we can see things flying around in the air, that is normal when you get a hot cautery or a hot tool. A little bit of particulate matter will flow around. A little bleeder on the backside there; we are going to have to take care of that. The surgeon will have to figure it out and say alright; maybe those are short gastric vessels from the stomach toward the spleen. Again, so oftentimes in surgery we are nervous about fatty patients, it's hard to see. Stomach to the left and spleen and pancreas to the right; a little blood vessel going in or out of the splenic tissue. Transected, we've got our specimen in the bag; there it goes very nicely without the spleen. We got just the specimen and hopefully this is a benign lump and the patient will go home in a couple of days.

Answers to Pancreas Challenge Questions

12.1. Periumbilical (Cullen) or flank (Grey Turner) ecchymosis due to underlying pancreatitis.
12.2. Idiopathic, ERCP, sphincteroplasty, virus, bacteria, hypercalcemia, or drugs.
12.3. It contracts the sphincter of Oddi.
12.4. Laparoscopic cholecystectomy to eliminate further gallstone creation.
12.5. Fibrotic scarred pancreas, chain-of-lakes pancreatic duct with calcifications.
12.6. Multimodality efforts ranging from observation, antibiotics, percutaneous drainage, endoscopy, to necrosectomy.
12.7. A surgeon from Rochester, New York, who performed, studied, and wrote about his efforts to relieve jaundice related to malignant peri-ampullary tumors.
12.8. GI continuity reestablished with 1) duodenojejunostomy, 2) hepatojejunostomy, and 3) pancreatojejunostomy.
12.9. The spleen.

13

Parathyroid Glands

Embryology

The parathyroid glands develop from the endoderm: the superior glands from the fourth pharyngeal pouch, and the inferior glands from the third pharyngeal pouch.

Anatomy

Parathyroid glands are usually found on the posterior surface of the thyroid gland. While the superior glands are consistently near the genu of the RLN or within the tracheoesophageal groove, the inferior glands are more varied in location (Video 13.1). The inferior thyroid artery (Figure 13.1) usually provides blood supply to both superior and inferior glands.

Physiology

Chief cells secrete PTH (Video 13.2), which has a half-life of 3 to 6 minutes. Intraoperative assessment of PTH values 10 to 30 minutes after successful parathyroidectomy will show a drop of PTH by at least 50% and transition into the normal PTH range (10-60 IU/dL).

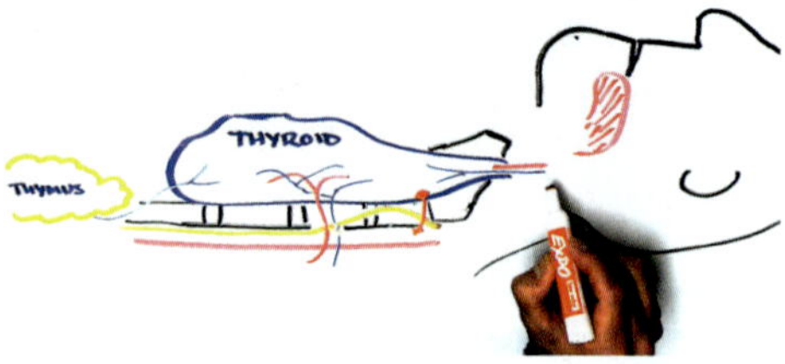

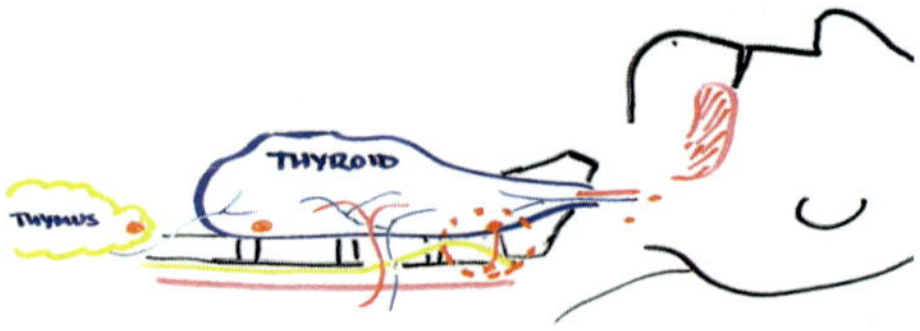

VIDEO 13.1. Location of the Parathyroid Glands.
Transcript: Parathyroid glands come from the pharyngeal pouches and, embryologically, the base of the skull and the back of the tongue in this region. They drift with embryology and the development of the fetus. The superior glands are typically posterior to the line that the recurrent laryngeal nerve draws for us here. So, invariably, they are on the backside of the thyroid gland or they will drop down into what is called the TE groove. This is the trachea, this is the esophagus; a fairly consistent location for superior parathyroid glands.

The inferior parathyroid glands, the third pharyngeal pouches, join the thymus and descend. They can be at the base of the tongue, the base of the skull, or (more likely) on the backside of the thyroid gland, or (commonly) within the thymus. If they go further, they can be in the anterior mediastinum within the chest. So the variability of parathyroid glands—the inferior parathyroid glands—has a significant distance. The superior glands are fairly consistently located on the backside of the thyroid gland.

Clinical Presentation

Primary HPT (Video 13.3) is most often asymptomatic and serendipitously found when the serum calcium value (Video 13.4) is increased on routine testing. Seventy-five percent of patients are postmenopausal women. Symptoms may include fatigue, memory loss, pain (kidney stones), and constipation. Parathyroid cancer (Video 13.5) is rare; it is associated with high calcium levels (>12 mg/dL), and 50% of patients have a palpable mass or vocal cord paralysis.

Imaging

The parathyroid glands can be evaluated with US, CT, MRI, or sestamibi scanning (Video 13.6).

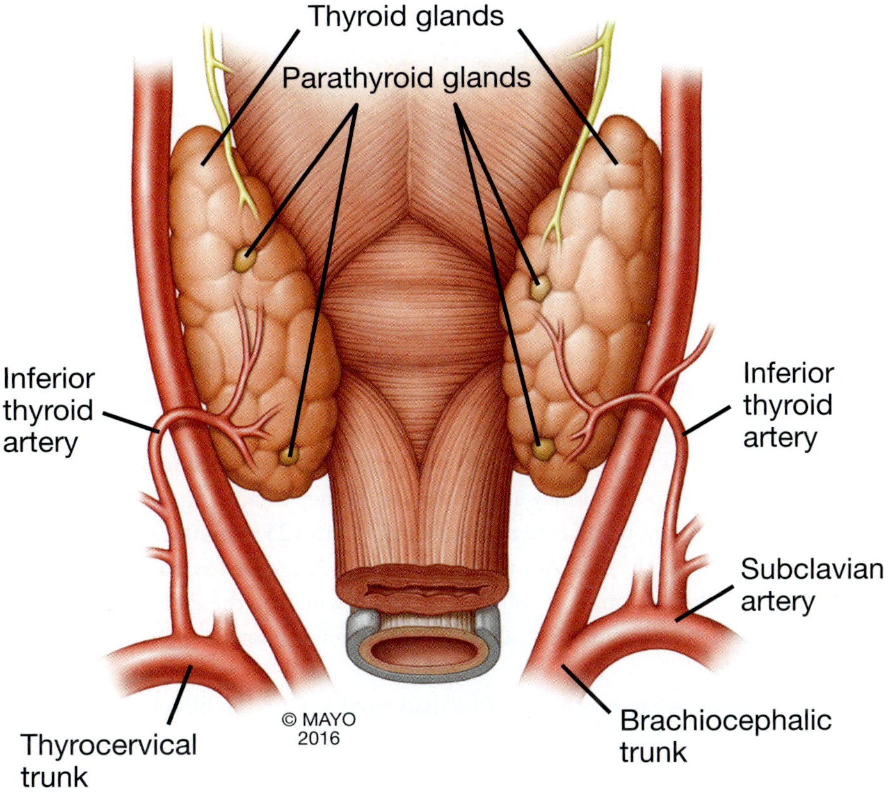

FIGURE 13.1. Anatomy of the Thyroid and Parathyroid Glands.

Operation

Cervical exploration for primary HPT involves resection of a solitary adenoma in approximately 85% of patients. From 10% to 15% of patients require a 3.5-gland resection because of 4-gland hyperplasia. Patients with secondary HPT require a 3.5-gland resection or 4-gland resection with reimplantation of parathyroid tissue to the forearm, pectoralis muscle, or subcutaneous fat. Patients with parathyroid cancer are best served by complete resection of the malignancy and the ipsilateral thyroid lobe and lymph nodes. Video 13.7 shows a right parathyroidectomy.

Complications

Injury to the RLN (Video 13.8) (hoarseness) and superior laryngeal nerve (Figure 13.2) (voice fatigue) does occur. Neck hematomas are uncommon but should be evaluated and treated immediately. Transient postoperative hypocalcemia confirms a curative procedure, but severe hypocalcemia may be caused by the hungry bone syndrome (Video 13.9).

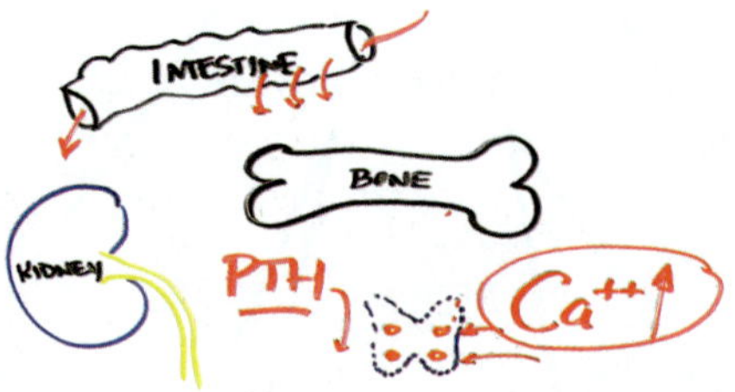

VIDEO 13.2. Function of PTH.

Transcript: Parathyroid hormone, or so-called parathormone, is an 84–amino acid metabolite that allows the parathyroid glands to have amazing influence over the bone, the intestine, and the kidney, and basically increases calcium in the body, in the bloodstream, if you will.

An amazing system! The PTH acts on bone, tells the bone to give up calcium and phosphate and raise the levels in the blood. It goes to the kidney and it tells the kidney to hold on to calcium, don't lose it in the urine. Also, within the kidney, it will convert the vitamin D to 125 vitamin D, which better allows the body to absorb the calcium from the diet. As calcium goes up, the negative feedback affects the parathyroid glands when the calcium is high enough, it will inhibit, and it will drop the PTH and reverse this system.

It is a tightly-regulated system because calcium is such an important metabolite and element in our body.

The parathyroid hormone, what does it do? More than anything it raises bloodstream levels of calcium.

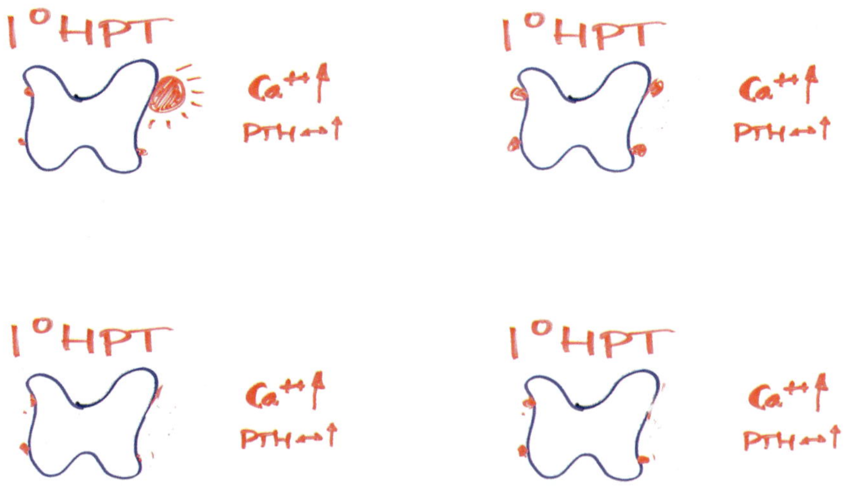

VIDEO 13.3. Primary HPT.

Transcript: Primary hyperparathyroidism is a disorder where calcium levels are elevated and PTH is normal or elevated. Importantly, remember that hypercalcemia coupled with PTH that is either high or normal. When the calcium is high in the bloodstream, the PTH is lower. How does this happen? Typically it happens instead of 4 normal little glands (about 80% to 90% of the time), 1 of the glands get bigger,

VIDEO 13.3. Continued

a so-called parathyroid adenoma. It's not a cancer; it's not a malignancy; and it's a benign growth that secretes PTH. And that PTH tells the bones and the kidneys and the intestines to raise calcium levels, and it does it effectively. No longer is this under negative feedback control, and so the PTH will be either high or normal. In a normal person with calcium high levels, the PTH will be undetectable. So 80% to 90% of the time it's 1 gland getting big. Well 10% to 15% of the time, it's all 4 glands that are a little bigger and more active than they should be. They can be of different sizes, but they are all 4 active and this is called 4-gland hyperplasia. The treatment for this is to remove 3 1/2 glands and leave a small portion behind. The treatment for an adenoma, 1 large gland, is to simply remove that gland and leave the normal 3 remaining glands behind.

This is wonderfully successful operation. It typically most commonly occurs in women, and it is postmenopausal women. Perhaps 1 in 200 women that are postmenopausal have primary hyperparathyroidism. It certainly does occur in men, but it is less common.

The symptoms from high calcium levels—about half the time at least patients have no symptoms whatsoever. Most patients are detected by a simple blood test. But if people do have symptoms, it's the classic stones, bones, moans, groans, and psychiatric overtones. What do we mean by that? Bone pain, because the bones are getting weak and losing calcium; groans from nausea, vomiting, constipation, and pancreatitis; and psychiatric overtones are anxiety and depression. It's a subtle thing, but as things get worse, it's a real problem when calcium levels are high. Primary hyperparathyroidism—common in postmenopausal women.

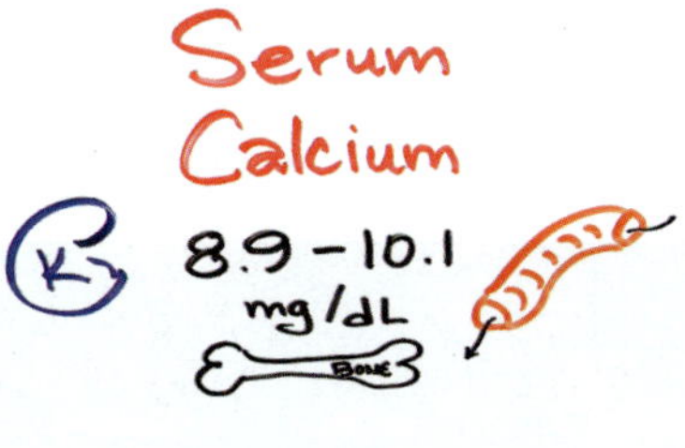

VIDEO 13.4. Serum Calcium.

Transcript: Serum calcium is exquisitely protected in the human body. Values range between 9 and 10 mg/dL. At our own institution, it's 8.9 to 10.1 mg/dL. Ninety-eight plus percent of all people will be tightly regulated. Calcium is a crucial element for cardiac contraction, muscle contraction, and a variety of other different functions within the body.

Regulating this calcium is directly under the control of the parathyroid glands. The parathormone affects the kidney. It creates vitamin D that is active and helps us absorb from the intestine the calcium. It tells the bone to give up calcium. Everything is related to calcium with PTH. But it's a wonderful negative feedback system, as so many things are in endocrinology. So when the calcium level slides up, the parathyroid glands and the chief cells within the parathyroid glands see the calcium is high and immediately shut off the PTH. So if you find yourself with somebody with a calcium on the high side (10.4, 10.5, 11.1), the PTH will be the opposite; the body will correct that and slide this number back into the middle. Negative feedback is crucial, and never more so than with serum calcium regulation.

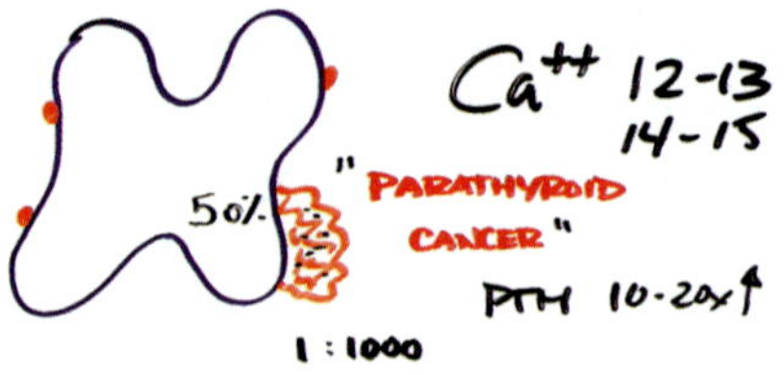

VIDEO 13.5. Parathyroid Cancer.

Transcript: Parathyroid cancer is decidedly uncommon. Of those people with parathyroid problems, less than 1 in 1,000 will likely have parathyroid cancer. Adenoma is the most common. Four-gland hyperplasia is 10%. This (parathyroid cancer) is less than 1%—more likely less than 0.1%.

Parathyroid cancer, how do we know it? Calcium levels will be extraordinarily high. Normal calcium is 9 to 10 mg/dL. People with parathyroid cancer, oftentimes 12, 13, 14, 15, or higher. These are emergent dangerous sort of levels of calcium. Parathyroid cancers—high calcium levels.

PTH levels, normal at our institution 10 to 65 IU. Here double, triple, 10, 20 times or more higher. PTH values extraordinarily high, calcium levels high.

The other thing worrisome about parathyroid cancer is if you meet somebody with a lump in the neck, invariably that is a thyroid nodule. But with parathyroid cancer, 50% of those people will have a palpable nodule and perhaps as many as 50% of them will have recurrent laryngeal nerve injury or dysfunction and they will have a hoarse voice.

So when you meet someone with high calcium, high PTH, heaven forbid a mass, or a voice change, you need to be thinking about parathyroid cancer. It's uncommon, thankfully. Having said that, when we do see it, it is treatable. And for those patients we typically remove that lobe of the thyroid gland, that parathyroid abnormality, and any lymph nodes that may be involved on that side.

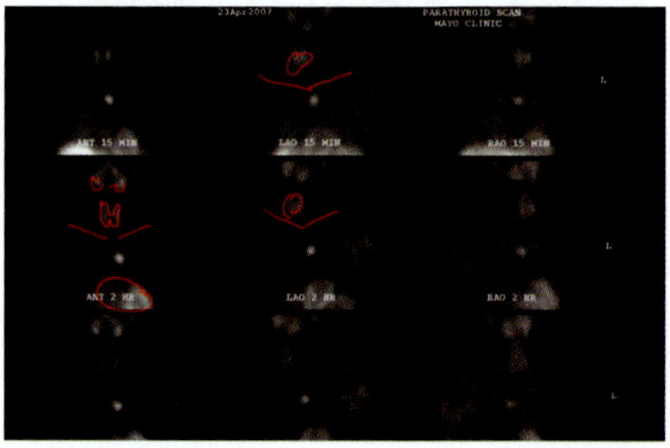

VIDEO 13.6. Sestamibi Scanning.

Transcript: This is a sestamibi scan, its amazing sort of stuff; inject this dye that goes into the blood and swirls around and any place with good blood flow lights up, including the heart and the thyroid glands.

We have got 9 pictures up here. It is a young woman and they have an anterior picture at 15 minutes and 2 hours, and several hours later of seeing what is happening. That is an anterior view, left anterioral oblique, so coming in from the side a little bit, and right anterioral oblique. It allows the radiologist to tell us where the abnormalities are.

VIDEO 13.6. Continued

I think you can see thyroid gland here in the neck. The collarbones are below that thyroid gland. And I am going to focus on this picture here because we have got a nice picture of the thyroid, sort of a butterfly shape, if you will; we have got submandibular glands above. We don't see much blood flow to the bones here but what we do see is the heart below and some sort of an abnormality in the mediastinum. The question is, is it the anterior mediastinum or the posterior mediastinum?

Now this is a sestamibi scan looking at a young woman with high calcium levels. This is primary hyperparathyroidism. So most times everything is in the neck, but maybe 1% of the time you get an ectopic gland and that is likely in the anterior mediastinum within the thymus. Unfortunately, the story is not exactly true for this young woman, she actually went to the operating room where her surgeons took out 3 1/2 glands and couldn't find an abnormality. And now after surgery is done, this lights up bright. She had those glands taken out erroneously. This is the culprit, we need to go into the chest and take that out and she will be cured.

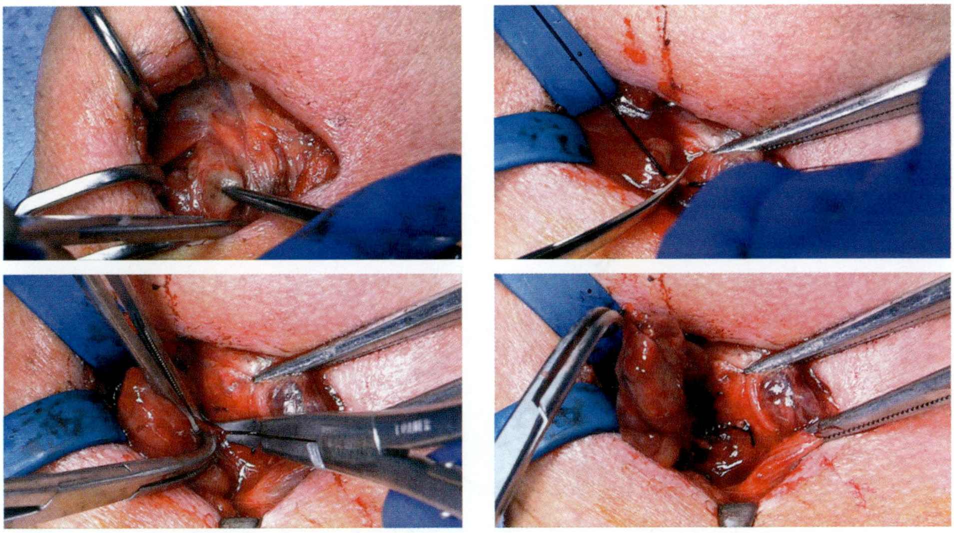

VIDEO 13.7. Right Parathyroidectomy: Intraoperative.

Transcript: Parathyroidectomy is oftentimes an easy procedure unless you can't find the doggone abnormality. You make a little curvilinear incision on the top of neck, maybe 2 cm above the sternal notch, usually in a skin crease. This incision looks like it is 3 or 4 cm in length. We have to divide through the platysma; you will usually see that by seeing the muscle contract. The key thing about the platysma is the anterior jugular veins are just deep to them, 2 on either side. Once we get through the skin and the fatty tissue and the platysma, then we have got to find the midline, we have to get in-between the strap muscles in what is called the median raphe, it's a bloodless plain and here it is. The surgeon is sneaking through, it's a young surgeon. We are trying to get through and we've got to see thyroid below us. We see the strap muscle that is the sternohyoid to the left. And we are working on the patient's right side and we are looking from below. Muscle above, thyroid vessel just below—got to be careful with that cautery. Sometimes turn it off and just paddle it. That's it, nice! Kocher clamp is on the thyroid gland now, there are 2 of them and we are rotating it medial. And we have got a funny little structure hanging off the back side of the thyroid. And it looks like a lima bean, if you will. It is to the left side underneath a little bit of bloody tissue. We have got a little vessel that we took, ligate in continuity with little 3-O silk sutures. We have

VIDEO 13.7. Continued

got funny little blood vessels going in and typically, the parathyroid gland has an artery and a vein. And once you can get those cut, usually, you can just sort of pull this business out. You have got to be careful; you don't want to tear the parathyroid gland. Those cells can live and grow and then you have a problem.

This person has primary hyperparathyroidism. High calcium levels and inappropriately high PTH levels.

The structure to the left is a parathyroid adenoma. That is a little vessel being clipped and we should be able to divide that vein and then this gland will be able to come out. A little right angle clamp holding things to the side. And most times there is very few vessels coming off the backside of the thyroid gland. We can see clearly here 1 small little vessel and hopefully this will do it. Maybe something else. Be careful with that cautery. Deep to the gland will likely be the recurrent laryngeal nerve and you don't want to hurt that. A light touch with the buzzer, be careful that you don't touch the metal. If the metal is touching something bad, that is a problem. Like so many parathyroid adenomas, it keeps getting bigger. The more we dissect, it keeps coming out. Instead of being a little lima bean it maybe is half of a golf ball or more. This 1 weighed almost a 1,000 mg. A normal gland weighs 35 mg.

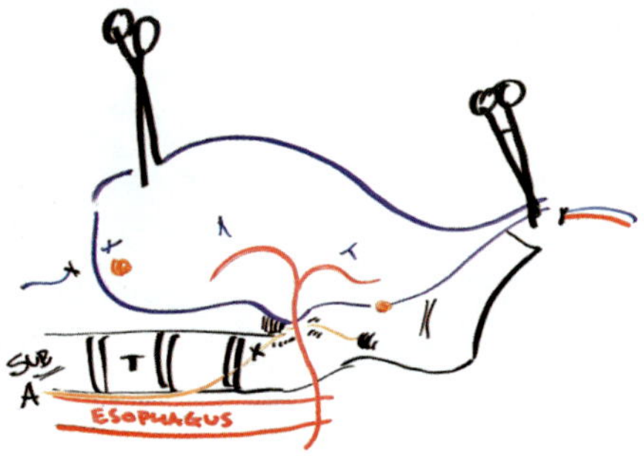

VIDEO 13.8. RLN.

Transcript: This is a side drawing. I am thinking that this is a drawing with the head here and the body here. This is the upper pole of the thyroid gland. The thyroid is being rotated off the esophagus and the trachea. The inferior thyroid artery sneaks up, supplies blood to both parathyroid glands. The trachea underneath, just posterior, the so-called ligament of Berry, and the tubercle of Zuckerkandl, the little bump where the genu of the recurrent laryngeal nerve, the little curve, curves together. The recurrent laryngeal nerve lies within the tracheoesophageal groove. On the left side, it wraps around the aorta. On the right side, it's the subclavian artery. We don't want to hurt this nerve because it innervates all the intrinsic muscles except the cricothyroid muscle within the larynx. It is key to voice control. If you knock out 1 nerve on 1 side, you will end up with a hoarse voice. If you knock out both nerves, on either side, you will end up with obstruction or wide open for aspiration. We just can't afford that. So we want to preserve this. We find it in the TE groove and it sneaks along the trachea and it curves into the laryngeal musculature to innervate the vocal cords that lie underneath the thyroid cartilage. There is 1 on each side. One percent of people will have a nonrecurrent laryngeal nerve that is typically on the right side where it doesn't wrap around the subclavian, it just goes straight into the larynx.

VIDEO 13.8. Continued

About 1% to 2% of all thyroid operations end up in an injury somehow. Either a permanent injury because of a thermal burn or cutting the nerve, or a transient injury, so-called neuropraxia. And if we push on this thyroid hard enough and we stretch that nerve, it may not work for several months and this happens from time-to-time.

Take-home messages: the recurrent laryngeal nerve lies within the TE groove (tracheoesophageal groove), it bumps up against the tubercle of Zuckerkandl, and makes a curve the genu of the nerve, and it innervates the vocal cords. The inferior thyroid artery typically lies anterior to it, but sometimes the artery can be posterior. Find the artery; find the tubercle of Zuckerkandl, the ligament of Berry, and that is where the recurrent laryngeal nerve will be.

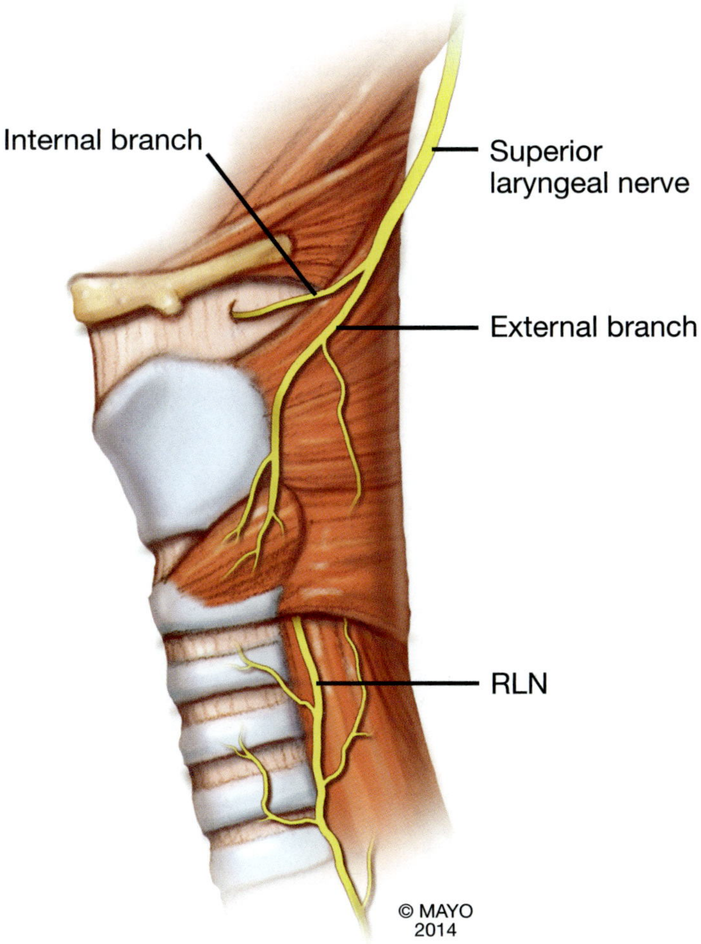

FIGURE 13.2. Location of RLN and Superior Laryngeal Nerve.

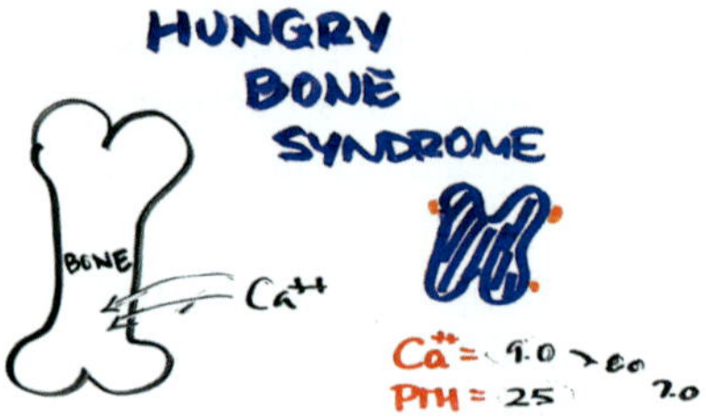

VIDEO 13.9. Hungry Bone Syndrome.

Transcript: The hungry bone syndrome is rather uncommon, but frequently can happen in elderly women that have high calcium levels, high PTHs, and have been living with a parathyroid adenoma unbeknownst to them for a long, long time. The PTH from the adenoma tells that bone to give up calcium and give up phosphate. It tells the kidney to produce vitamin D better and absorb and make calcium higher. You can imagine that if an elderly woman undergoes a parathyroidectomy, and instead of now having calcium of 12, it now becomes 9.0 and her PTH is now normal at perhaps 25, she has had years where these bones have been giving up calcium. And the negative feedback is gone and so instead of giving up calcium, this elderly woman will actually try to help make her bones stronger. So, calcium, even after the operation is done, will be absorbed by the bone and try to create better function of the bones. And this calcium might plummet. It might go to 8, it might go to 7. And some people get tingling around the mouth, the fingertips, and the toes. Usually oral calcium will remediate that. But, there are some people that can get tetany and that is where the muscles lock up and it's a miserable state and it's dangerous. As calcium drops lower, people can have cardiac problems.

So when you hear the word hungry bone syndrome it's likely an elderly person that has had high calcium levels and high PTHs for a long time and their bones are finally willing to fight back. And not only does the surgeon correct the calcium, but now their body overcorrects, and now you have hypocalcemia with symptoms, and laboratory studies will show you low calcium levels.

Parathyroid Gland Challenge Questions

13.1. What is the half-life of PTH?
13.2. Who was Captain Martell?
13.3. Where are adenomas usually hiding?
13.4. What is benign familial hypocalciuric hypercalcemia?
13.5. Who gets primary HPT?
13.6. What does a normal parathyroid gland look like?
13.7. What are secondary HPT and tertiary HPT?
13.8. When might the superior parathyroid gland reside inferior to the inferior parathyroid gland?

Answers to Parathyroid Gland Challenge Questions

13.1. PTH is an 84–amino acid peptide that is broken down in most humans within 3 to 6 minutes.

13.2. An American sea captain in the 1910s requiring multiple neck explorations for persistent primary HPT.

13.3. Deep to the thyroid gland, but they can be found throughout the neck or chest. Failure of the inferior parathyroids to migrate normally, or separate from the thymus, gives rise to most variances in anatomy (eg, base of tongue or skull, intrathyroidal, carotid sheath, thymus).

13.4. An autosomal dominant condition in which affected family members often have mild hypercalcemia and normal PTH levels. Parathyroidectomy is not useful.

13.5. Mostly women (75%), but people of all ages can have this benign disorder. Children may have primary HPT, sometimes as an early feature of MEN-1 or MEN-2.

13.6. The tongue of a jaundiced hummingbird: A tannish, orange, yellowish 35-mg soft bit of tissue, roughly the size of a grain of rice.

13.7. Secondary HPT usually develops with renal failure. Calcium levels lower, but PTH levels rise. Sometimes 3.5-gland parathyroidectomy is useful when calcium metabolism is dysfunctional. Tertiary HPT is usually the development of primary HPT after years of secondary HPT (due to renal failure) and a successful kidney transplant.

13.8. When it is located within the tracheoesophageal groove.

14

Rectum

Embryology

The rectum develops from endoderm, emerging from the distal tip of the hindgut (cloaca). The dentate line (Figure 14.1) marks the transition of endoderm into ectoderm in the anal canal.

Anatomy

The rectum measures 12 to 15 cm (rectosigmoid junction to anal canal). The upper one-third of the rectum is mostly intraperitoneal, and the distal one-third is extraperitoneal. Three distinct mucosal folds (Houston valves) (Figure 14.1) separate the lower, middle, and upper thirds. Posteriorly, the mesorectum (Figure 14.2) is invested by the fascia propria. The rectum is perfused by the 3 rectal arteries (Figure 14.1): superior (branch of IMA), middle (from internal iliac artery), and inferior (internal pudendal). There is extensive collateral circulation. Hemorrhoidal tissue (Figure 14.1) is located in the anal canal.

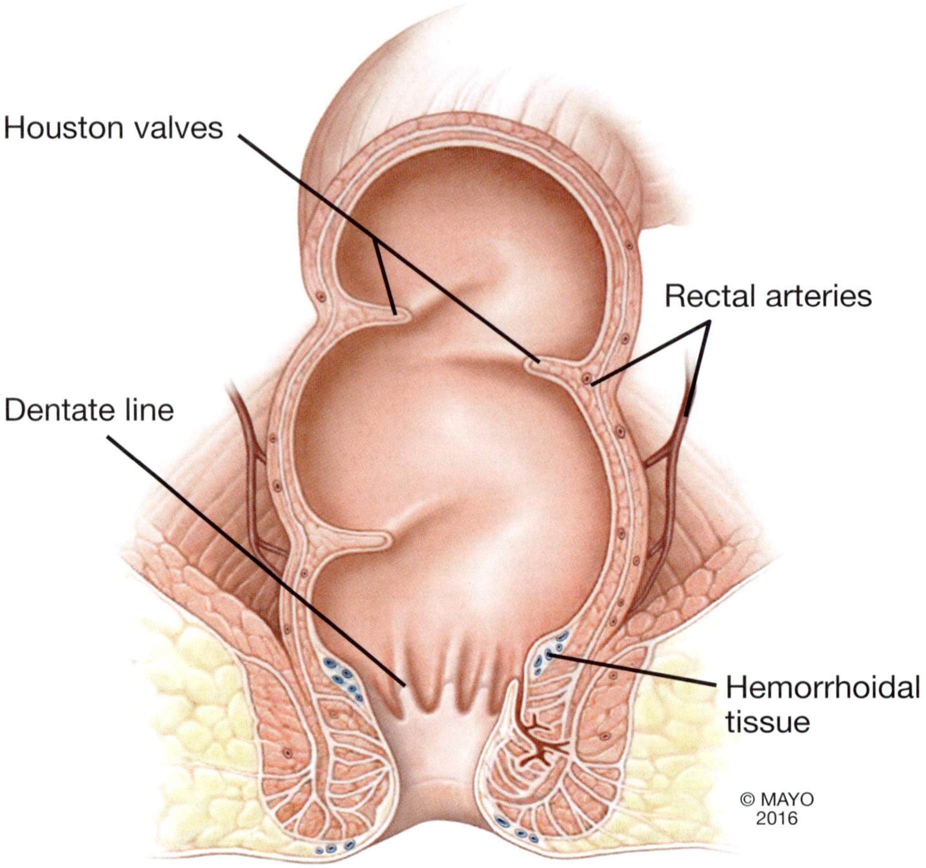

FIGURE 14.1. Anatomy of Rectum.

Physiology

Resting rectal pressure is approximately 10 mm Hg. During defecation, Valsalva pressure increases rectal pressure and causes relaxation of the external anal sphincter to result in expulsion of stool. Chronic straining with defecation may lead to engorged hemorrhoidal tissue.

Clinical Presentation

Internal hemorrhoids (Video 14.1) cause painless bright-red bleeding. External hemorrhoids become painful acute intravascular thrombi. Rectal cancers may present with bleeding, tenesmus, or a change in stool caliber. Most perianal abscesses can be drained with the patient under local anesthesia.

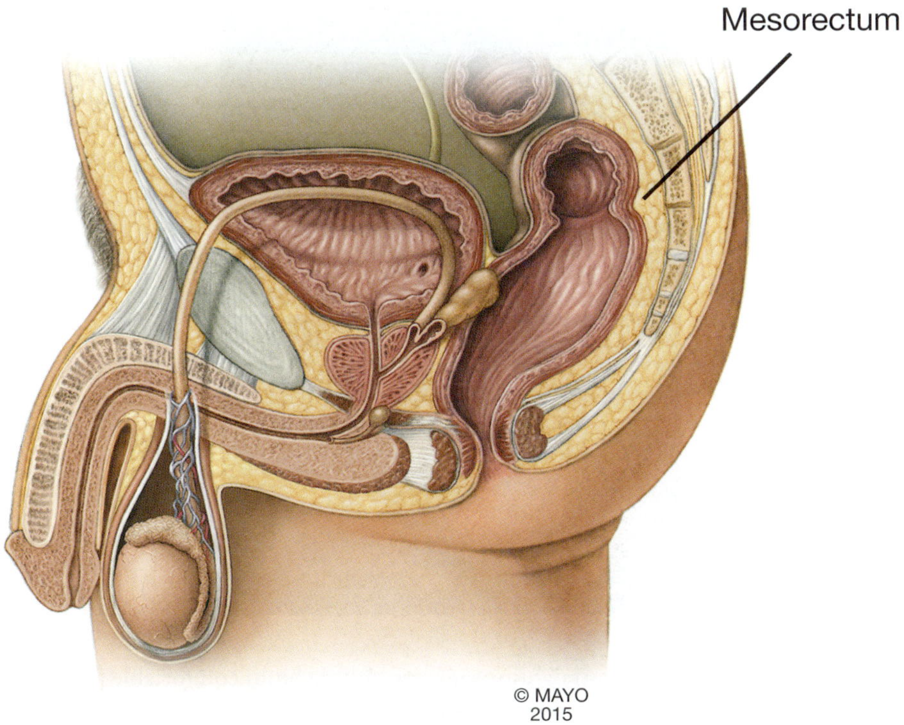

FIGURE 14.2. Location of Mesorectum.

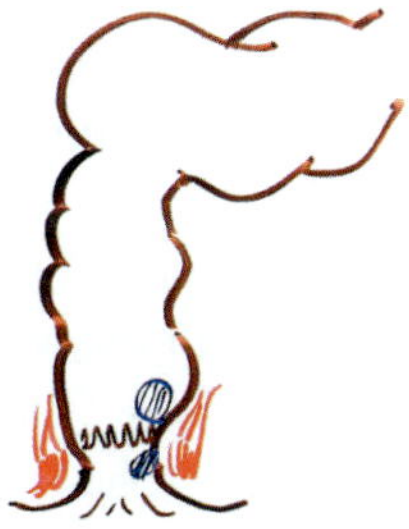

VIDEO 14.1. External and Internal Hemorrhoids.

Transcript: So this is the anus, rectum, sigmoid colon, muscles, and making a sphincter at the anus. This is what is called the dentate line. It is the difference between ectoderm that is innervated and endoderm which is not innervated for pain fibers. So if you have an external hemorrhoid, a little blood clot and some funny tissue that is below that dentate line, it is exquisitely painful. Whereas you can have a bulge above that, an internal hemorrhoid that has no pain fibers and it doesn't hurt at all. And we can see patients with these 2 structures.

External hemorrhoids, they will present with pain and sometimes bleeding when they go to the bathroom or wipe their bottom.

Internal hemorrhoids, not painful but there can be blood per rectum. It's an important difference between ectoderm, endoderm, and the dentate line between them.

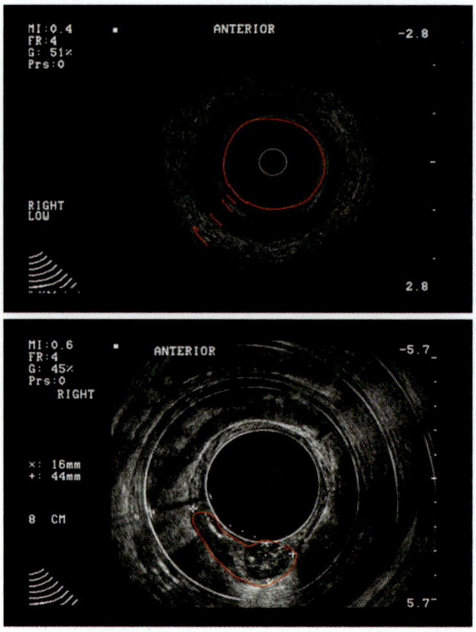

VIDEO 14.2. Endorectal US.

Transcript: Endorectal ultrasound is a straightforward test. A little bit uncomfortable for the patient, but the nice thing about this test is that it is dynamic. You can look up and down and look at what is inside the walls of the rectum. It is not terribly expensive. It has no radiation as opposed to other imaging. So this is an endorectal ultrasound and the probe is in the rectum. Anterior is above, so in a man the prostate gland might be there, or the bladder in a woman, depending on what level. And then each of the layers outside becomes a defined tissue category: mucosa, submucosa, muscularis, and the fat on the outside. And the important thing is we must have found something on a digital rectal exam or colonoscopy or whatnot—so we are looking at the rectum.

Let me show you an abnormal endorectal ultrasound. Again the key thing here is normal, is concentric circles, they should all be sort of the same width all the way around. But we can see something that is abnormal down here posteriorly. This is anterior above. They measure it for us. It is 1.6 cm in depth by 4.4 cm. This is a potential cancer, and importantly it has a depth to it of 1.6 cm. That may be a cancer that is advanced through the mucosa, through the submucosa, and the muscularis. And it may be into the lymph nodes. And we can move this probe up and down to find out might there be a lymph node back here and might we even be able to biopsy it?

Endorectal ultrasound is a very useful test for rectal pathology.

Imaging

Surgeons evaluate the rectum mainly by performing a digital rectal examination, anoscopy, endorectal US (Video 14.2), and MRI to determine the extent of disease. CT is used to evaluate distant disease.

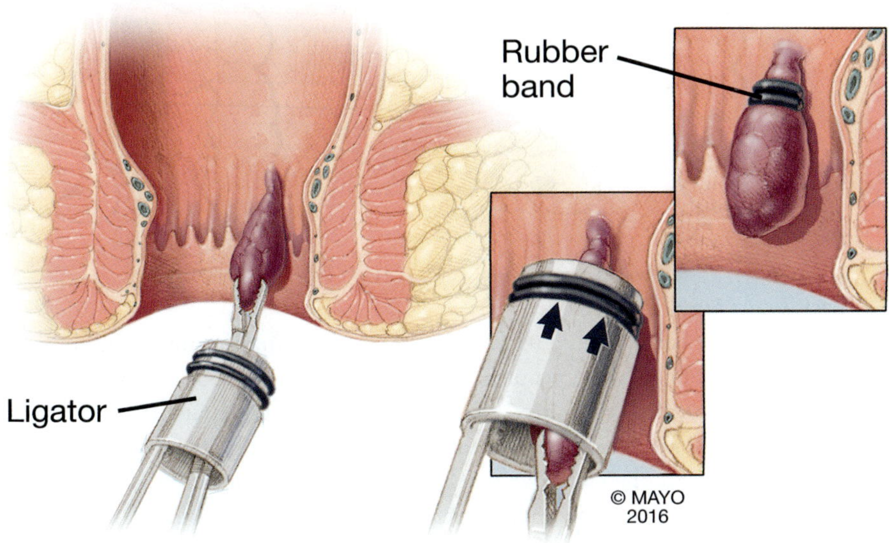

FIGURE 14.3. Steps for Rubber Band Ligation. Left, Location of hemorrhoid in rectum. Middle, Application of ligator. Right, Rubber band in place on hemorrhoid.

Operation

The choice between rubber band ligation (Figure 14.3) and excisional hemorrhoidectomy (Video 14.3) depends on the location (internal vs external) and degree of internal hemorrhoids. Low anterior resection (Videos 14.4 and 14.5) is used for proximal rectal cancers (12-16 cm from the anal verge). Abdominoperineal resection (Video 14.6) is indicated for distal rectal cancer (7-8 cm from the anal verge) that is not amenable to sphincter-preserving surgery. Neoadjuvant chemoradiotherapy is used for locally advanced rectal cancer (stages II and III).

Complications

Complications from excisional hemorrhoidectomy may include bleeding, urinary retention, and severe pain. Anastomotic leakage and pelvic sepsis are potential postoperative complications of rectal surgery.

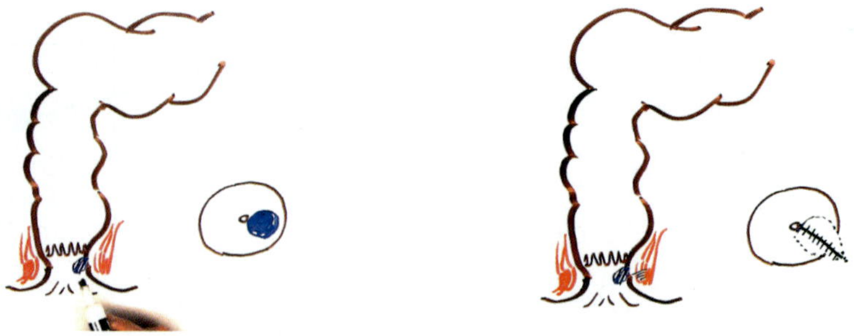

VIDEO 14.3. Excisional Hemorrhoidectomy.
Transcript: So now we have been asked to remove this hemorrhoid that is painful and throbbing. Usually we don't have to operate, but in some people it is exquisitely painful and it starts to necrose and skin becomes problematic. So touching this hurts. So it is typically done under anesthesia. If this was the anal sphincter, this is the area of the buttock around the side. A surgeon oftentimes will make a little incision around the outside of it, excise the clot, take that tissue out of there, and then depending on who it is, they might sew it back together again or leave it open with a little gauze dressing. The key thing here is to not cut the muscle and go deep enough, because if you go too deep you can cause problems with incontinence. People can't control their defecation.

So external hemorrhoidectomy—simple little operation, get rid of the clot and usually excise that tissue, sometimes can be a little bloody. But it is a simple outpatient procedure, but it hurts like heck.

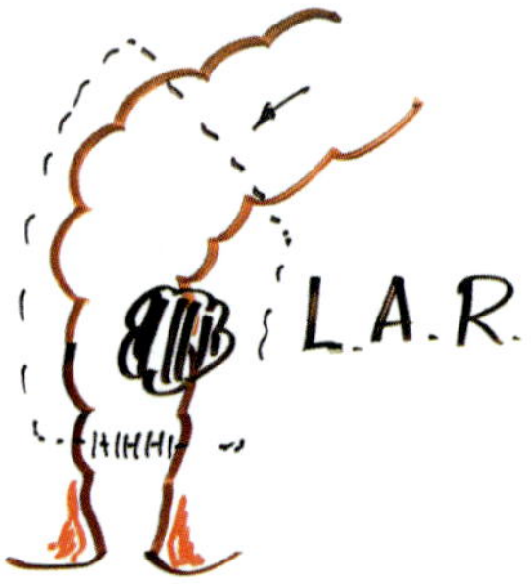

VIDEO 14.4. Low Anterior Resection.
Transcript: Low anterior resection is a surgical procedure that involves removing a cancer that is 10 to 18 cm from the anal verge. The muscles would be intact down below. What we want to do is resect the tumor with a wide margin and all this tissue will come out in a low anterior resection. And we now bring the sigmoid colon down to the rectum for an anastomosis. And that will be a viable anastomosis because the anoderm and the anal sphincter are intact. This is an operation that is used when you have a tumor that 12 to 16 to 18 cm from the anal verge.

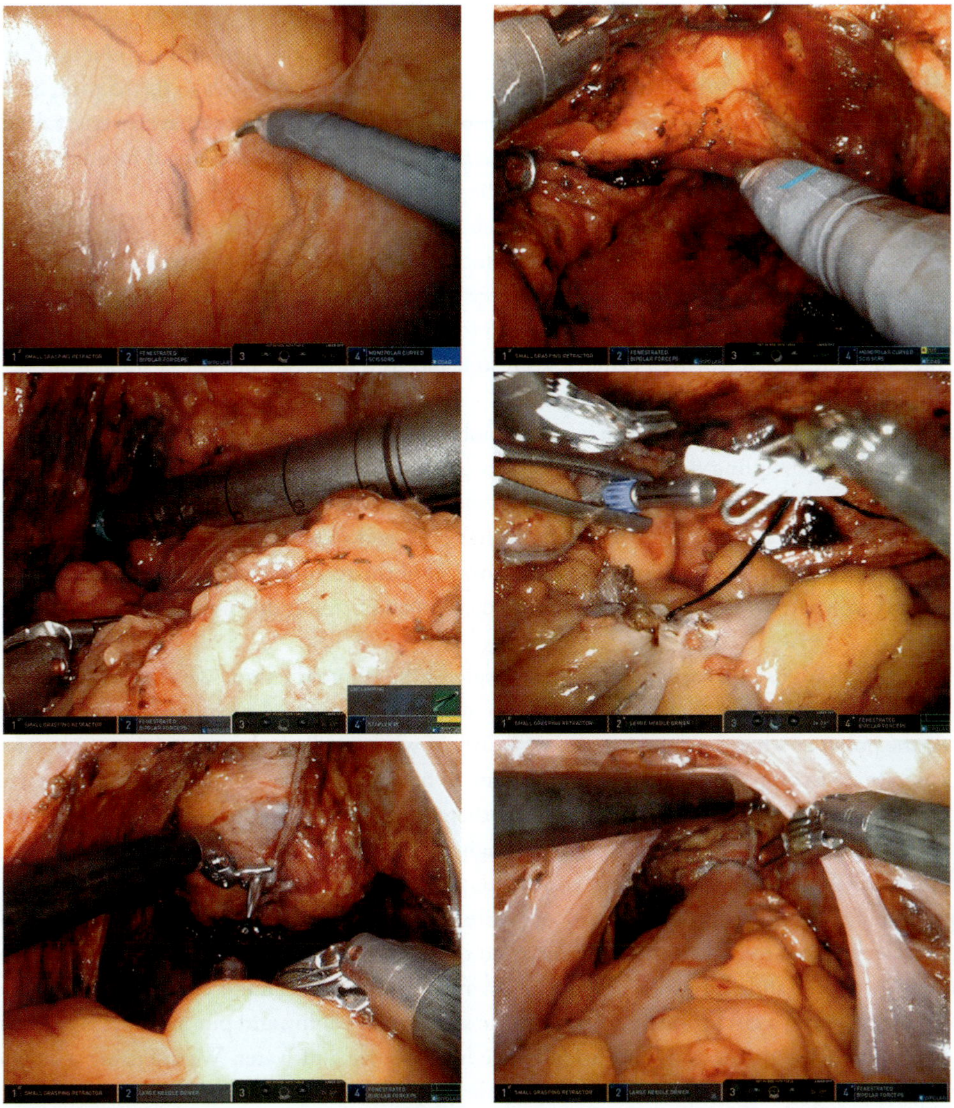

VIDEO 14.5. Low Anterior Resection: Intraoperative.

Transcript: This is a robotic low anterior resection, meaning that we are going to remove the rectum and sew the sigmoid down near the anus. We are looking from the belly button down into the pelvis in a man. And there is a right inguinal hernia way up high on the right of the screen.

Now we are looking down into that pelvis. The rectum is mobile, sigmoid colon here and we have got a lot of gadgets, they are robotic gadgets. And we are trying to find the ureter. It is marked there, and it is a white little thing and it will vermiculate, it will squeeze urine from time to time. Iliac vessels and other structures are sitting underneath so we have got to be careful with the use of electric cautery. Somebody that has done this hundreds of times, it is a piece of cake. Somebody that is doing it for the first or the tenth time needs a little help and that is what is going here. We've got the robotic scissors and it is hooked up to the cautery so it can be hot. And what the staff person wants is a light little touch on the peritoneum. And you can see that this trainee is just missing the peritoneum. But now is just cutting through it and seeing little blood vessels underneath. So what we are going to try to do is stay away from the iliacs,

VIDEO 14.5. Continued

mobilize the mesentery, the sigmoid, and the rectum. We have got some noncrushing clamps that are elevating that sigmoid and rectum anteriorly, and trying to find the blood vessels to the rectum. So we have got to think about superior hemorrhoidals and inferior hemorrhoidals. And we have a variety of different structures that we have to be careful to. This is done robotically and there are lots of numbers and things down below that you can look at the gadgets and the orientation of the camera.

But again, somebody that has done this a bunch, it is pretty straightforward. We are getting down near the bottom heading toward the anus. A little suction, a little scissors, a little cautery. We have got it mobilized on the backside of the rectum. We can see a little blood vessel coming from left to right from 3 o'clock to 9 o'clock. The scissors is about ready to touch it. The staff person says that it is a small blood vessel you can come across it with a cautery. And so it bleeds a little bit, but it is a small little vessel and they know what they are doing.

Now we have got a stapler in because we have mobilized the bottom of that rectum freely and we are going to try to put a stapling device that has 6 sets of clips and 3 rows on 1 side, 3 rows on the other, squeeze it down and then cut between them to divide this rectum. So now this stapler has squished the rectum, cut it, and just a little bit of the rectum is left on 1 end so we will have to divide that and free it up. So that line represents the anus and the lower portion of the rectum and we need to get things cleared off above now so where we could divide the sigmoid colon and bring it down to that lower portion of the rectum.

We have got an anvil, a little gadget that goes inside of the sigmoid colon. We've got the rectum down below and we can attach the sigmoid colon to the rectum. We've already removed the rectum with the cancer or the polyp or whatever reason and now we've got what is called a low anterior resection done and we are going to do a colorectostomy. And this is going to be a stapled anastomosis. So we have got an anvil inside the sigmoid colon that is that metal business there. And now from the bottom, we are going to take a little spear through the anus, carefully put it through near the middle of that stapler, and dial it through, push through and now it is going to join inside this other gadget, it's an engineering wonder. Put these 2 things together and then crank it back the opposite way and pull that sigmoid colon back down to the rectum. The key here is to make sure that there is no tension. So now we are going to slide that anvil over that post and gauge it and you will see it spin down and it will get closer and closer and closer, and there is a circle on 1 side and a circle on the other. And the stapler will deploy and put multiple layers of staples, a couple of squeezes and it is good and we now we have got air and water. We are using a colonoscope or a rectoproctoscopy and we can see that it is not leaking and there are no bubbles. We put some fluid in there and this is a beautiful tension-free anastomosis. So rectum has been removed and now it is sewn together. That is a low anterior resection.

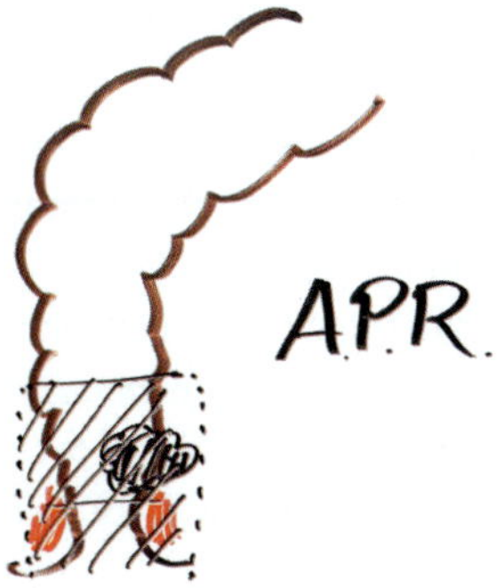

VIDEO 14.6. Abdominoperineal Resection.

Transcript: The sigmoid colon joins the rectum down into the anus. A cancer of the lower rectum, something that we can feel usually within 7 or 8 cm of the anus, is a low cancer. If you try to take that out, and sew the tissues together, the muscle will be destroyed and the person becomes incontinent. And that is just not possible; it is just not a way to live because an ostomy that goes out your bottom, you cannot control it. So the unfortunate thing is, a low rectal cancer needs what is called an abdominoperineal resection.

You make an abdominal incision and a perineal incision and you take this out and you bring out the sigmoid colon as an ostomy.

Abdominoperineal resection, so-called Miles procedure, means that you can feel the cancer, eradicate it, but they no longer defecate from below. They need an abdominal colostomy.

Rectum Challenge Questions

14.1. What is the name of the peritoneal reflection anterior to the rectum?
14.2. Where do taeniae coli fuse?
14.3. Superior, middle, and inferior rectal veins drain into what circulation?
14.4. Which is better for assessing rectal cancer: CT or MRI? Why?
14.5. What is the most common reason for performing endorectal US?
14.6. What is a J pouch?

Answers to Rectum Challenge Questions

14.1. Rectovesicular space in males; rectouterine space in females.

14.2. Taeniae coli are located where the sigmoid colon becomes upper rectum, just anterior to the sacrum.

14.3. They drain into the inferior mesenteric vein of the portal system.

14.4. MRI is better for evaluating the extent of the primary tumor (T stage) and nodal involvement (N stage). CT is better for detecting liver metastases (M stage).

14.5. Endorectal US is likely best for T+N assessment. It is less costly, it is dynamic, and there is no radiation exposure.

14.6. A modified portion of ileum created in the shape of a *J* to become a reservoir for stool in patients undergoing an ileoanal pouch anastomosis.

15

Soft Tissue

Embryology

The integumentary system is formed from the mesoderm.

Anatomy

Skin and its appendages compose the largest bodily organ. Skin covers up to 2 m^2 and is 15% to 20% of total body weight. Skin is composed of epidermis and dermis (Figure 15.1); the layers are connected through interpapillary ridges at the dermal-epidermal junction (Figure 15.1). The epidermis of thin skin is composed of 4 layers (5 layers in thick skin), but it does not contain blood vessels. The dermis is about 25 times thicker than the epidermis; it contains nerves, blood vessels, and lymphatic drainage. Appendages of the integumentary system include hair, nails (Figure 15.2), and sebaceous, eccrine, and apocrine glands (Figure 15.1).

Physiology

The integumentary system and underlying soft tissue (fat, fascia, and muscle) protect the body from damage and infection. The skin and its appendages maintain homeostasis and thermoregulation and have secretory and excretory functions.

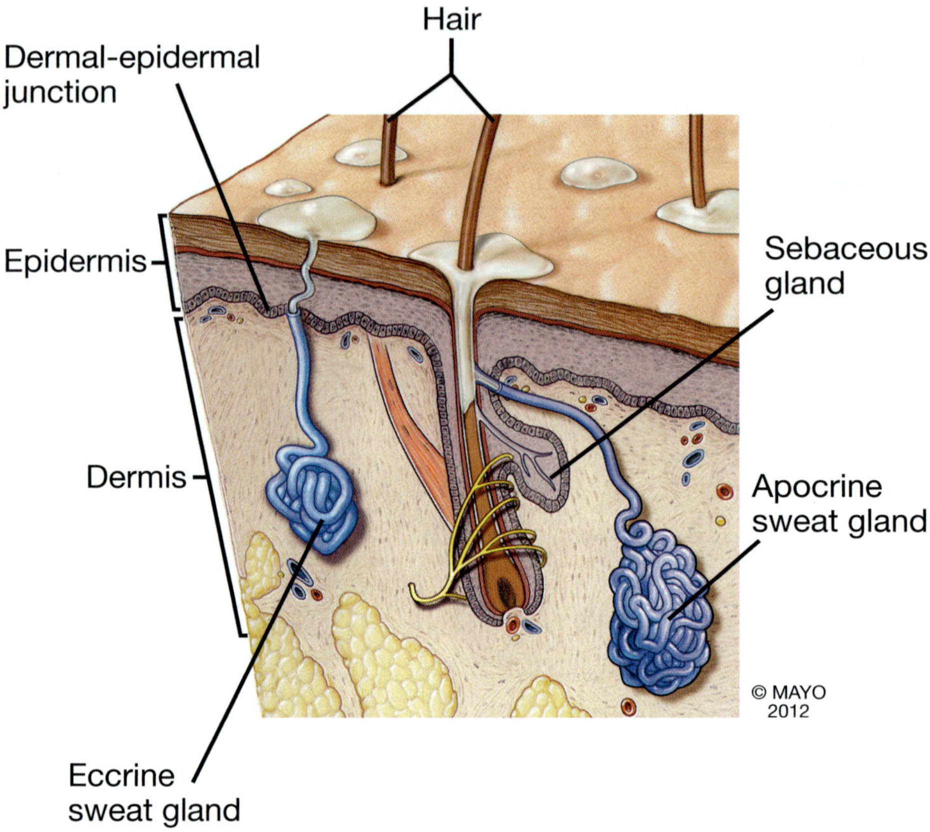

FIGURE 15.1. Skin Layers and Appendages of the Integumentary System.

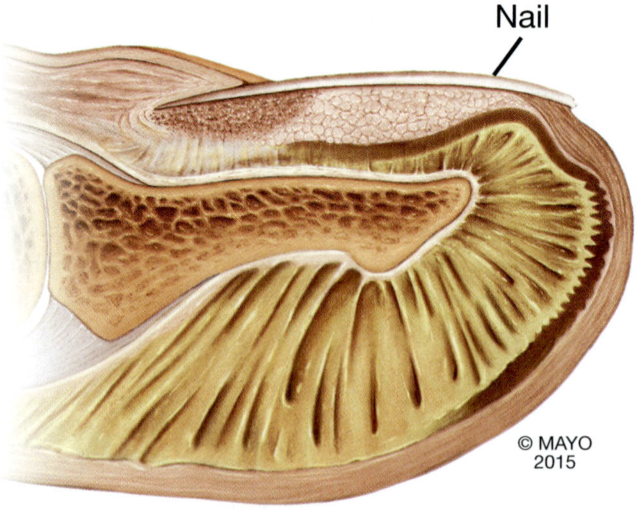

FIGURE 15.2. Cross-Section of Nail Bed.

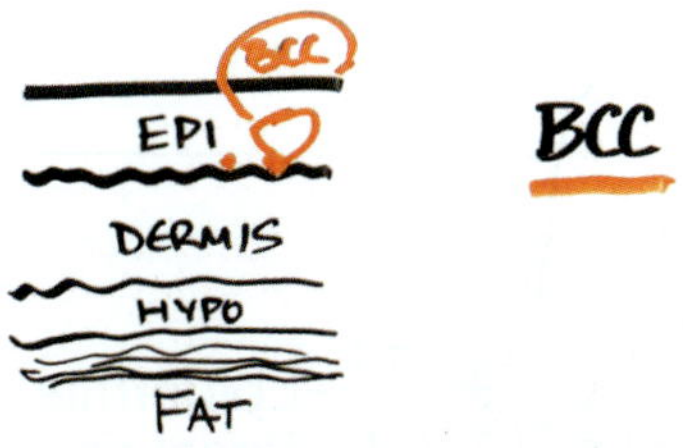

VIDEO 15.1. Basal Cell Carcinoma. HYPO indicates hypodermis.
Transcript: Basal cell carcinoma (BCC) is the most common type of skin malignancy. It comes from the epidermis; the cells right on the basement membrane. And as they grow over time, they tend to be roundish. Most basal cell carcinomas are round protuberances that people can see and oftentimes will have them removed. It is readily curable.

Fortunately, 75% of all skin cancers are basal cell cancers. They typically occur the older we get. If you find those lumps and bumps, see your physician and likely get them excised.

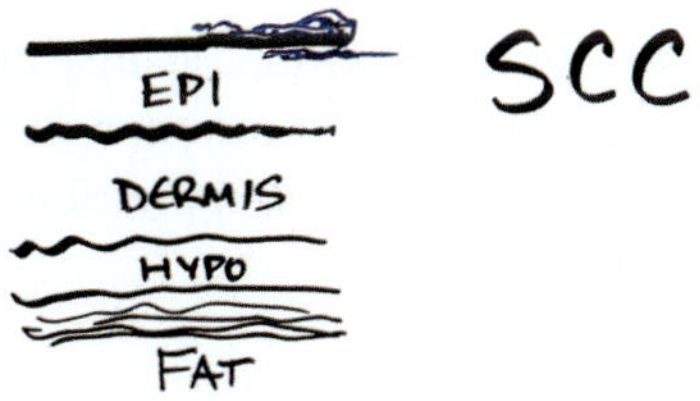

VIDEO 15.2. SCC. HYPO indicates hypodermis.
Transcript: Squamous cell cancer is the second most common type of skin malignancy. Roughly 20% of all skin cancers in the United States are squamous cell. And they typically come from the epidermis. They tend to run a little bit and sometimes they can be flat and other times they can be elevated and discolored. Sometimes they are tough to see and unlike basal cell, which tends to be round and easier to see, squamous cells for some reason look like freckles at some point in some patients. And they tend to be a little bit more delayed.

Take a look, if there are skin changes, raised, altered, it could be a squamous cell cancer. It is readily curable if caught early—simple skin excision. The older you get the more likely it is that you can have squamous cell cancers.

Clinical Presentations

Skin lesions are typically asymptomatic, but they occasionally itch, bleed, or ulcerate. The most common malignant tumor of the skin is basal cell carcinoma (about 75%) (Video 15.1), second is SCC (20%) (Video 15.2), and third is malignant melanoma (3%) (Figure 15.3 and Video 15.3).

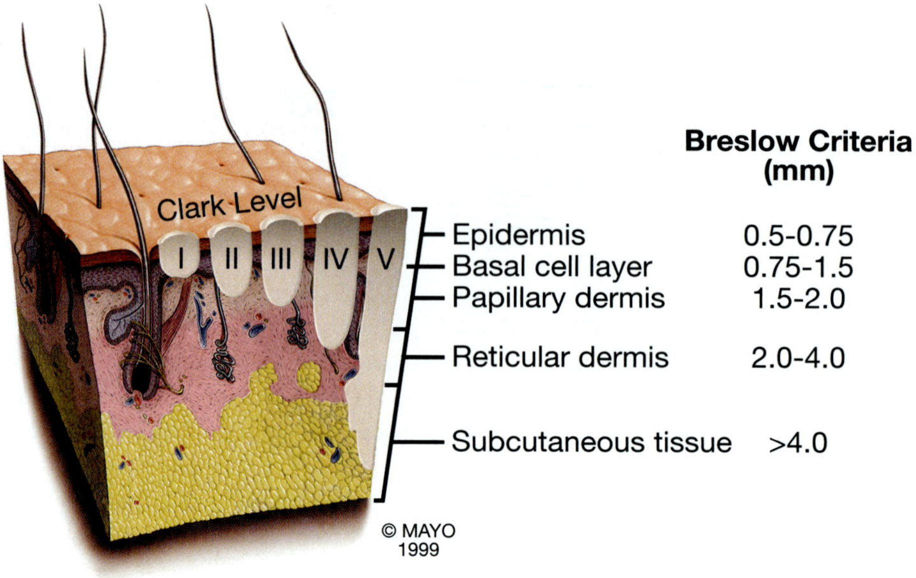

FIGURE 15.3. Clark Level and Breslow Criteria for Melanoma in Relation to Skin Layers.

Soft tissue sarcomas develop and are usually painless until large. Soft tissue sarcomas can metastasize hematogenously (most common site is the liver). Risk factors for soft tissue sarcomas are radiation, immunosuppression, lymphedema, chemical exposure, chronic wounds, and burn scars.

Imaging

Work-up for diagnosis of soft tissue sarcomas includes CT, MRI, and biopsy. Imaging work-up for metastases includes CXR (Video 15.4), chest CT (Video 15.5), and liver function tests.

Operation

First-line treatment for symptomatic benign lipomas is surgical resection (Video 15.6). Treatment of malignant soft tissue sarcomas includes surgical resection (ideally with negative margins) and often radiation with or without chemotherapy. Basal cell carcinoma, SCC, and malignant melanoma treatment options are excision, ablation, Mohs micrographic surgery, and radiation (Video 15.7). The treatment of choice for metastases isolated to the lungs or liver is resection.

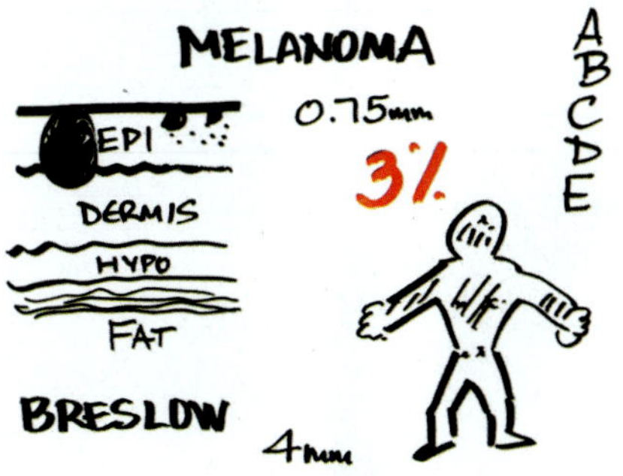

VIDEO 15.3. Malignant Melanoma. HYPO indicates hypodermis.
Transcript: Melanoma only represents only 3% of the skin cancers. But perhaps more than 50% of the deaths related to skin cancer. Melanoma comes from the melanocytes that sit with inside the epidermis. Sun-exposed regions increase the risk of melanoma. People on the chest, arms, face, and back have higher risk of melanoma. Having said that, melanoma is a tumor that can grow almost anywhere; in the eyes, in the anus, in the skin, all over the place. And it can metastasize to lymph nodes, to lung, to brain, and bone. It is a very aggressive tumor. Having said that, caught early, it's readily treatable.

One of the key factors nowadays is to know about the Breslow scoring system, or the Breslow criteria, the depth of this lesion. When these melanocytes grow they get to a certain depth and the deeper they become, the more dangerous they are. So something that is <0.75 mm has a low risk of spreading to lymph nodes and is readily cured. As these melanomas get bigger, and invade into the dermis and get into blood vessels, the risk becomes exceptional. If the thickness is 4 mm or greater, it is very likely that person already has lymph node–positive disease, and will likely die from melanoma.

Melanoma. What do we need to know from a medical student standpoint? A, B, C, D, E. We need to know if it is asymmetric, does it bleed, is there a color change, is the diameter bigger than 6 mm, and is it elevated or raised from the skin—a variety of early signs. But any sort of skin change that is getting bigger, changing colors, bleeding or ulcerating, should be carefully looked at by a physician and most likely excised.

Complications

Complications of surgical treatment of malignant tumors of the skin and soft tissue are postoperative bleeding, infection, hematoma, and recurrence. Wound breakdown or dehiscence can occur, especially in previously irradiated surgical sites.

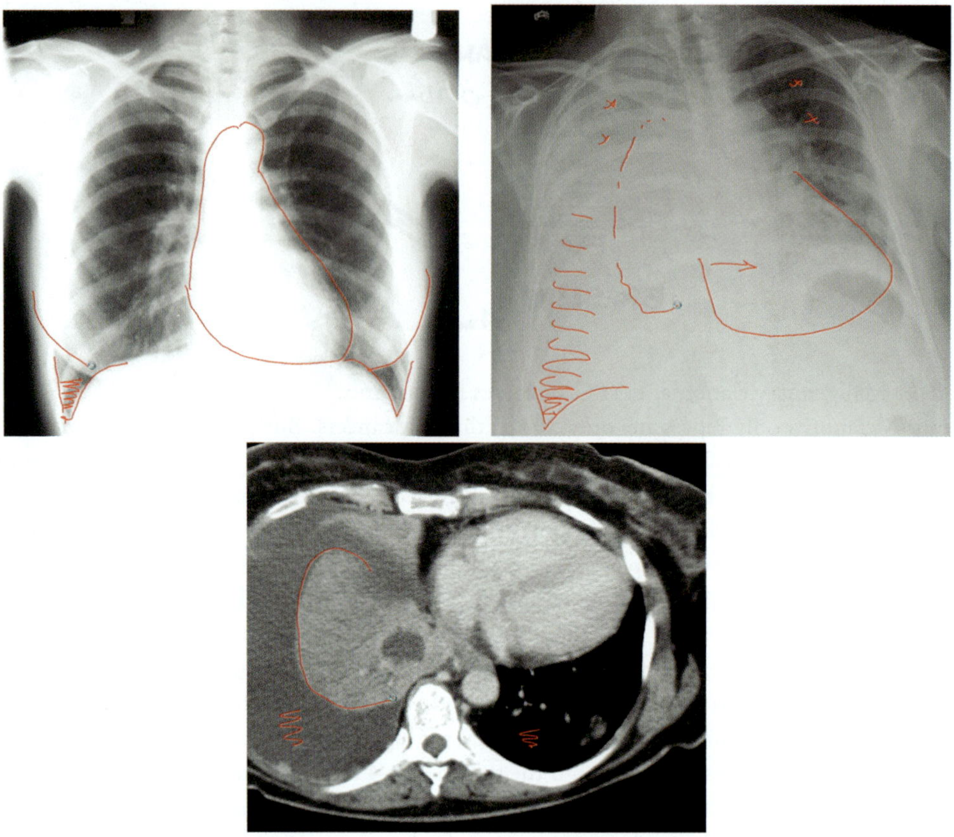

VIDEO 15.4. CXR Showing Metastasis.

Transcript: Chest x-ray is very useful for looking at the lungs, and the heart, nice normal-looking heart, aortic knob that is the heart in the middle. We can see the lungs on either side. Good inspiration, we have got diaphragms down at the bottom that are nice and clear, there is no fluid sitting down here. Same thing on the other side, this is a woman with breast tissue. But we can see the rest of the lung; it looks the same on 1 side versus the other. There should be symmetry in the density when you look at this. This is a normal-looking chest x-ray. No evidence of metastatic disease.

In contrast, let's take a peek at this chest x-ray. Couple of different things to think about: 1) Where is the heart? It is hard to see but an actual fact, it is sitting over here, it is pushed over this way a little bit. And why is that? Well, this is normal-looking lung here, but everything is whiter on this side. There is an extensive amount of fluid. And how do we know that? Well, I can't see any diaphragms down here, this is all water, and this is all blood. This is something in the right chest and it is tough to know where the lung is. Looking at it right now I can get a sense that maybe the lung looks something like that. We've got a bubble of air over here. We have got potential densities.

If we would use a CT scan for this patient in particular, we would actually see lots of fluid here on the side, this is normal lung. But, this is lung that is compressed. A normal-looking heart. So, we are going back to this chest x-ray. What do we look at this? We can see normal-looking lung here, and it is opacified, whitish on this side. There is likely something here, that is fluid. This is likely somebody with metastatic cancer; sarcoid, squamous cell, this is an advanced lesion. The chest x-ray shows us that this person is in trouble.

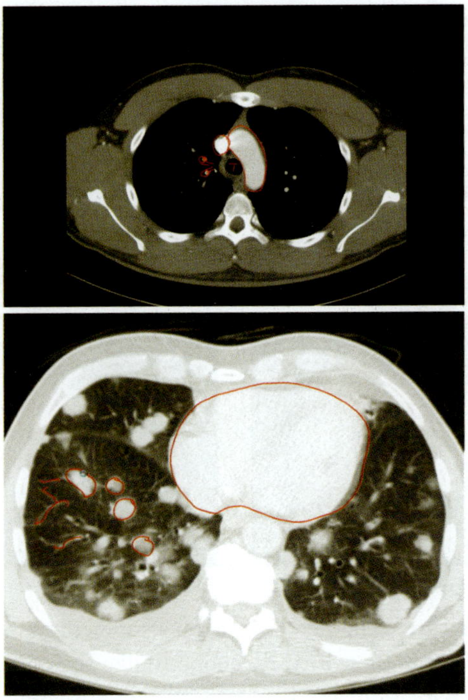

VIDEO 15.5. CT Showing Metastasis.

Transcript: CT scanning of the head, chest, abdomen, and pelvis is a great way to stage patients with cancer. We are looking here the lungs, the chest if you will. This is a beautiful CT scan. A couple of things to note: Contrast is being given, the superior vena cava, the aorta, they have contrast in it. We can see the trachea and then we look to the lungs and we look for metastatic problems, what about these little circles here, those are not metastatic things, those are blood vessels eventually going to be leading us back to the heart. And what we want to do is to see these circles get bigger and bigger as they close in toward the heart and they should be tiny out here. And in fact, with this patient it is a normal CT scan, there is nothing evil, these are all sorts of normal little blood vessels.

So let's contrast that to this CT scan. It is pretty obvious right off the get-go. We can see there is our heart, and this is what is called a pulmonary window, so the lungs are not black and we get to see actual little blood vessels out here. The problem is, these little grapes that sit out here are all metastatic cancer. In this person it is squamous cell cancer. It could be a sarcoma; it could be a variety of things. But this is a CT scan showing us florid metastatic disease within the lung perimeter.

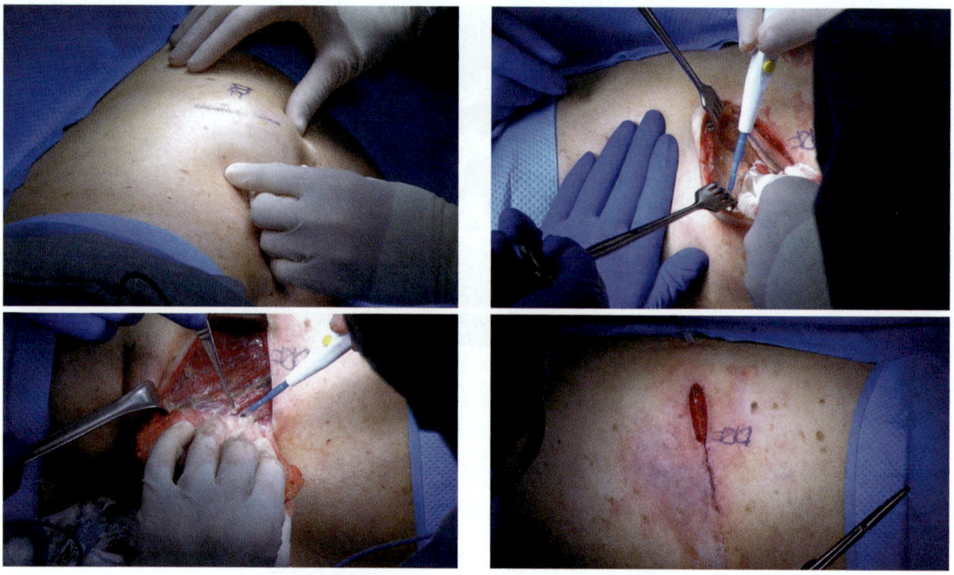

VIDEO 15.6. Recurrent Lipoma Excision: Intraoperative.
Transcript: This patient had a recurrent lipoma. That happens sometimes when you don't get it all out the first time. Lipomas sometimes create these little pseudopods, like arms of an octopus.

We are now going to make an incision, and I am nervous that it is going to recur again so we go widely around the past incision. We are going to slide under the fatty tissue underneath the skin and then ideally get around the lipoma and not leave any of those fatty cells that can grow back again.

So we have got an island of tissue, we are into the fatty tissue, hands there, the blue hand pulling cephalad, the white hand pulling toward the buttocks, more traction, more tension, the better. Things pull apart. Those are Murphy rakes and we are working on the inferior caudal side. The surgeon is pulling hard with their index finger trying to stay away from the fatty tissue, sneaking in and raising the flap. It is a lot like a mastectomy flap. The idea is to stay away from the yellowish lipomatous tissue. This lipoma sticks to the backside of the muscles. And so at some point we have to get down to the muscles. Oftentimes we don't take fascia, but for a recurrence like this, I think the best thing is to take the fascia. So the whitish thing under the specimen is fascia. You can see the muscle contract with the electrocautery working next to it. The lipoma is just on the other side or our side of that fascia. Got to be careful here, tension is the key. The more tension, the faster you can work. The specimen comes out. There is a little perforating blood vessel; don't be afraid to go back and tie that off—we did that.

Now we need to close up this wound, and usually the best way to do it is a couple of deep sutures and then maybe run some sutures below the skin. The more you can take the tension off, the narrower the skin will be at the end. Here is a nice subcuticular closure. It came together nicely. We used an ellipse of skin and at least a 3:1 ratio length to width, so the skin comes back together. Nice job!

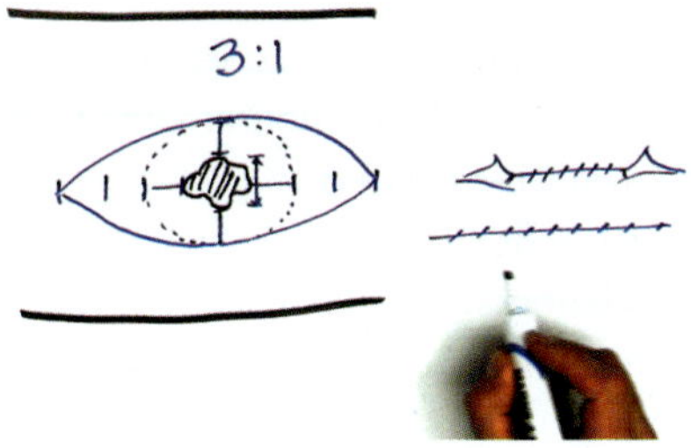

VIDEO 15.7. Surgical Resection of Melanoma.

Transcript: Surgically resecting a skin abnormality; maybe this is on the abdomen, or the thigh, or the forearm. Let's say this is 1 cm in length. If this is a cancer, we would like to get negative margins. If it is a melanoma, we will get margins based on the Breslow depth. Basically, we need at least 1 cm margins for these skin cancers. And 1 cm on each side means that his 1-cm diameter object is going to be 3 cm by 3 cm. The problem with that is, when you get ready to close this, circles don't close up very well. They come together what are called dog ears. So if we were going to close something up, it might have a funny sort of a look to it on either end. It is bumped up because there is too much tension.

So what I would like to teach you is what is called a 3:1 ratio or greater. So if we have got negative margins, we want 3:1 ratio length to width, so the width is 3 cm. We need that to be more on this. We actually need, well let's extend out, how many are we going to make? One cm, 3 cm margins here. This ellipse will be more likely to heal up without a dog ear. It will be a longer incision, but it will be more difficult to see, it will be more cosmetic. So when you think about taking out an abnormality, you can cut it out as a circle, but don't set your patient up for dog ears. Typically, make the ratio 3:1 or greater. Sometimes when the skin is under great tension, it needs to be 4:1 or 5:1. This will allow the wound to come back together primarily and make a very cosmetic incision.

Soft Tissue Challenge Questions

15.1. Name 2 distinct staging systems to determine the depth of melanoma.
15.2. Name the 3 most common malignant soft tissue sarcomas in adults.
15.3. What is the most common type of soft tissue sarcoma to metastasize to the lymph nodes?
15.4. What is the classic cell type associated with Hodgkin disease?
15.5. What is the most aggressive and fatal skin cancer?
15.6. What are the most common sites of basal cell carcinoma and SCC?
15.7. What are the signs of SCC metastases?
15.8. What is Bowen disease of the skin?
15.9. Where does melanoma occur?
15.10. What malignancy is most likely to metastasize to the bowel?

Answers to Soft Tissue Challenge Questions

15.1. The Clark level and the Breslow criteria.
15.2. Fibrous histiocytoma (25%), liposarcoma (20%), and leiomyosarcoma (15%).
15.3. Malignant fibrous histiocytoma.
15.4. Reed-Sternberg cells.
15.5. Malignant melanoma.
15.6. The most common sites are the head, neck, and hands (sun-exposed areas).
15.7. Enlarged LNs.
15.8. SCC in situ.
15.9. Melanoma can occur in the skin, eyes, or anus.
15.10. Melanoma.

16

Spleen

Embryology

The spleen develops from mesoderm during the fifth week of gestation.

Anatomy

Eighty-five percent of humans have 1 spleen, and 15% have accessory spleens. The spleen sits adjacent to the diaphragm in the left upper quadrant of the abdomen. It spans the 9th, 10th, and 11th ribs. Arterial blood is supplied through a tortuous splenic artery (from the celiac artery) and small, short gastric vessels from the left gastroepiploic artery (Figure 16.1). Venous blood drains from the splenic vein into the portal vein, and the short gastric veins drain into the left gastroepiploic vein (Figure 16.1). The spleen is attached to the stomach, colon, kidney, and diaphragm by suspensory ligaments (Video 16.1). The tail of the pancreas lies within the hilum of the spleen.

Physiology

The spleen cleans the blood by trapping and breaking down dysfunctional or old red blood cells. The spleen acts as a major lymphatic warehouse providing lymphocytes for immune function.

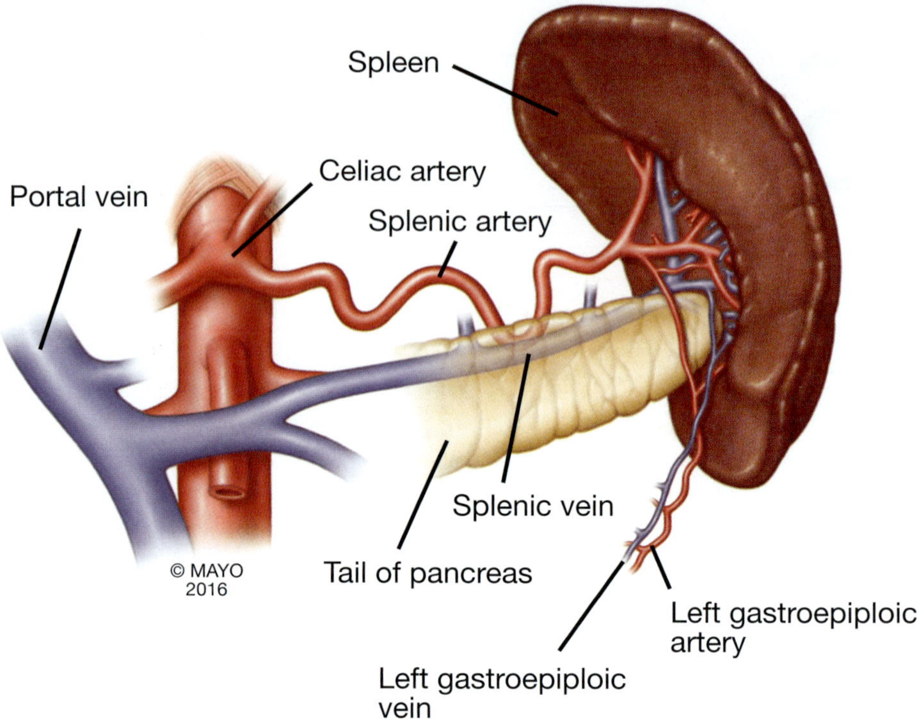

FIGURE 16.1. Anatomy and Blood Flow of the Spleen.

Clinical Presentation

Splenic problems most commonly arise with trauma, lymphoma, benign cysts, and hematologic disorders (Video 16.2).

Imaging

Surgeons evaluate the spleen using plain radiography (CXR; kidney, ureter, bladder), CT (Video 16.3), MRI, angiography (Video 16.3), and nuclear studies. Hemodynamically unstable patients who have had traumatic injuries receive a FAST examination (Video 16.4).

Operation

Open splenectomy (Video 16.5) for trauma or splenomegaly is at times dangerous and difficult with the need for speed, blood transfusion, and hemodynamic support. Laparoscopic splenectomy (Videos 16.6 and 16.7) is elective, and careful transection of the splenic attachments and vasculature leads to straightforward removal.

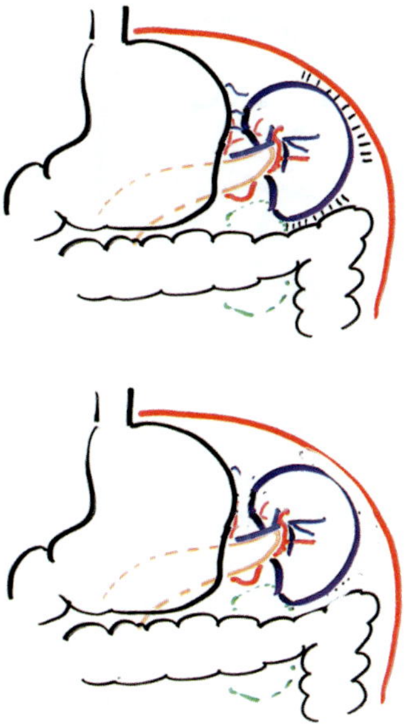

VIDEO 16.1. Suspensory Ligaments.
Transcript: The spleen is housed in the left upper quadrant of the abdomen protected by the rib cage, and it is attached to the colon, the splenocolic ligaments, the phrenicocolic ligaments, the short gastric vessels (mostly little veins that go from the stomach to the spleen, but sometimes a little artery), and then deeper down, hidden underneath, is an attachment to the kidney that sits underneath; the so-called splenorenal. So when trauma surgeons have to take out the spleen quickly, they need to divide the gastrocolic ligament, the diaphragmatic attachments, the so-called splenophrenic, they have to carefully get through the blood supply, the short gastrics, and make sure it doesn't bleed and then this spleen is allowed up, release the attachments to the kidney, and then a safe splenectomy can be performed.

These are all basically avascular ligaments, except for the short gastrics.

Complications

Potential early postoperative complications include abscess, pancreatic injury, pneumonia, and wound infection. Delayed gastric perforation, overwhelming postsplenectomy sepsis (Video 16.8), and portal vein thrombosis can occur weeks, months, or years later.

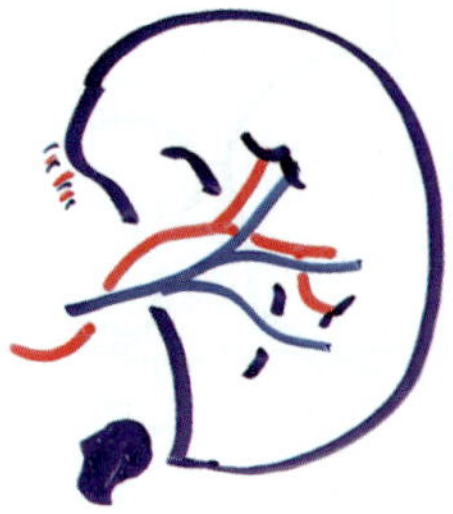

VIDEO 16.2. Hematologic Disorders.
Transcript: The spleen has a fantastic blood flow through this tortuous splenic artery, and then subsequent drainage from the splenic vein and also short gastric vessels into the stomach. From time to time, hematologic disorders can happen. Probably the most common for surgeons to deal with is what is called idiopathic thrombocytopenic purpura (ITP). Basically, the spleen and the body make antibodies against the platelets. And therefore, the spleen tackles those platelets and people's platelet counts drop. And oftentimes we are asked as surgeons to remove the entire spleen because this is a blood-cleaning organ and the platelets are removed and destroyed here. Typically the spleen does not get big from ITP and it is a normal size, about the size of your fist. From a surgical standpoint it is a great opportunity to help patients out because about 50% to 60% of the time people are benefited.

One key factor is to remember is that some people will have an accessory spleen and if you take this spleen out for ITP and you leave the little baby spleen behind, it will grow large, and in fact I know this to be true. I saw a gentleman 50 years after a splenectomy as a child come back; he had basically a normal-looking spleen to me and it was nothing more than an accessory spleen.

Other hematologic disorders that would be useful sometimes for surgeons to take out the spleen is hereditary spherocytosis. The red blood cells are no longer in a beautiful flexible shape and they get destroyed in the spleen and it eradicates those red blood cells.

Sickle cell disease—sometimes we get infarction and terrible pain that people will need the spleen out.

Thalassemia at some point can cause problems with blood counts low enough, patients require blood transfusions.

Splenectomy for warm autoimmune hemolytic anemia and other problems like TTP also will benefit patients.

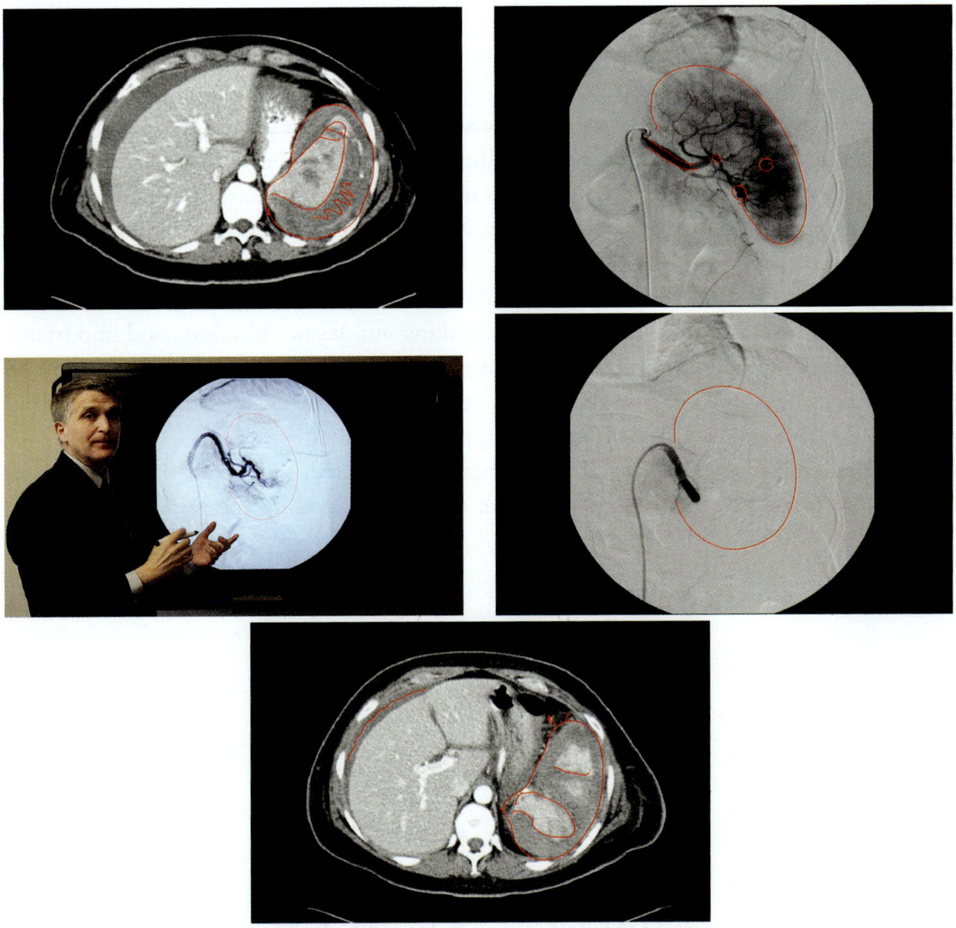

VIDEO 16.3. CT and Angiography of the Spleen.
Transcript: This is a CT scan of the abdomen in a young patient involved in a motor vehicle accident. It shows some significant trauma. We see importantly it is a CT scan with oral contrast with dye in the stomach and also intravenous or arterial contrast in the aorta and also in the portal vein.

So this dye has been circulating around. And for trauma surgeons, or medical students, or anybody looking at it, immediately I hope you can see the liver is well perfused, but then there is this fluid density off to the side. That is likely blood. That is a lot of blood in the abdomen. When we sneak over here to look at the spleen, which is the most common traumatic injury that causes would go to the operating room for, we can see that it is no longer homogeneous, it is broken up. In fact, there is blood around the outside of it or within the confines of the spleen. There is some viable spleen, but it has got some cuts in it and it's got a lot of blood. So this is a spleen that has been shattered, if you will. Now this patient to get this scan must have been hemodynamically stable. So the surgeons and the emergency medicine physicians give them fluid, give them some blood, and if they are doing okay, they might take them to angiography.

Let me show you what 1 of those pictures looks like. So here is the catheter sliding in, up from the aorta from the groin into the splenic artery. So this is our spleen that is perfused with blood from the splenic artery. Interestingly to note, big accident, lots of pseudoaneurysms, breaks within the blood vessels in the spleen. Now you might imagine our interventional radiologist, if they could put some material in and clot

VIDEO 16.3. Continued

off the artery, instead of having blood flow out of here, it would stop the bleeding. Unfortunately, it may stop the entire blood flow to the spleen.

This is the same catheter and we are starting to put some clot in, some gel foam, thrombotic agents, and we can see there is less perfusion here. If we wait a little bit longer and let this clot, watch what happens. Now we have no blood flow to the spleen. The good news is, there is no bleeding, and this patient doesn't need to go to the operating room for a splenectomy. Now they have a remnant there and we will see if it becomes viable or not.

Let's take a peek at a CT scan 24 hours later. Again, we can see blood in the abdomen, and we can see that there is a spleen here, and there is no contrast sneaking out, it's not bleeding, and importantly there is some viable tissue. Hopefully with time that splenic tissue will work from an immunologic standpoint and help this patient fight infection. So this person got a real bang for their buck—no big operation, no surgical scar, and yet we still have some functioning spleen at the end.

Splenic injuries are graded from 1 to 5; 5 is completely shattered, that is not this, this is more like a grade 4 splenic laceration and the patient avoided an operation. Good for the patient.

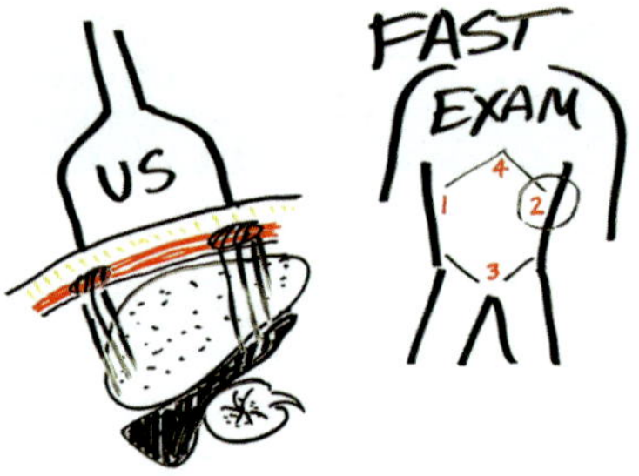

VIDEO 16.4. FAST Examination (EXAM).

Transcript: A FAST exam is the focus assessment with sonography for trauma; "F-A-S-T." You put the probe bar in the right upper quadrant, the left upper quadrant, on the bladder, and in the xiphoid, looking for blood or fluid, perforated bowel, or liquid in the abdomen. If we are talking about the spleen, we want to put the probe on the chest wall in the left upper quadrant in the flank and ideally see the spleen and the kidney. And what we are looking for is the ultrasound to show us a blackened layer—that is fluid. It's harder to see the spleen on a FAST exam than it is the gallbladder or some other place. So oftentimes there are ribs in our way. And you will see with this video right here that there is shadowing because of the ribs, it blocks it off. But you can get a sense of the underlying spleen and the underlying kidney.

The FAST exam is useful for trauma evaluation to find out if people are bleeding or have intra-abdominal problems; especially for the spleen. It is the number 1 reason that surgeons go to the operating room for blunt trauma—an injured spleen. So taking a look in that left upper quadrant through the ribs to find the spleen and the left kidney and sense is there any fluid which will be hypoechoic or black on a FAST exam.

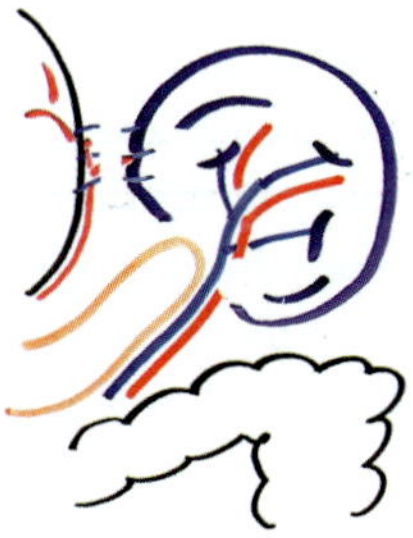

VIDEO 16.5. Open Splenectomy.
Transcript: Open splenectomy should be a straightforward operation; but it may be difficult to a really enlarged spleen or because of trauma and bleeding. But the pearls of wisdom about taking the spleen out remain the same. You can imagine the subcostal margin and the rib in your way. Good exposure is important. Getting the spleen up and out of the abdomen is crucial. To do that you need to transect the ligaments; the splenocolic, the splenophrenic, and then carefully divide the short gastric vessels with either gadgets or clamps and ties, and the short gastric is carefully taken apart. Now with these attachments, the spleen can be lifted up and out of the abdomen. Releasing the attachments to the kidney basically leaves us on a stalk, and it is important to remember what is in the stalk; the splenic vein, the splenic artery, and the tail of the pancreas. You want to divide 2 of the 3. Don't hurt the tail of the pancreas. Ideally, when you think about taking the spleen out, think about which 1 you want to take out first, the artery or the vein.

I pause for a second, if I could divide the artery first and tie that off, then the drainage to the spleen through the splenic vein, the blood would slide out and the gland would be smaller and safer and that is what you want to do. Take out the splenic artery first and divide the splenic vein, and then be very careful that you don't injure the tail of the pancreas.

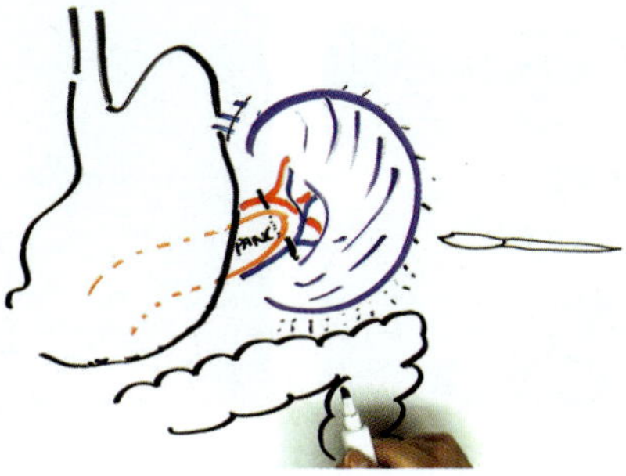

VIDEO 16.6. Laparoscopic Splenectomy.
Transcript: Laparoscopic splenectomy is often done with a patient in the lateral decubitus position, on their side. So the spleen is up and everything else is going to fall down. And the key to getting the spleen out safely through abdominal incisions laparoscopically is to release the attachments to the diaphragm and the musculature and the colon. These little things can be incised, and it allows this spleen to be freed up and mobile. But there are still multiple attachments; the splenic artery, the splenic vein, and the short gastric vessels—some arteries but mostly veins.

Several different ways to do it. Some folks like to go up front early and take these big blood vessels. Others, like myself, like to incise, make this mobile and wobbly, and then be careful of the pancreas. The pancreas sits in the hilum. And so, when you are dividing blood vessels, the splenic vein or the splenic

VIDEO 16.6. Continued

artery with a stapler, it is possible that you might injure the tail of the pancreas and get a leak. There are some nice gadgets, the ligature, the Harmonic scalpel, and others, that will allow you to easily divide the short gastric vessels. In an open operation these are the deepest structures and sometimes the hardest to get. Laparoscopically they can sometimes be very fun. And once this spleen is mobile, and then you can flop it either way. Then ideally what you would like to do is stop or transect or ligate the splenic artery first. Why the splenic artery first? Because the blood flow goes into the artery, it's cut off, and now the blood in the spleen can empty through the splenic vein and actually allow the spleen to shrink, make it smaller, and you can actually autotransfuse the patient. They get their own blood back. Never transect the splenic vein first, always the artery, usually with a stapling device.

Once you get the spleen free, now you can put it in a bag. And if it is through a little bitty incision, how do you get that spleen through there? Either you have to make a larger incision or you can morsalize it, basically go in with a ring forceps and crush it inside the bag, and it comes out in chunks. It is a wonderful way to take out a spleen through small incisions. It is very useful to our patients, but you have got to be careful of the tail of the pancreas and the order of the blood vessels how you take them.

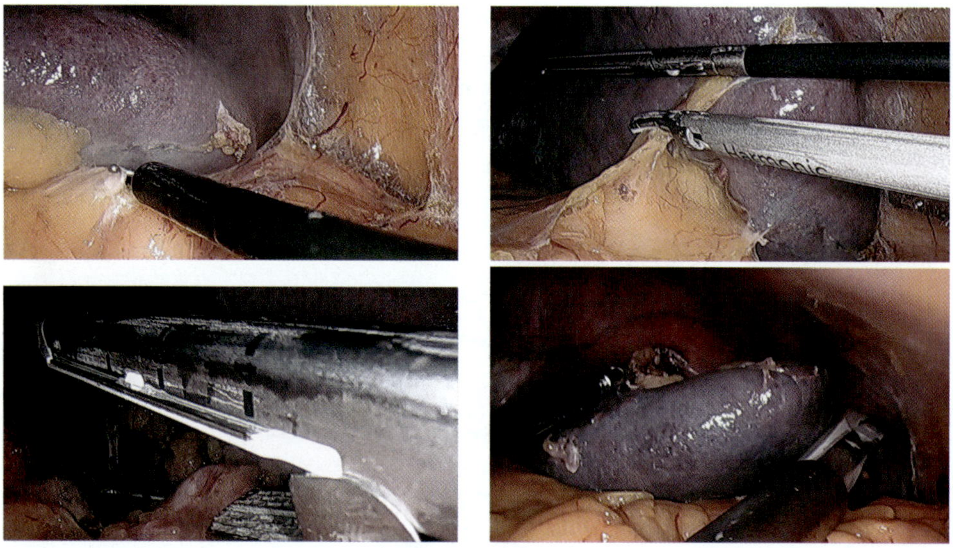

VIDEO 16.7. Splenectomy: Intraoperative.

Transcript: Splenectomy—putting the patient in the right side down, left side up, the head is to the left. And we put the laparoscope in and we are going to take a spleen. Somebody that may have lymphoma, somebody that may have some sort of bleeding disorder, some sort of abnormality, we are looking in the patient's left upper quadrant and we have got a hook cautery that is taking down some adhesions. The spleen is tethered to the retroperitoneum with a variety of different fascial attachments, and here just some omentum is being stuck to the spleen. And this is a good-sized spleen. The normal spleen is about a fist size. This is more like a mini volleyball, a big grapefruit.

We are sitting behind the spleen and we are looking up toward the head and the diaphragm is up above and we are releasing the retroperitoneal attachments. Once we get that released we push the spleen laterally and now we see where the hilum is. We have got some gadgets, an electrocautery, a Harmonic scalpel,

VIDEO 16.7. Continued

and a Ligature device that divide blood vessels. And you can see a few blood vessels going into the spleen. The stomach is to the left. These are beating vessels that come in and out of the spleen that may go to the short gastric vessels of the stomach. This gadget divides those blood vessels very nicely and we can lift up the spleen. And we can see parts of the spleen are now blue, they have lost their blood supply.

Now we are going to get closer to the hilum and I think you can suggest and see the splenic artery beating there. There will be a splenic vein. Both of those are dangerous. We want to take those carefully. And the tail of the pancreas will be somewhere close. Using a grasper and a hook cautery we are sneaking down underneath. It is going to be the splenic vein to the left. The spleen is up above us. We are mobilizing this thing up. Stomach to the left of the screen, spleen to the right, short gastric vessels visualized. Those all need to be taken down to get the spleen out.

Here using the Harmonic scalpel to do that with heating a device. It's nice with this splenectomy, it's nice time, it doesn't take a lot of time, but we don't have to be in a hurry unlike a trauma case where somebody might be bleeding out and this would have to be all done in a matter of seconds to minutes. A lot of the times just to get to the spleen out and then take care of the bleeding. We have mobilized the stomach away from the spleen. These are short gastric vessels that are being divided. About the only thing left holding the spleen in place is the hilum and that is the splenic artery and the splenic vein. You can see the splenic artery pounding away. There is one vessel, sometimes there will be a couple of them, and it depends on how they branch. You have got to be really careful, and in an ideal world, we take the splenic artery first, that way the blood flow is decreased, the blood drains out of the spleen, and the patient can actually get an autotransfusion. Here comes a stapling device. We are going to put 3 different rows of staples on 1 side, 3 rows of staples on the other, and then cut between them. Crimps down, deploy that stapler, and hopefully it makes it bloodless. Cuts through—let's take a look and see what we have. We have got to be careful, it gets stuck. Take your time. There are our little staples and not a drop of blood that is beautifully done. It's a great instrument, it's a great gadget.

Now we need to get the splenic vein and we will be ready to take this out. So somewhere hidden underneath is the splenic vein in that fatty tissue. Using the electrocautery, we can dissect a little bit and we get a sense that the grayish structure, blueish structure to the left of the screen is the splenic vein. And it is probably more dangerous as a bleeding organ than the splenic artery. But now that it is pretty much cleaned off, we take the stapling device again; the splenic vein is a little better seen. Widely across that we have got all the retroperitoneal attachments done. We deploy the stapler, fire it, cut it, and carefully release it. And at this point it needs to be put in a bag and taken out. First things first, it looks like it is done very nicely with no bleeding.

Now this spleen that is as big as a grapefruit or bigger needs to be put in a bag and then brought out through these tiny little incisions. You might ask, how is that done? Well you can either make a big incision and take it out or, the advantage of laparoscopic surgery is that you can actually morsalize the spleen. Put it up next to the incisions and put a little grasping tool that breaks up the spleen and it can be taken out through a 1- or 2-cm incision and the patient can go home either that day or the next.

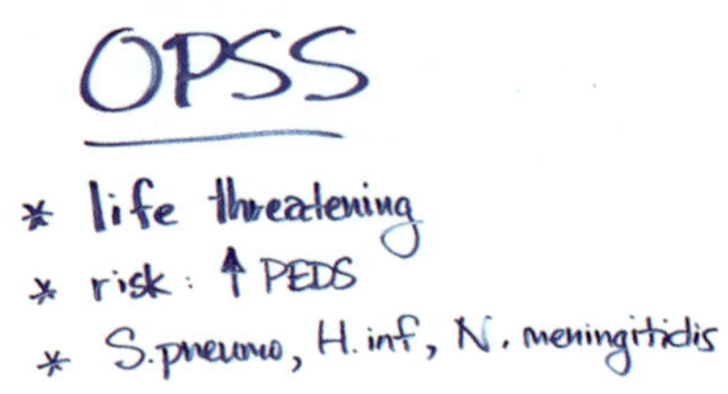

VIDEO 16.8. Overwhelming Postsplencectomy Sepsis. S pneumo indicates *Streptococcus pneumoniae.* Transcript: Overwhelming postsplenectomy sepsis, obviously occurs after you eradicate and remove the spleen. Without a spleen, adults, but more importantly pediatric patients, have a life-threatening risk from encapsulated bacteria. The spleen is fantastic for eradicating *Streptococcus pneumoniae*, *Haemophilus influenzae*, *Neisseria meningitidis*; these 3 organisms can be deadly. So this isn't anything to laugh about. The risk is real. One percent or 2% of people that have this will die from it, especially young patients. The older we are as adults, we have been exposed to more bacteria and the rest of the body can handle some of these infections. But young tots, 1, 2, 3, and 4 years old, have a real risk. So when in doubt, if you can preserve the spleen, you want to preserve the spleen. If you know you are going to have to take out the spleen in someone, if you can give the vaccine for *S pneumoniae*, *H influenzae*, and *Neisseria* preoperatively, a couple weeks in advance that would be useful. So you have trained your spleen and the rest of the body to be prepared for that, then take the spleen out. If you can't give someone a vaccine, a 4 year old in a bicycle accident needs their spleen out, then shortly after surgery, within a week or 2 vaccinations are given. Antibiotics are typically given for the teenage years through the teenage years of a child, and then careful education for the family and the patient. The lifelong risk of OPSS is real. It is a life-threatening problem.

Spleen Challenge Questions

16.1. Where are the splenic vessels located?
16.2. Why do deceleration injuries cause splenic trauma?
16.3. What is the Rule of Odds for the spleen?
16.4. How do you detect a pancreatic leak?
16.5. Which vessel is preferably ligated first during splenectomy?
16.6. Which traumatized spleens must be removed?
16.7. What are the indications for elective splenectomy?
16.8. Where are accessory spleens located?
16.9. How might an endoscopist damage the spleen?
16.10. Which children may require splenectomy for pain relief?

Answers to Spleen Challenge Questions

16.1. In the retroperitoneum. The splenic vein is just posterior to the pancreas. The splenic artery meanders but is close to the pancreas.

16.2. The body stops, the spleen moves forward, the splenic attachments hold tight, and these forces cause tears in the fragile spleen.

16.3. The normal spleen is 1×3×5 inches in size, weighs 7 ounces, and lies between ribs 9 and 11 in the left upper abdominal quadrant.

16.4. A pancreatic leak is eventually confirmed with sampling a fluid collection showing high amylase levels.

16.5. The splenic artery. Ligation allows the spleen to empty of blood (autotransfusion).

16.6. Those leading to severe instability (hypotension, tachycardia) or unresponsiveness to fluid resuscitation or blood. Often, they must be removed in patients with severe head injuries or others requiring anticoagulation. Most patients with injured spleens can be observed (IV fluids, rest, blood transfusion as needed) or have embolization if a vascular blush is noted on CT.

16.7. The 3 Ps: Pain, -Penias (eg, thrombocytopenia, leukopenia), and Pallor (anemia).

16.8. Perisplenic area, omentum, retroperitoneum, or perigonadal area.

16.9. Applying torque on the splenic flexure during colonoscopy.

16.10. Children with spherocytosis and idiopathic thrombocytopenic purpura can have painful splenic infarctions.

17

Stomach

Embryology

The stomach develops during the fifth week of gestation from the dilated caudal portion of the foregut.

Anatomy

The gastric cardia is just distal to the gastroesophageal junction, the fundus is the upper curvature to the left of the cardia, the body is the central region between the fundus and antrum, and the antrum tapers into the pylorus. The stomach receives its blood supply (Figure 17.1) through the right and left gastric, right and left gastroepiploic, and splenic arteries, all of which have extensive collaterals that protect the stomach against ischemia. Veins mirror the arterial pathways.

Physiology

Gastric parietal cells (Video 17.1) secrete hydrochloric acid and intrinsic factor, chief cells secrete pepsinogen (Video 17.2), and G cells secrete gastrin (Video 17.3).

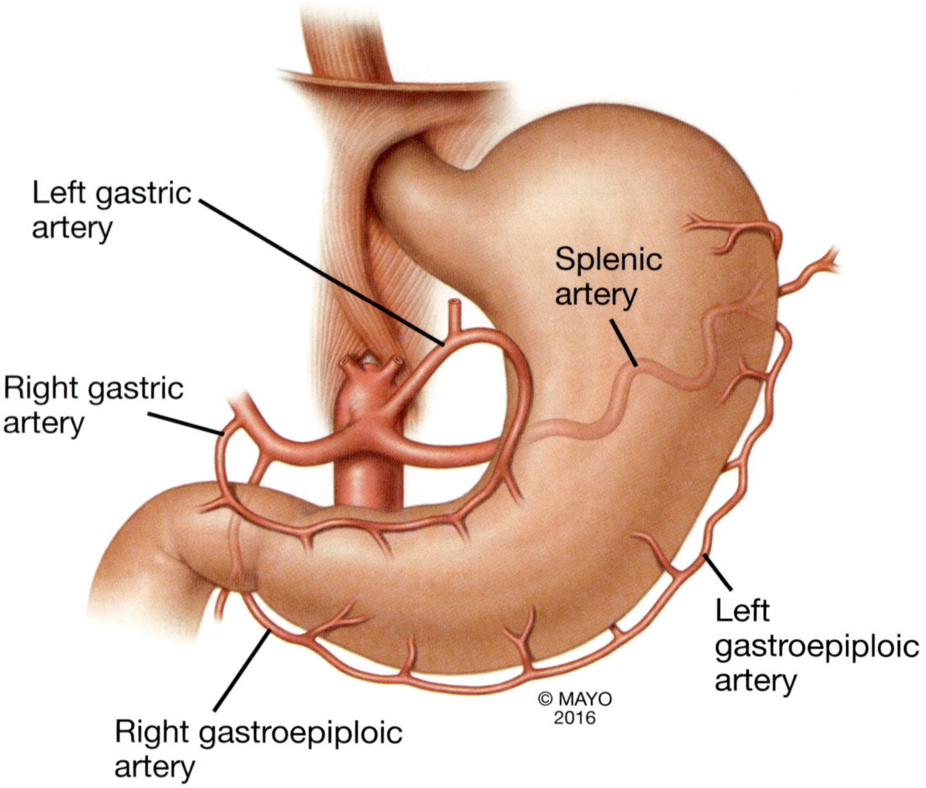

FIGURE 17.1. Arterial Blood Supply for the Stomach.

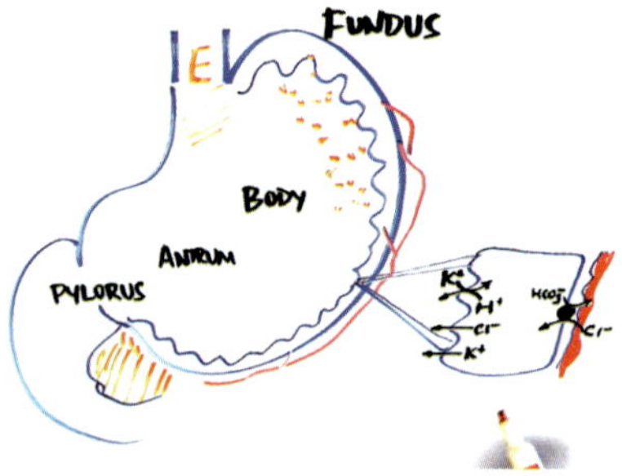

VIDEO 17.1. Parietal Cells in the Stomach.
Transcript: So the human stomach is broken up into the cardia right near the esophagus and the gastric junction. That is the cardia, this region here. The fundus is above the cardia and it can expand to accommodate food. The body is the middle portion of the stomach. The antrum, a little bit more muscular and thicker, and the pylorus gives way to the duodenum.

It is important to note that within the fundus and the body, the parietal cells are dominant. We have got lots of parietal cells throughout the stomach wall and these parietal cells are great at doing 2 things: making hydrochloric acid and secreting and creating intrinsic factor. Both of those things are crucial to digestion as well as red blood cell production.

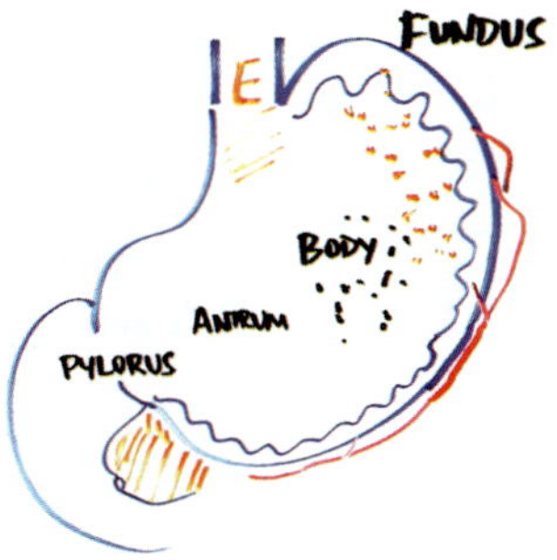

VIDEO 17.2. Chief Cells in the Stomach.
Transcript: Chief cells are located throughout the stomach and the chief cells are important and they create a zymogen or proenzyme called pepsinogen. It is secreted by the chief cells and that pepsinogen gets cleaved by hydrochloric acid in the stomach. And pepsinogen becomes pepsin and pepsin becomes crucial to breaking down protein, a vital function of the stomach.

Clinical Presentation

PUD (Video 17.4) is the most common cause of massive UGI bleeding. Pain is invariably the presenting symptom, which worsens with food in patients with gastric ulcers (Video 17.5). Severe PUD and diarrhea from acid hypersecretion occur in Zollinger-Ellison syndrome (Video 17.6). Violent retching in alcoholics can tear the mucosa and submucosa of the stomach near the gastroesophageal junction, resulting in bleeding from Mallory-Weiss tears (Figure 17.2). Neoplasms of the stomach include cancer (most commonly ACA, Video 17.7), GIST (most common benign gastric tumor, Video 17.8), mucosa-associated lymphoid tissue lymphoma (Video 17.9), gastric lymphoma, and carcinoid, among many others.

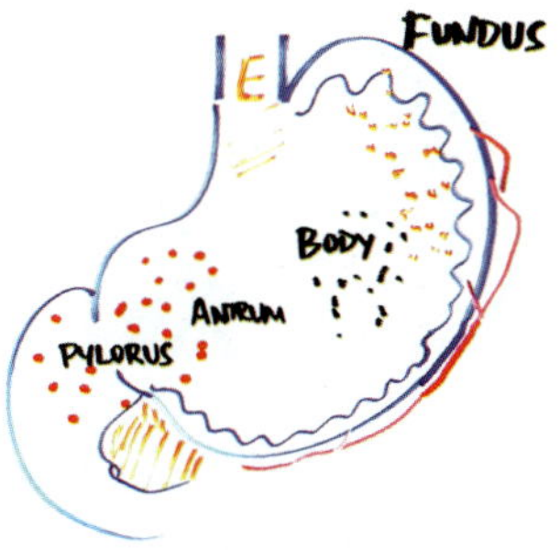

VIDEO 17.3. G Cells in the Stomach.
Transcript: The stomach also secretes and creates gastrin, usually from the antrum, and also parts of the duodenum will do that as well. Gastrin is an important hormone. It will affect the stomach, increasing acid secretion with a direct effect on the parietal cells to make more acid.

It also senses to make more acid when the antrum gets distended when food comes down. Or, when there is no acid in the stomach, the gastrin cells will kick into gear. Gastrin is important for food breakdown.

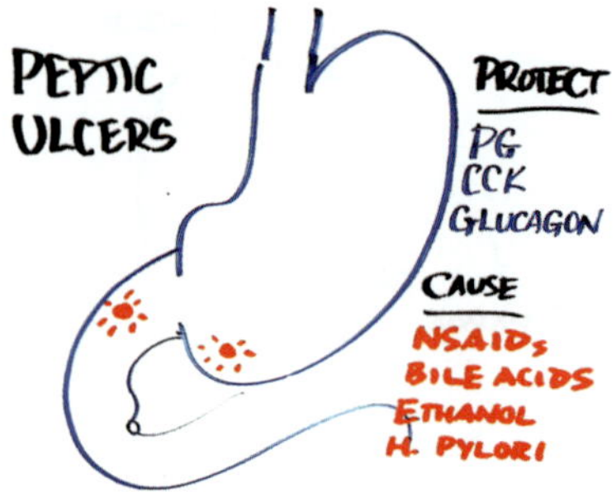

VIDEO 17.4. PUD.

Transcript: Peptic ulcers are common. They typically are caused when too much acid and not enough protection from the mucosa. Things that protect against peptic ulcers are prostaglandins, cholecystokinin, and glucagon. Things that help cause peptic ulcers, which usually mean duodenal ulcers, are nonsteroidal anti-inflammatory drugs, bile acids, ethanol or alcohol, and definitely in this day and age, *H pylori*. Peptic ulcers are frequently in the duodenum.

Gastric ulcers are a little bit different, usually occur on the lesser curvature of the stomach. They tend to have a nice clean smooth base as opposed to a malignant ulcer related to gastric cancer. The risk for gastric ulcers is smoking, alcohol, *H pylori*, uremia, and steroids.

Imaging

Although a UGI series (Video 17.10) can be used for diagnosis of gastric lesions, some are indistinguishable from benign peptic ulcers; all patients with a new gastric ulcer should undergo EGD with biopsy (Video 17.11). Supine and erect radiographs (Video 17.12) should be ordered if ulcer perforation is suspected; it may show free air.

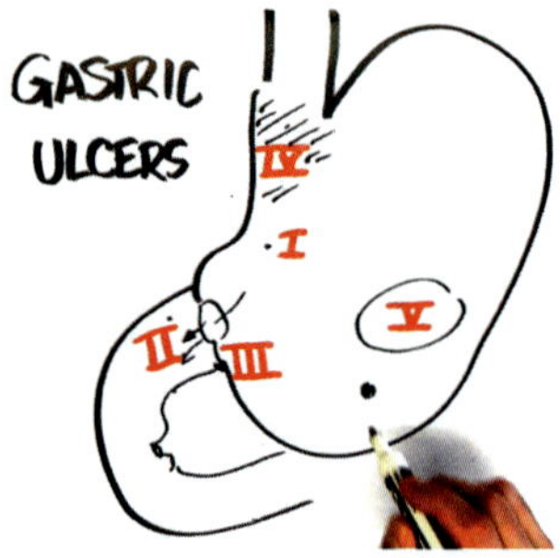

VIDEO 17.5. Gastric Ulcers.

Transcript: Gastric ulcers often happen in malnourished, immunocompromised, or critically ill patients. They are most common on the lesser curvature of the stomach as opposed to the greater curvature. In a type I gastric ulcer, is along the lesser curvature within the body of the stomach. Type II is a lesser curvature ulcer with a duodenal ulcer. So these people actually have not 1, but 2 ulcers. Type III is a prepyloric ulcer not far from the opening where food empties into the duodenum. Type IV is high on the lesser curvature near the cardia. The cardia is that portion of the stomach near the esophagus. And Type V is related to nonsteroidal anti-inflammatory agents. Those pills go down into the stomach and they cause problems locally where they sit.

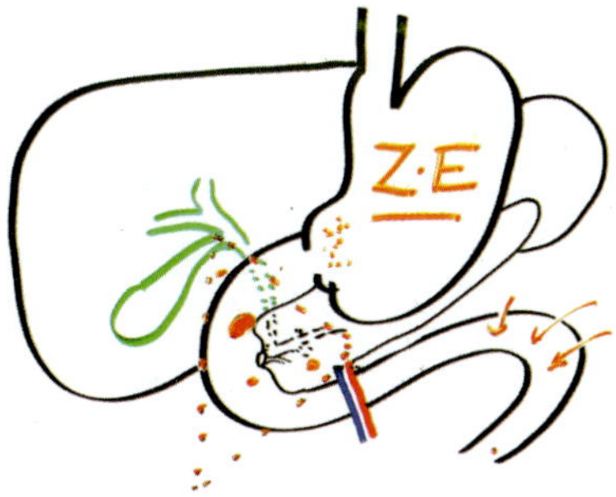

VIDEO 17.6. Zollinger-Ellison Syndrome.

Transcript: Zollinger-Ellison syndrome is a rare disorder and it's a disorder of gastrinemia. Too much gastrin is being generated and that is because there are lumps or bumps, either within the pancreas, in the duodenum, or lymph nodes in what is so-called the gastrinoma triangle. The cystic duct, the neck of the pancreas, the junctions of the second and third portions of the duodenum; there is a funny tumor here that secretes gastrin and tells the antrum to make extra acid. And if it is making extra acid, people develop ulcers not only in the duodenum but downstream in the ileum or the jejunum, or stomach ulcers. Massive diarrhea is common because the body is trying to counteract this acid and puts water into the intestine. So people with peptic ulcer disease and diarrhea, we need to think about this rare syndrome called Zollinger-Ellison syndrome. Two surgeons back in the middle 1900s from Ohio State detected this and treated this. It happens sometimes in patients with MEN syndrome—Zollinger-Ellison syndrome.

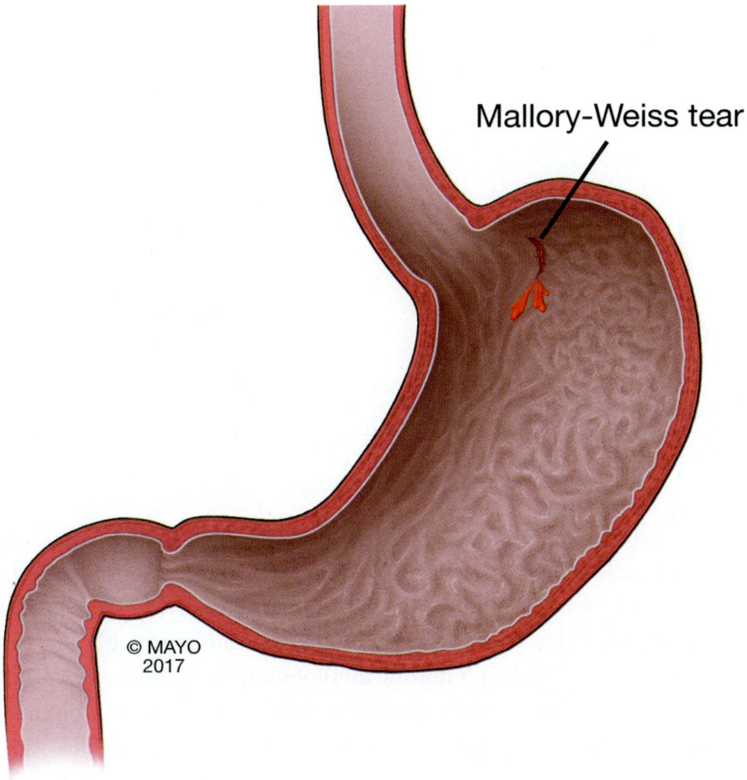

FIGURE 17.2. Location of a Mallory-Weiss Tear.

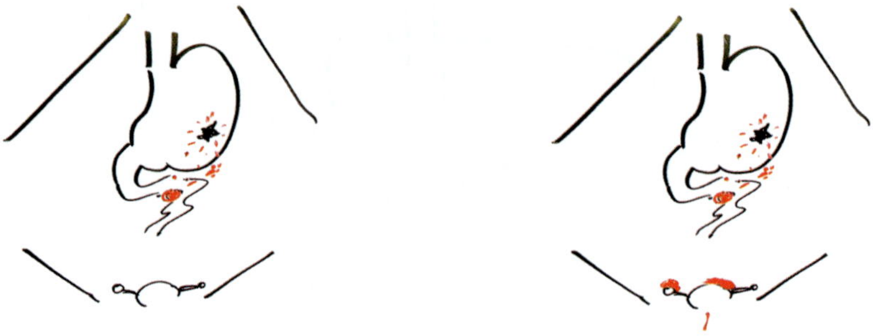

VIDEO 17.7. ACA.

Transcript: Gastric cancer sometimes gives detection on physical examination. A tumor within the stomach may spread, and may spread to a lymph node near the stomach or to the belly button, the umbilicus, and that is often called a Sister Mary Joseph sign. Sister Mary Joseph was a scrub nurse for Dr William Mayo in the late 1890s and early 1900s. She did a lot of stomach surgery and he would comment that she would say, "I feel a lump in the umbilicus, I don't think you will be able to do anything." And he finally asked her, "How do you know that this cancer is going to be advanced?" "I can feel a spot in the umbilicus." That is usually a very rapidly advancing tumor and we don't see that very often nowadays.

On rectal examination, especially in a woman, or man, feeling through the rectum, sometimes firmness, especially near the vagina in a woman, is what is called a Blumer's shelf, a thickening that you would not normally expect. Or on physical examination, a mass in an ovary, so-called a Krukenberg tumor. Those would be 3 separate things showing advanced cancer; a Sister Mary Joseph sign, a Blumer's shelf palpation, or a Krukenberg tumor.

VIDEO 17.8. GIST.

Transcript: Gastrointestinal stromal tumors, or mesenchymal tumors, are rare lesions of the stomach that occur from the smooth muscle cells within the wall of the stomach or other spots in the GI tract. These cells are called interstitial cells of Cajal. The problem is a mutation in the C-kit gene. A majority of these tumors will stain positively for C-kit. Most of these tumors are readily treatable and curable. As they get larger with higher mitotic rates, more than 5 mitotic divisions within 50 high-power cells will let us know that we have a worrisome lesion. Most times resection, simple wedge resection, or enucleation will solve the problem. But larger tumors will require formal resection and Gleevec and imatinib, 2 chemotherapy agents, are effective against treating these tumors, oftentimes dissolving them even with evidence of liver metastasis.

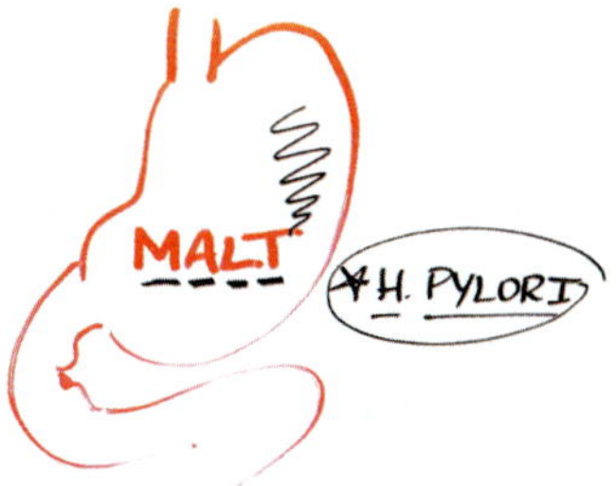

VIDEO 17.9. Mucosa-associated Lymphoid Tissue.

Transcript: Lymphoma of the stomach can happen. It is usually a rare type of lymphoma called mucosa-associated lymphoid tissue or so-called MALT lymphoma. It's unusual, when you get a biopsy of this lesion, pathologists can tell you that it is there and they can tell you that it is related to *Helicobacter pylori*. And if you treat the *Helicobacter pylori*, the MALT lymphoma melts away. If the entire stomach is involved and we can't get this treated, resecting the entire stomach is possible. But what I want you to remember are when you see MALT lymphoma, think about treating that with simple antibiotics of *H pylori* and watch this so-called cancer melt away.

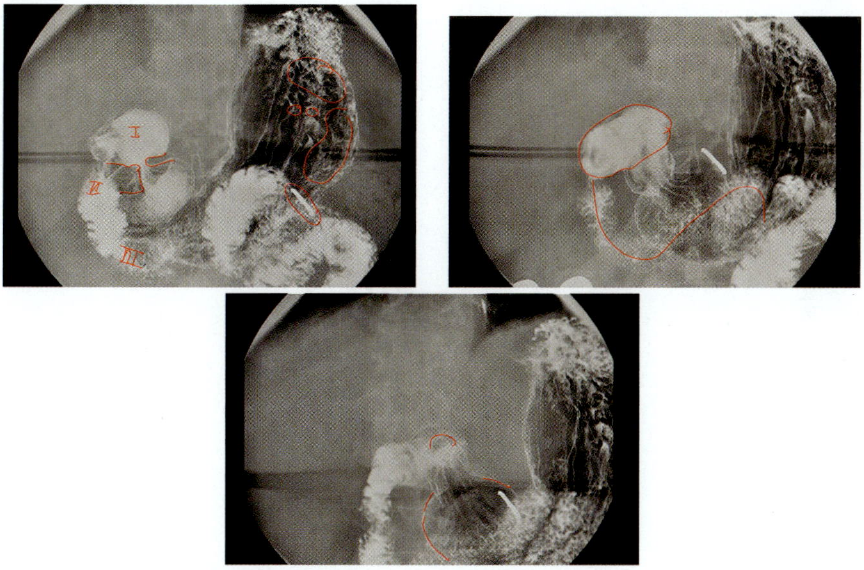

VIDEO 17.10. UGI Series Radiographs.

Transcript: An upper GI series, that is upper gastrointestinal tract series, is nothing more than a patient swallowing some material, either gastrografin or barium, and outlining the stomach, the antrum, the pylorus, the first portion of the duodenum, and then the second, third, and fourth portions as it moves on. This is a test done with a radiologist in the room. And the reason I know that is this thing right here. It's a wooden paddle with a little piece of metal on the top. And the radiologist actually taps on the abdomen and kind of squishes things around. So this is an upper GI study that actually shows a patient that swallowed some barium and has a couple tiny little polyps here, nothing terribly worrisome. The dye has moved on. Maybe there is a little bit of difference in the antrum, there are not quite so many rugae. And

VIDEO 17.10. Continued

this is the rugae that we see. Those are normal looking things. Maybe there is a little inflammation down here but the key thing for me to teach you are this little structure here, this is a pylorus; this is the muscular area where things are firing through from the stomach to the antrum. And then to the first portion of the duodenum, then the second portion, and the third portion, and then the fourth as it sneaks up. This is a relatively normal study; I don't see any big ulcers or erosions.

Let's take a look at a couple of other normal pictures. So again, we can see that the radiologist's paddle, we know that they are at the helm. This is a nice picture. It doesn't show us the fundus as well; the body, the antrum, the pylorus is down here as the stomach makes waves and you can see things sort of moving through. This is a big bulb of the duodenum, the first portion of the duodenum. And we get a sense again, stomach curving up to the duodenum, and then the second, third, and fourth portions of the duodenum and eventually become part of the jejunum.

Let's take another picture. So now this radiologist is clearly fixating and focused on, is there an ulcer here in the duodenum? Is the antrum normal? And there is maybe some mild inflammation. I am not a radiologist, but I can see their paddle and poking here. They have got their paddle pushing and trying to clear things out, get gas out of the way, get the dye moving around, and give them the best look. Then these become static images. And then we get a chance to decide alright is there a problem or not.

Upper GI series is useful for bowel obstructions, polyps downstream; but, in this day and age, most people are doing endoscopic evaluations.

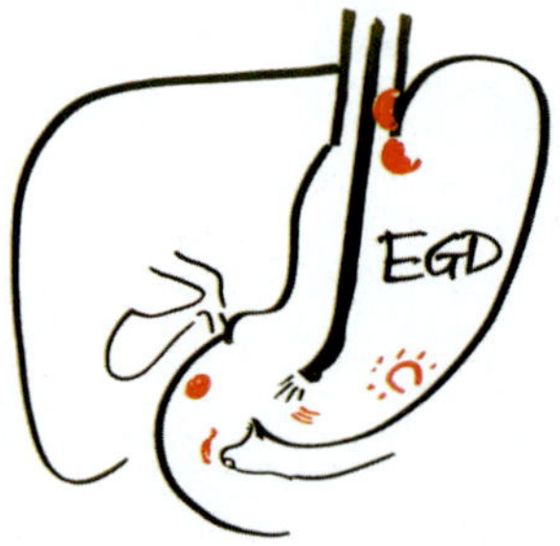

VIDEO 17.11. EGD.

Transcript: We can't talk about the stomach and stomach surgery without talking about endoscopic biopsy, so-called esophagogastroduodenoscopy (EGD). When the person performing this, whether they are a surgeon, gastroenterologist, internist, a variety of reasons to do this; looking for tumors, lumps and bumps, looking for healing ulcers, looking for ulcers, and looking for bleeding. A variety of other accesses can be obtained through the pancreas looking at the biliary tree, downstream in the small bowel. But most times EGD is to look at the stomach and the first portion of the duodenum; looking for neoplasia, looking for healing, looking for ulcers, looking for bleeding. The nice thing about EGD, it can also sometimes be therapeutic. It can band gastric or esophageal varices. It can treat bleeding episodes. It is a wonderful tool if used well; it's incredibly helpful to our patients.

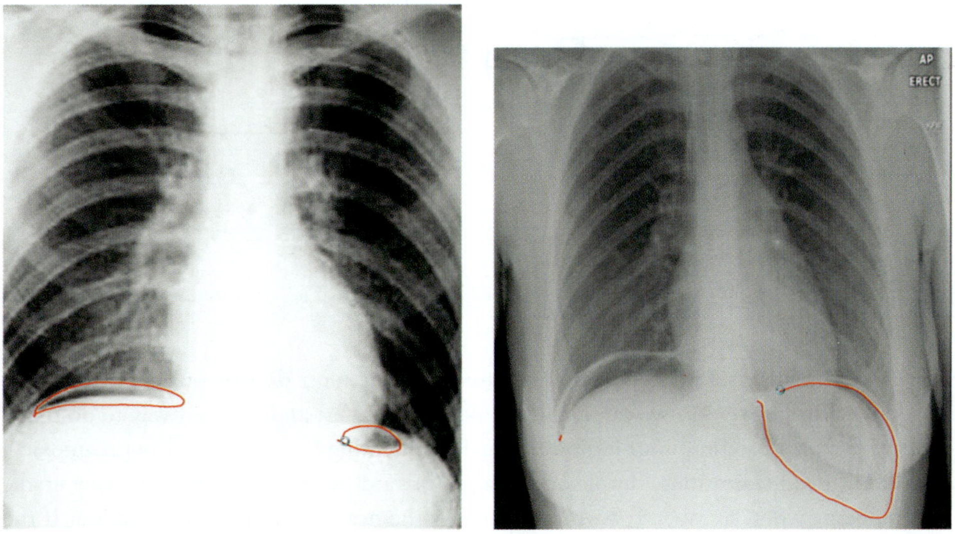

VIDEO 17.12. Chest Radiograph.
Transcript: A chest x-ray isn't the greatest film to look at the stomach. In fact, it is terrible! Having said that, medical students and trainees will look at this, and I am hopeful on an upright chest x-ray, you see this spot and this spot. Now a gastric air bubble is fairly normal, but air underneath the diaphragm above the liver, that is free air, that's a perforation. It usually happens in the duodenum or the stomach. That would be something to be nervous about. This is a little more modern picture in a healthier younger person; but here we see far more free air. Take a look at this spot. There is a lot of air underneath there. Same thing on this spot, there may be huge amounts of air. This is somebody that likely has a larger hole, a gastric ulcer, and it's pouring bile and whatnot; but air underneath the diaphragm and they come in with severe pain. An x-ray like this typically means we are going to the operating room and we don't need all of these other tests. A chest x-ray is useful for gastric problems.

Operation

Surgery for ulcers is now uncommon; most benign gastric ulcers respond well to proton pump inhibitors and *Helicobacter pylori* eradication (Video 17.13). Truncal vagotomy and antrectomy are reserved for PUD complications (bleeding, perforation, and obstruction) (Video 17.14). Near total or total gastrectomy is indicated for resectable gastric cancers (Video 17.15). The most common gastric surgery is now bariatric (Video 17.16).

Complications

Possible complications of gastric surgery include bleeding, anastomotic leak or stricture, or reflux esophagitis (Video 17.17).

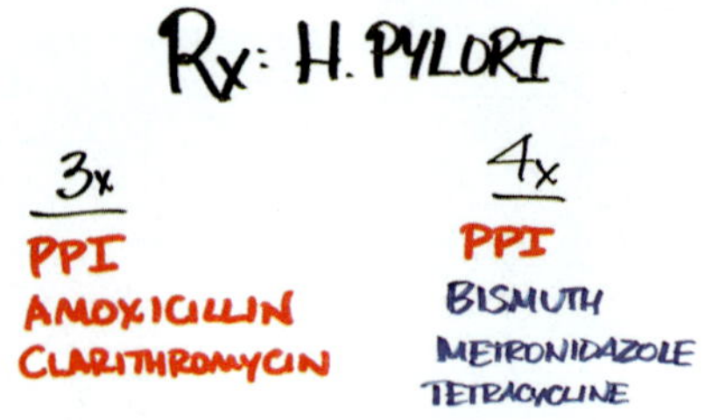

VIDEO 17.13. *Helicobacter pylori* Eradication.
Transcript: *H pylori* remains a high incidence of causing peptic ulcer disease—ulcers within the duodenum. If we can eradicate *H pylori* we can eradicate ulcers. The safest and quickest way to do that and the least expensive is with a proton pump inhibitor, usually something like omeprazole with amoxicillin and clarithromycin. Three medications, simple and straightforward, over 7 to 10 days, usually eradicates *H pylori*. If this doesn't work, number 1, I would ponder is the person taking the medication. If they truly did it, and we don't get rid of *H pylori* then we would go with a PPI, bismuth, metronidazole, and tetracycline. One of these 2 methods typically will eradicate *H pylori* in nearly 95 or more percent of the time.

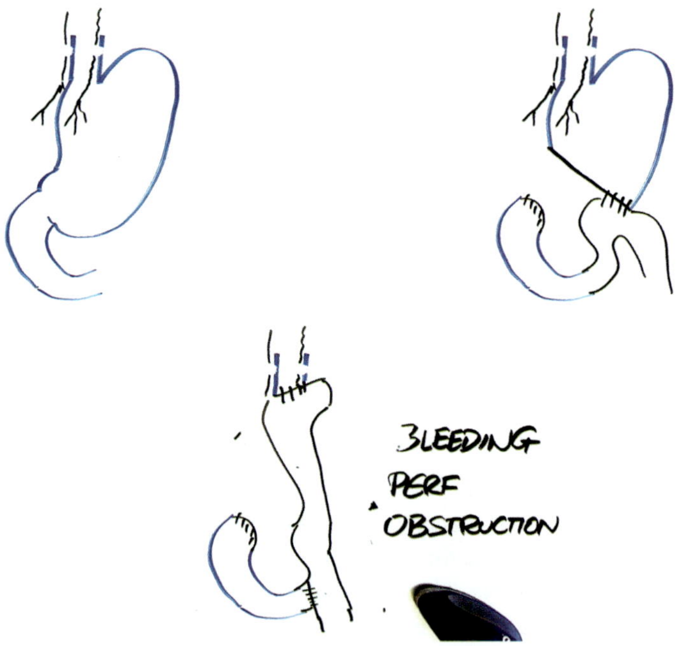

VIDEO 17.14. Truncal Vagotomy, Antrectomy, and Surgery for PUD Complications.
Transcript: If medical therapy doesn't eradicate peptic ulcer disease, then we can start thinking about potentially aggressive surgical intervention. If we cut the vagus nerves, the left and the right, that will decrease acid production. But it also affects the motility of the GI tract that is a big thing to do. We could also remove the antrum, get rid of the gastrin secretion; that, too, is a big move. Now we need some sort of anastomosis to hook up and that may cause reflux and other problems. But if need be, those are reasonable options. This is what is called a truncal vagotomy or vagectomy and antrectomy, with either

VIDEO 17.14. Continued

a Billroth I or a Billroth II gastrojejunostomy. These are effective on decreasing the acid secretion in the stomach. More likely nowadays, we are not treating patients with problems like this with surgery, we do it with medicine; proton pump inhibitors, H_2 blockers, antacids, and so forth.

Where we start thinking about bigger aggressive operations like this we think about major problems with bleeding, perforation, or obstruction. And these are complex problems. Bleeding from throughout the stomach that can be a terminal event or a massive ulcer or a cancer. Perforation—an actual hole with acid and succus secreting out can be a septic event and a life-threatening one. Surgical intervention sometimes simple repair versus resection. Obstruction—terrible ulcer disease or a malignancy, and that is when we start to need to think about antrectomy, subtotal gastrectomy, which leaves some cuff of stomach versus total gastrectomy. Total is exactly that, we lose the entire stomach and we bring up a Roux limb, this is jejunum, and people no longer have a stomach. And as you well know vitamin B_{12} intrinsic factor, those will be important medications or shots to give postoperatively. And life is completely different without that stomach, there is no reservoir, people immediately fill up quickly, and this becomes a weight-losing problem or a malnutrition problem. People can live nicely, but it takes a very motivated and dedicated patient to do it. But when you think of big problems of bleeding, perforation, or obstruction, we think of bigger gastric surgery.

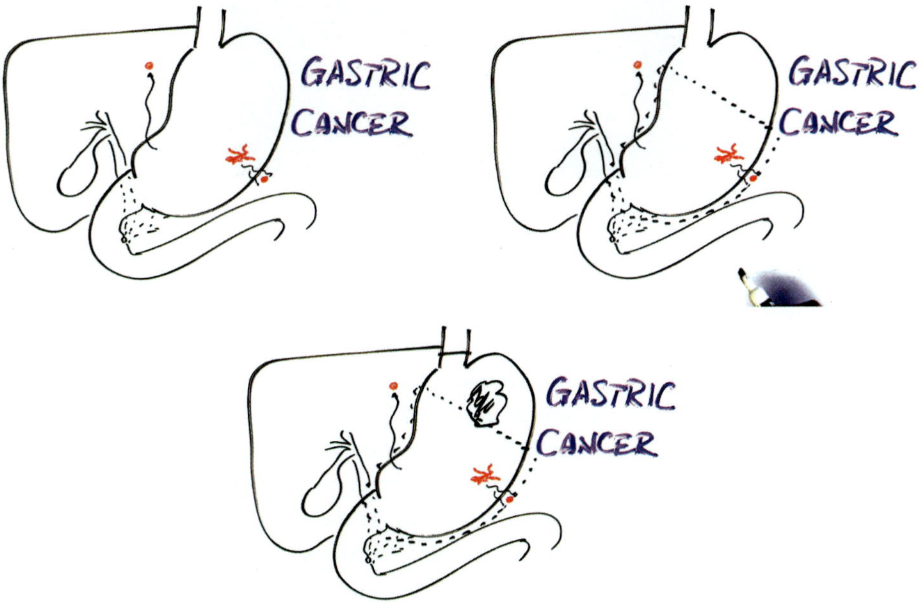

VIDEO 17.15. Gastric Cancer.

Transcript: Gastric cancer is fortuitously decreasing in the United States. Incidences are still high in Japan, or Chile, or Finland. Places perhaps where smoked fish or raw fish, and other forms of environmental toxins, may increase the risk of gastric cancer. In the United States it is decreasing but it is still a deadly disease. It often forms in the body or the antrum of the stomach. It often invades lymph nodes early on and metastatic disease to the liver, it makes it unresectable. Oftentimes tumors now can be treated with chemotherapy with some evidence of benefit, but in an ideal world with a tumor in the body, most

VIDEO 17.15. Continued
surgeons will do a subtotal gastrectomy, removing the lymph nodes and removing most of the stomach. If the tumor itself is much higher up in the stomach, then the entire stomach, what is called a total gastrectomy, this entire stomach will be removed. These are big operations that carry some risk, but patients if caught early enough can be cured with gastric cancer.

Numerous Japanese articles talk about early screening, catching early cancers and treating them endoscopically, and biopsying, and removing lesions.

Unfortunately, in the United States when cancers develop in the stomach they are usually detected late, often with lymph node and metastatic involvement, so the risk of mortality is very high.

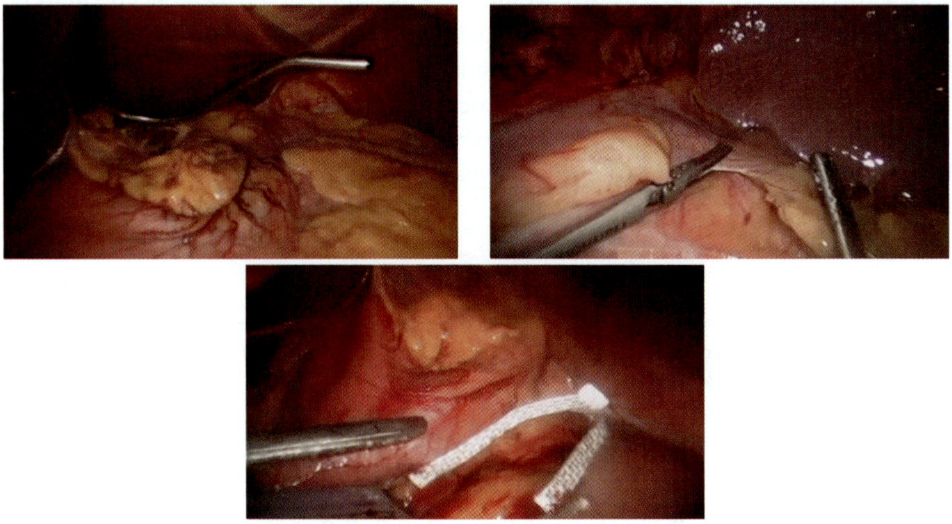

VIDEO 17.16. Laparoscopic Sleeve Gastrectomy: Intraoperative.
Transcript: There are numerous bariatric operations. This one is showing the left lateral sector of the liver being moved out of the way to show us the stomach underneath so we can do what is called a sleeve gastrectomy. We are looking from the belly button up toward the head. The heart will be beating in the background. Grasper in the left hand, hook cautery, it is actually an L hook, releasing these attachments up underneath the liver, the lesser omentum, the stomach down below. This is going to be the greater omentum. We are going to get into the retrostomach space and basically at that point we will get to be able to see the pancreas. The colon is below us, the stomach is above us. And we are dividing those attachments that head out toward the spleen, and we will chase this greater curvature all the way up. This Harmonic scalpel, a wonderful tool that goes through little blood vessels and fatty tissue without any difficulty.

The spleen is to the right. The liver is above the screen. The stomach is to the left. The pancreas is deep to us. We want to make sure that we don't cut off the stomach; we are right on the edge. Short gastric vessels, these are vessels, typically veins that go from the stomach to the spleen and we want to take care of those. We are eventually going to divide this entire stomach and take a big strip of it all the way along from the antrum all the way up to the GE junction. So the antrum and pylorus is to the left, the body of the stomach is sitting in front of us. We are going to start in the antrum with a big stapling device. We are along the gastric curve, the greater omentum, the greater curvature, and this stapler is going to fire 6 staple lines and cut in the middle of it. Beautiful!

Oftentimes there will be a bougie or a tube in the stomach to know just how much stomach we are going to take. So instead of having a big water bottle type of stomach, we are going to end up with a long

VIDEO 17.16. Continued

tube. And there is a tube in the stomach to the left of that stapler. We are just methodically marching up, and we are going to cut off a huge section of the stomach. We are up near the GE junction now and we can see the spleen up behind us. The stapler is being deployed. Are we going to get to the entire thing? It is going to be close. It doesn't look like we quite made it. We will need 1 more staple to divide it. And then once we get that divided, we can remove that with a plastic bag through 1 of the smaller incisions. The patient can go home the next day or day after. And this usually generates significant weight loss without some of the other problems seen from a Roux-en-Y gastrojejunostomy.

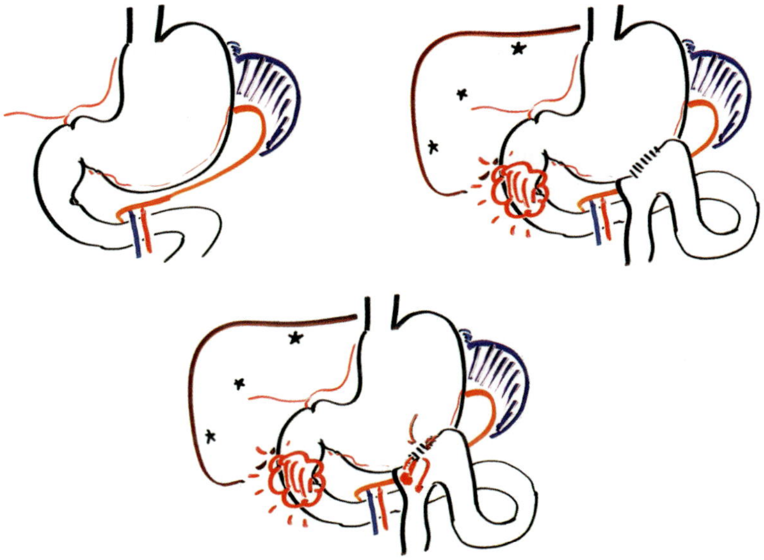

VIDEO 17.17. Complications After Gastric Surgery.

Transcript: Esophagus, stomach, duodenum, pancreas, and spleen. If you are going to operate on the stomach you just have to recognize what is close by it and what problems might you have. Injuring the short gastric veins, injuring the pancreas, tearing the spleen, and then the stomach has an amazing blood supply and if you are going to cut part of it off, bleeding, and if you are going to sew it to something else, potential stricture anastomosis or other problems.

Let me show you what I mean. So in this patient we have got liver metastasis from a duodenal cancer. The patient is obstructed and vomiting. Sometimes people do what is called a palliative bypass; hook up the stomach to the jejunum. The duodenum underneath, the jejunum comes around. When we sew this together, 2 nice layers and nice healthy anastomosis, it usually works well. A couple of things can go badly. You can bleed from this and the mucosa of the stomach has a great blood supply. So when you sew this together avoid bleeding postoperatively—careful anastomosis.

The stomach has acid. The jejunum is not ready to protect itself of that. The pancreas and biliary juice might be blocked, and so you could have an ulcer. And that would look something like downstream here, an ulcer, which might cause bleeding or it could stricture and narrow down this anastomosis so it would be hard for food to get through.

Complications after gastric surgery: we have to think about bleeding, ulceration, anastomotic stricture, and then some patients will have reflux with material that goes back up into the intestine—reflux esophagitis. The number 1 thing though, bleeding, stricture, and leaking after surgery. Technically you have to do a good job to avoid those problems.

Stomach Challenge Questions

17.1. What percentage of gastric and duodenal ulcers are associated with *Helicobacter pylori* infection in the United States?

17.2. Why is the left vagal trunk anterior to the stomach and the right vagal trunk posterior?

17.3. What is a Cushing ulcer? Curling ulcer?

17.4. What is a Virchow node?

17.5. When are GISTs considered malignant?

17.6. What are the steps for a Roux-en-Y gastric bypass?

17.7. What is a Borchardt triad?

17.8. What is a Heineke-Mikulicz pyloroplasty? Why is it important after a vagectomy?

17.9. What is a Sister Mary Joseph nodule?

17.10. Who was A. Theodore Billroth? Who was his famous musician friend?

(Answers appear on page 244)

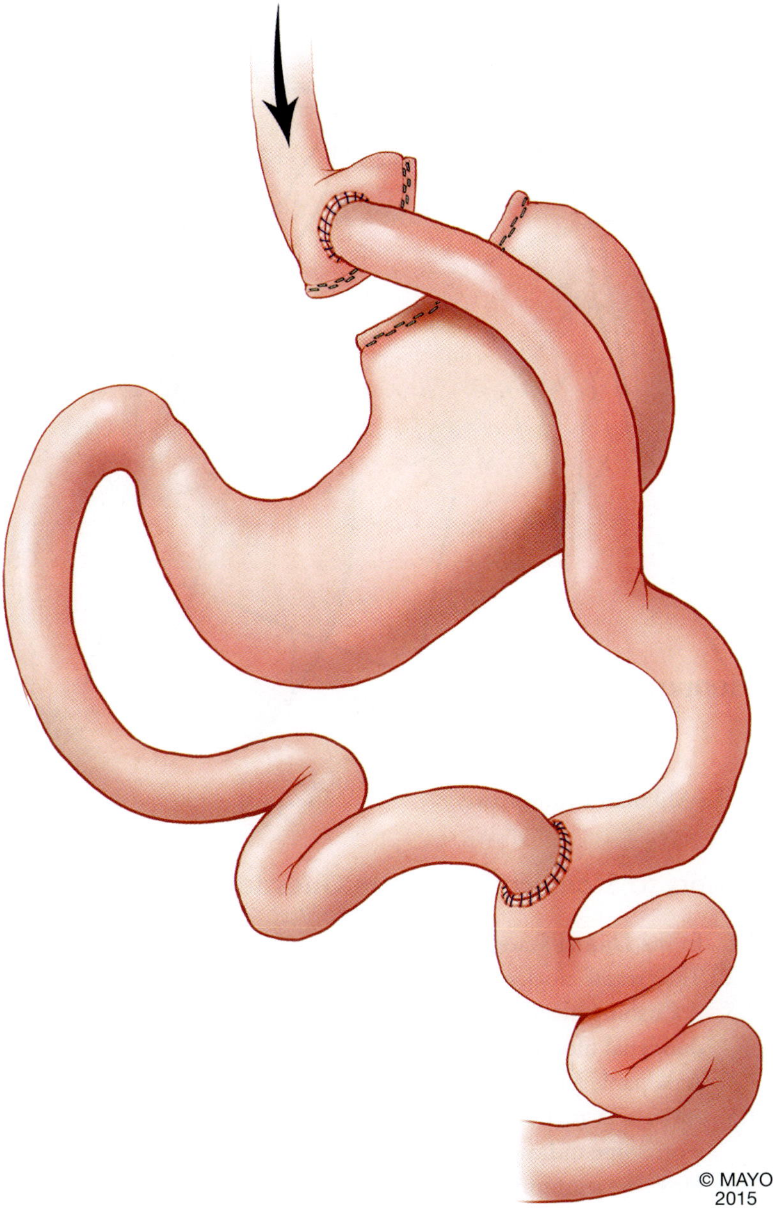

FIGURE 17.3. Roux-en-Y Gastric Bypass.

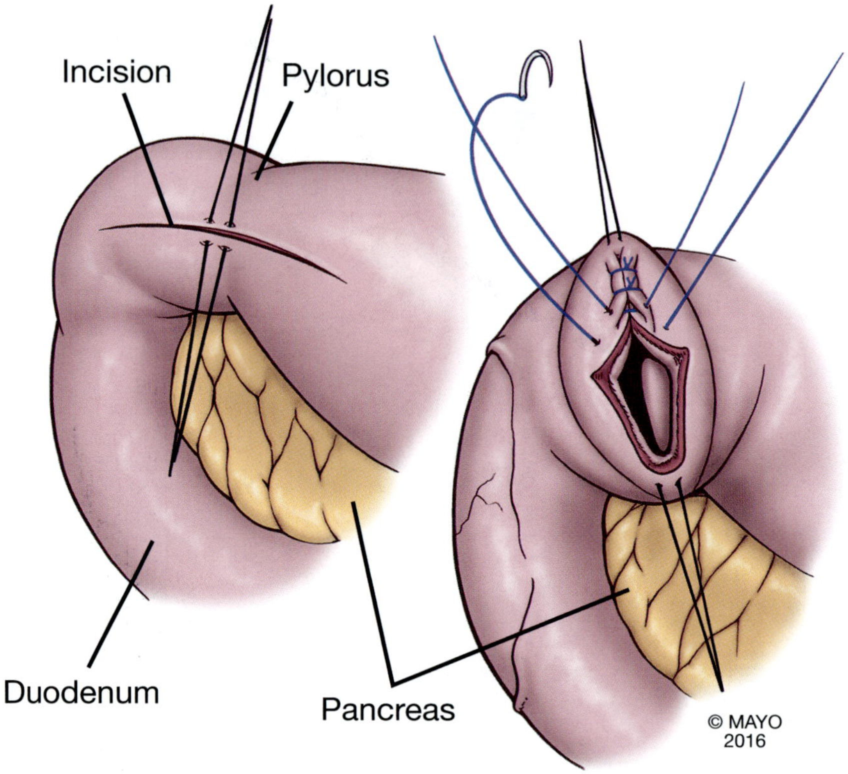

FIGURE 17.4. Heineke-Mikulicz Pyloroplasty.

Answers to Stomach Challenge Questions

17.1. In the United States the incidence is 1%, prevalence 2%.

17.2. They rotate clockwise as they progress along the esophagus and stomach.

17.3. A Cushing ulcer is a gastric ulcer related to neurologic injury. A Curling ulcer is a duodenal ulcer seen in patients with cutaneous burn injuries.

17.4. A palpable left supraclavicular neck node representing metastatic cancer.

17.5. All GISTs are potentially malignant, but greater size and more mitotic figures are worrisome indications.

17.6. First, the jejunum and cardia are transected. Next, the distal part of the transected jejunum is brought cephalad and sewn to the proximal stomach. The proximal jejunum (biliary limb) is sewn downstream to the jejunum (Figure 17.3).

17.7. The combination of epigastric pain, retching, and an inability to pass a nasogastric tube due to a gastric volvulus.

17.8. Longitudinal transection, repaired transversely to fix the pylorus in an open position (Figure 17.4). It is important because the pylorus may fail to empty after a vagotomy (properly termed a vagectomy) (>20%).

17.9. A palpable periumbilical mass (malignant lymph node) representing an advanced intra-abdominal malignancy.

17.10. Legendary German surgeon (1829-1894) and leader in modern abdominal surgery. His musician friend was Johannes Brahms.

18

Thyroid

Embryology

The thyroid gland forms from endoderm beginning at gestational week 5. Parafollicular cells (Video 18.1) develop from neural crest cells (Figure 18.1).

Anatomy

The butterfly-shaped thyroid gland wraps around the trachea, cricoid, and thyroid cartilages. Deep to the strap muscles, the thyroid gland is supplied by paired superior and inferior thyroid arteries (Figure 18.2) and drained by 3 thyroid veins (Figure 18.3). Parathyroid glands usually abut the thyroid on its posterior aspect.

Physiology

Excess thyroxine causes hyperthyroidism and suppression of the sensitive thyroid-stimulating hormone value (Video 18.2).

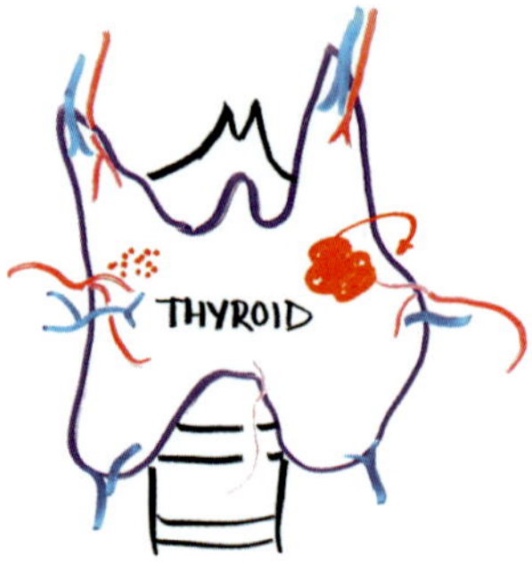

VIDEO 18.1. Parafollicular Cells.
Transcript: Parafollicular cells are cells on the back side of the thyroid gland, usually about a third of the way down, and they secrete calcitonin. Calcitonin regulates calcium levels in the body. Not crucially important, but parafollicular cells, if they get out of control, can turn into what's called medullary thyroid cancer. So, parafollicular cells, important for secreting calcitonin and potentially developing medullary thyroid cancer.

Clinical Presentation

Hyperthyroidism may cause sweating, irritability, weight loss, and atrial fibrillation. Thyroid nodules (Video 18.3) may cause voice changes and compressive symptoms with swallowing and breathing. Most thyroid nodules are benign and asymptomatic (95%), but as many as 100,000 thyroid cancers (Video 18.4) are diagnosed each year in the United States.

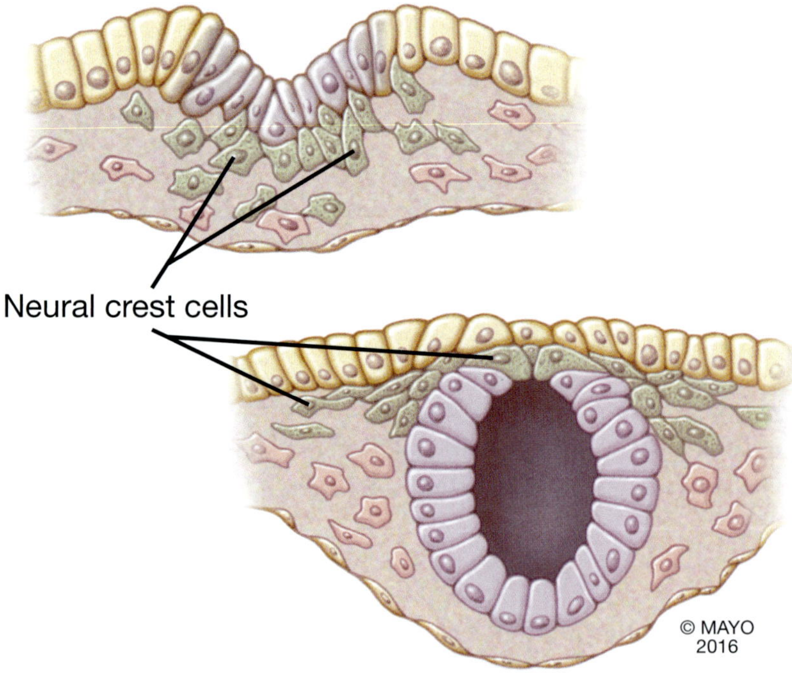

FIGURE 18.1. Neural Crest Cells.

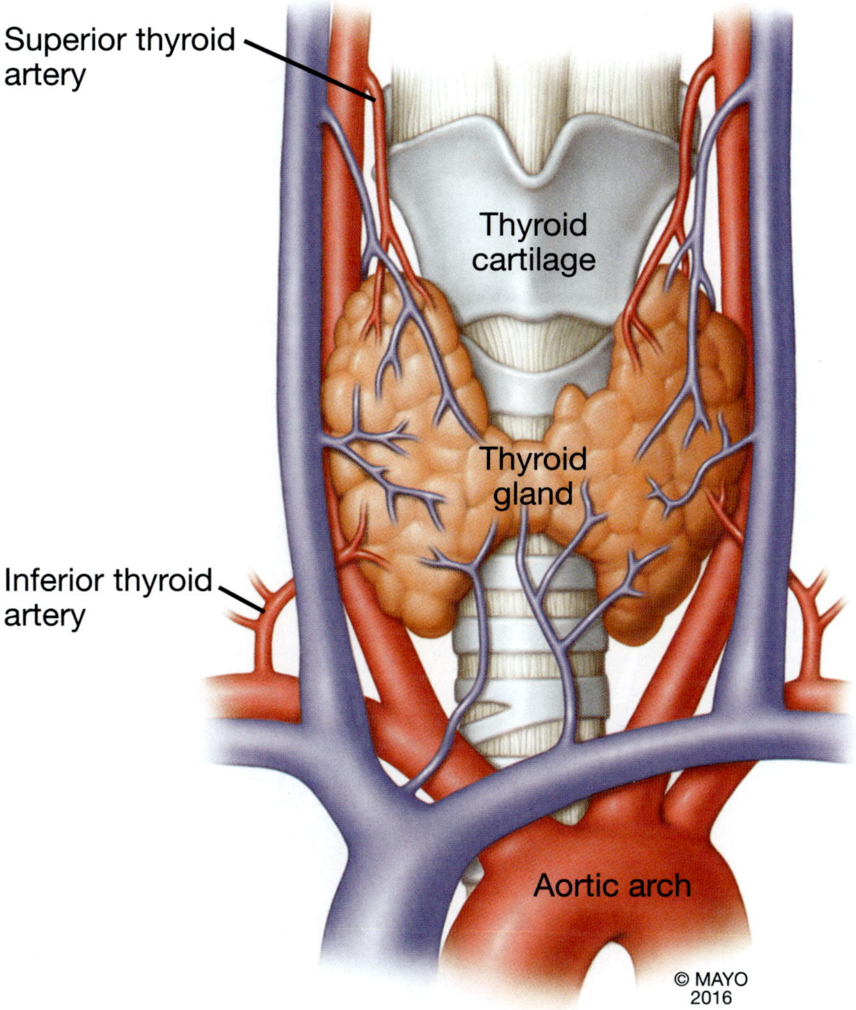

FIGURE 18.2. Blood Supply for the Thyroid Gland.

Imaging

US (Video 18.5), nuclear imaging (Video 18.6), and CT (Video 18.7) are useful. Fine-needle aspiration (Video 18.8) is critical for evaluation of thyroid nodules.

Operation

Collar incisions of the neck with transection of the platysma muscle (Figure 18.4), opening the median raphe (Video 18.9), and exposing the thyroid isthmus are straightforward steps (Video 18.10). Removing half (thyroid lobectomy and isthmectomy) or all (total or near-total thyroidectomy) (Videos 18.11 and 18.12) of the thyroid gland involves careful dissection, exposure, and transection of the arteries and veins of the gland. Layered wound closure involves loose reapproximation of the sternohyoid muscles and platysma.

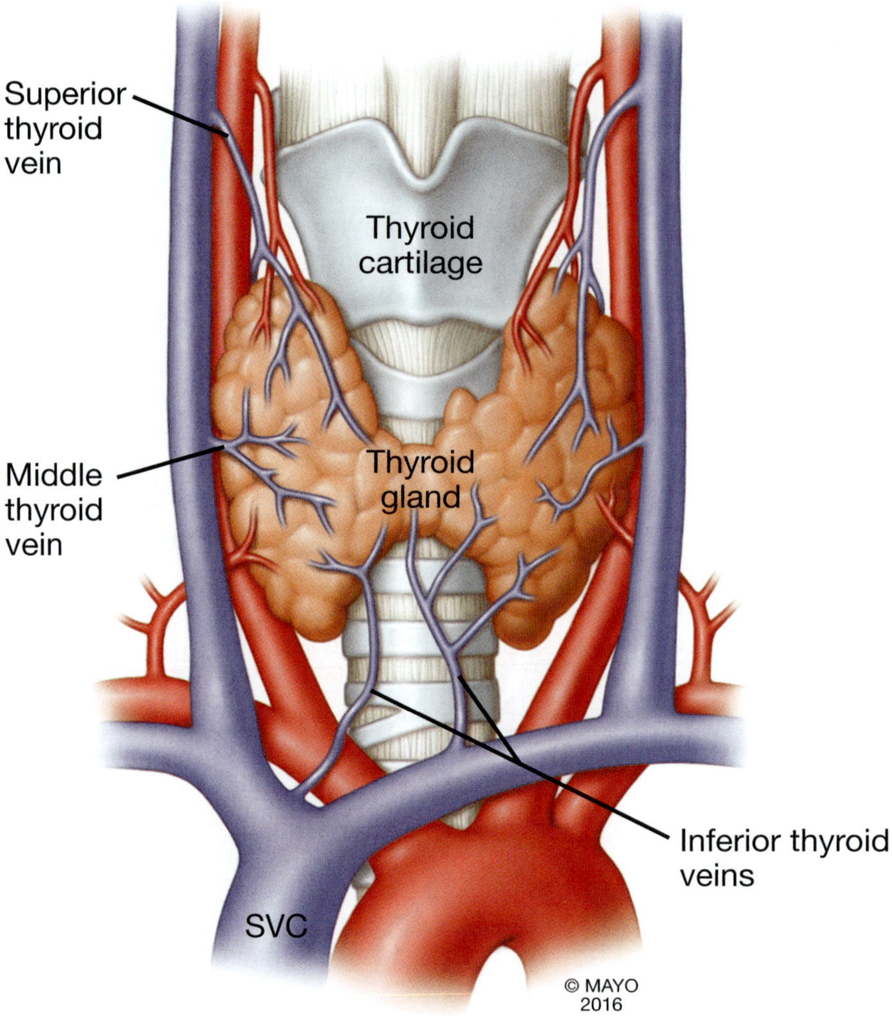

FIGURE 18.3. Veins Draining the Thyroid Gland. SVC indicates superior vena cava.

Complications

Possible surgical complications are postoperative hematoma (<1%) (Figure 18.5), RLN injury (about 1%) (Video 18.13), and temporary hypoparathyroidism (10%-20%), and they should be avoided at all costs. Early recognition of cervical hematoma and evacuation may be lifesaving.

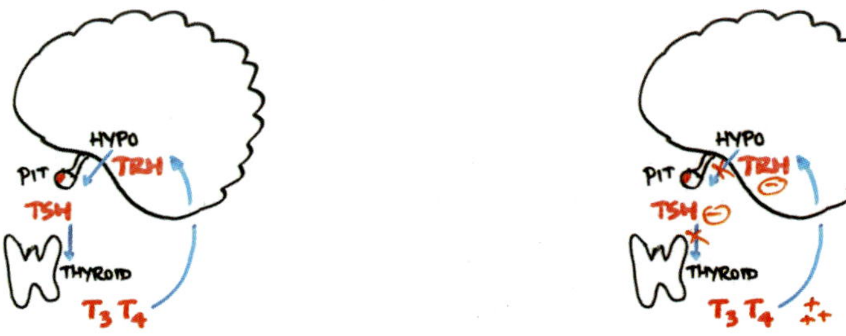

VIDEO 18.2. Sensitive Thyroid-Stimulating Hormone.

Transcript: The thyroid gland is regulated by the brain. Basically, the hypothalamus secretes thyroid-releasing hormone, and that tells the anterior part of the pituitary, make thyroid-stimulating hormone. The thyroid-stimulating hormone gets into the thyroid cells and tells it to produce triiodothyronine and tetraiodothyronine, T_3 and T_4. These are thyroid hormones that tell the body to rev up. It's the engine of the body, it's the furnace, if you will—be warmer, be more efficient, be more active.

These levels of hormones increase, and when they get in the positive, they will come back in the bloodstream, and the hypothalamus will say whoa, way too much thyroid hormone, and it'll stop the thyroid-releasing hormone, which will stop the thyroid-sensitizing hormone, which will basically shut this down as well. So, some unusual blood tests. When your thyroid hormones are really high and making a lot of it, these should be negative, they should be low. And so 1 of the tests you'll see is a TSH, a sensitive TSH. This is a staple of tests for endocrine surgeons and endocrinologists. If that TSH is really low, it means the body is making way too much because it's shutting this system off, and that means you're hyperthyroid, so it's a confusing thing. The TSH is low, but you're hyperthyroid, you've got too much thyroid. The other way around, if you're not making enough, then you'll stimulate this. The TSH will be high, and for some reason, as we age or have problems with radiation or something, we'll have low thyroid levels, it doesn't make enough, and so these all become negatives. If that's the case, there's not enough thyroid hormone, the brain, the hypothalamus, will tell that gland, pituitary, make more, and so the TSH will be very high. So these are confusing numbers, and this is what's called a negative feedback loop. If you make a lot of this, it shuts this off. If you don't make a lot of it, then it keeps this perpetuating. So, it's sensitive TSH as a baseline test to let us know whether you're hyper- or hypothyroid. It's the cheapest, easiest test to find out how well the thyroid gland is working and how well this axis works together.

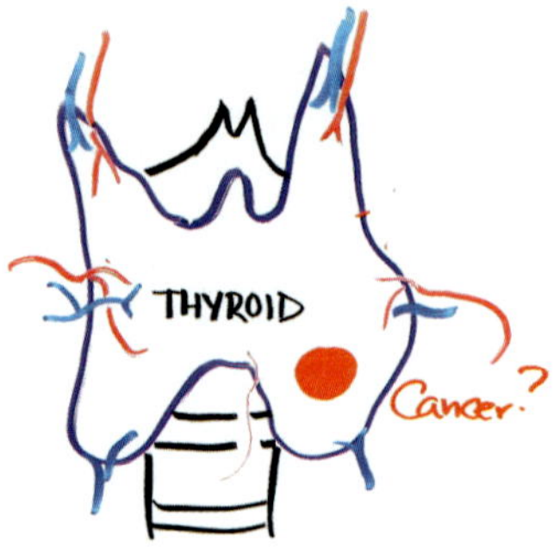

VIDEO 18.3. Thyroid Nodules.

Transcript: Thyroid nodules are common. However old you are, that's about the chance you have of having a thyroid nodule. Fifty-five-year-old people about 50% of the time will have a lump in the thyroid gland. Most of these are benign, probably 95%. What makes this likely to be a cancer? There are several different things that come into mind with cancer:

1. X-ray therapy, radiation treatment in the past, Chernobyl; higher incidence of people with thyroid cancers.
2. Children that have lumps in the thyroid gland; oftentimes when we think about a thyroid cancer.

Other risks: genetically, there are some families, multiple endocrine neoplasia type II, medullary thyroid cancer can be problematic.

Cancers tend to be firm, harder, they tend to get bigger with size. They don't come and go. Those would be more likely to be a cancerous problem. If you have a nodule in the thyroid gland, an ultrasound with physical exam, and then a fine-needle aspiration is the number 1 test. A little needle sneaks in and takes a slip of tissue out and an expert cytopathologist can tell us whether it's cancer or not.

So what to do with a thyroid bump? Number 1, 95% of the time it is benign, but a physician needs to see it usually with an ultrasound and if there is any concern about malignancy, fine-needle aspiration.

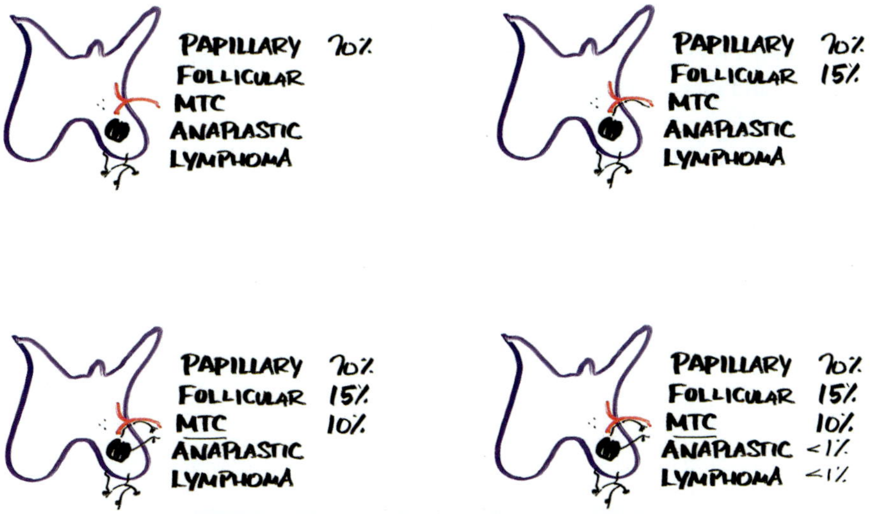

VIDEO 18.4. Thyroid Cancer.

Transcript: Thyroid cancer is common. There may be 100,000 cases this year in the United States, most of which are papillary thyroid cancer. Depending on whose data you look at, at least 70% of them are papillary thyroid cancer. It's an irritating disease. A lump grows, oftentimes in a younger woman, 20, 30, 40 years old. Men can get it, but it often happens in young women. The survival is excellent, 95% at 20 years. Virtually no cancers do we talk about 20-year survival, but patients do extraordinarily well. Take the cancer out. There oftentimes are lymph nodes involved with papillary thyroid cancer. We like to get those out, but even those tend not to be lethal. Somehow, the human body and papillary thyroid cancer get along relatively well. Surgery is useful unless they are really tiny little cancers, then maybe they can be observed. Take that gland out with a lobectomy and isthmectomy and maybe more if it's a bigger tumor.

The next most common is follicular. Maybe 15% of all thyroid cancers are follicular thyroid cancers. Now, most nodules in the thyroid gland will have some follicle cells in them and are benign, so it's rare that we get a follicular cancer, but they happen because follicular adenomas are common. Follicular cancers don't typically spread by the lymph nodes, they spread by the bloodstream, and so especially in young people we sometimes see lung metastasis. Again, these 2 tumors are readily treated. Surgery plus other therapies can make them basically curative. So follicular thyroid cancer spreads by hematogenous routes, but again, surgery usually eliminates that disease before it happens. Medullary thyroid cancer: Perhaps 10% of all cancers or less are medullary thyroid cancers. From the parafollicular cells, the ectopic-type cells, and they will typically be from an ectodermal origin and oftentimes in familial instances—MEN2 patients with medullary thyroid cancer. These go to lymph nodes. They're more aggressive, and we're nervous about medullary thyroid cancer hurting patients and shortening their lives. Some of these folks and families will have 2-year-old children or less, have surgical intervention to prevent a cancer that's known to develop.

The worst of all cancers is anaplastic. Fortunately, it's less than 1%. Oftentimes with a larger nodule that's been there for a long time, and for some reason it goes ballistic. These are rarely cured. They're rarely useful with surgery. I've taken out a couple myself, but eventually they came back with metastatic

VIDEO 18.4. Continued

disease. Ideally, neoadjuvant chemotherapy and XRT, radiation therapy, may help with that, but it's a brutal disease.

Thyroid lymphoma is extraordinarily uncommon as well, but it can happen, and usually a biopsy denotes what that is, and then radiation therapy is curative.

Thyroid cancers: Most commonly, the facts are, papillary thyroid cancers; at least 70%, if not 80% of cancers will be papillary. Patients do extraordinarily well. Follicular, a solid adenoma that can spread by bloodstream. It's good to get those out. Medullary, more dangerous and common in familial patients. Then less common, thankfully, anaplastic and, treated with radiation therapy, lymphoma.

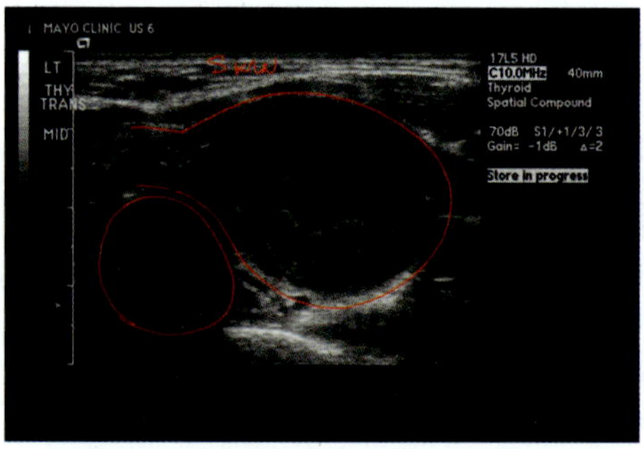

VIDEO 18.5. Thyroid US.

Transcript: This is an ultrasound of the thyroid gland. It doesn't look like much to the untrained eye, but we can take some information on the top here. It says, "Left side, thyroid gland, transverse, mid." So that means the ultrasound probe is transverse, we're in the mid-neck, trying to look at the thyroid gland, and the technologist or the radiologist is sort of scanning up and down and says, "Doggone-it, you're about in the middle of the thyroid gland." So the skin will be up top here. We've got the probe on the skin, fatty tissue and muscle. When we don't see things well, oftentimes there is trachea or air, and so I'm going to visualize this from the feet up. The trachea is here, the thyroid gland is here, the isthmus, and then there's a big blob here, and I suspect you can see that it's heterogeneous; it's hypoechoic, which oftentimes means fluid; and more dense tissue. It's likely a nodule, it's likely a benign, multicystic nodule in the left lobe of the thyroid gland. We didn't know that to start with, but there's a lot of information here. Look at the outside first, and then try to get your bearings. Looking from the feet up and saying, yep, that's going to be on the patient's left side. It looks like a benign thyroid nodule.

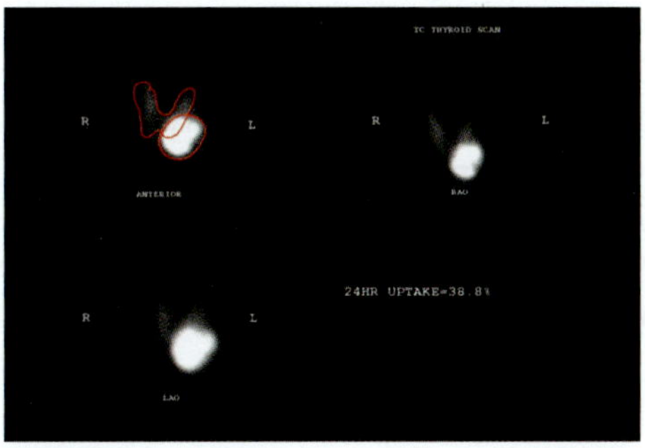

VIDEO 18.6. Nuclear Thyroid Scan.

Transcript: So this is a thyroid scan. I think you can take a look and hallucinate back and say, yeah, the thyroid is sort of a butterfly-shaped gland, it looks something like that. This person has been given some dye. You can give radioactive iodine, you can give pertechnetate, you can give a variety of different things, and depending on what it is, the thyroid will respond to it. The thyroid is a human vacuum cleaner when it comes to iodine. It loves to take up iodine and hold on to it. Iodine will circulate around the body, throughout the body, but really the thyroid gland is the only one that will really hold on to it. So what we see here is this amazingly high concentration of dye, and this is a nodule, likely within the thyroid gland. The important thing for endocrinologists and physicians and young trainees and surgeons is a hot nodule is usually benign; not a guarantee, but it's usually a benign problem. This focus is creating too much hormone, thyroid hormone. This young patient had excess thyroid hormone, hyperthyroidism, and if you remove this or radioablate this, they'll be cured. So this is a nice study to show it's not a whole problem with the thyroid gland, it's just one little nodule, and if you eradicate that, this patient will be cured.

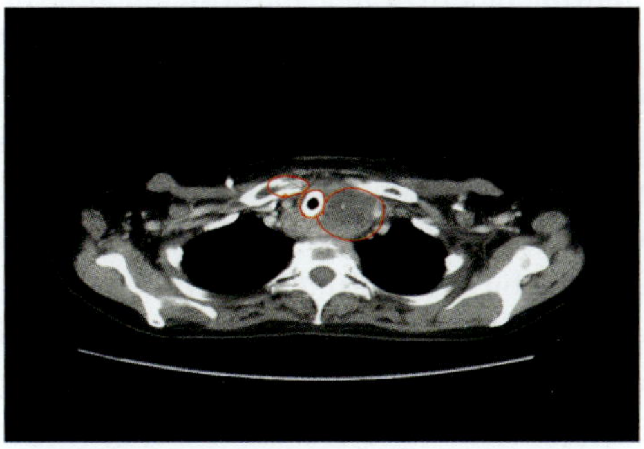

VIDEO 18.7. Thyroid CT.

Transcript: So this is a CT scan of the upper chest, and it is an amazing study with a very difficult and dangerous problem. So visualize again now, the patient is lying on their back, they're supine, the feet are toward us, the head is on the other side of the screen. So this is right, and that is left. We can see the spine in the background, and black is air. That's lung. These are the top of the lungs. We see skin on the top, and we see bones on either side. Things should be fairly symmetric in the human body. We can see a normal-looking clavicle here. I don't know, can you tell this business? There's something wrong with the right collarbone. There's a lytic lesion. That's a bony metastasis, and it's scary here because we've got a tube, it looks like, in the trachea. This is somebody that's in a critical problem. This is likely in an ICU. That trachea should just have a hole; there shouldn't be a big ring around it. And we see this other business here; there's a mass, a cystic mass that has less density, or less Hounsfield units. We may have a couple

VIDEO 18.7. Continued

lumps and bumps here as well. We've got lots of different circles. Some of these may be lymph nodes. This is likely a thyroid malignancy, and those that go to bone are typically either follicular thyroid cancers or metastatic medullary thyroid cancers or anaplastic cancers. So this could be either an anaplastic or follicular tumor in my mind, but this is a problem of normal-looking lungs, bone here looks good, skinny sort of person, but we've got a goiter, we've got a mass, an intrathoracic, mediastinal goiter, and the goiter likely is a cancerous process showing at least a metastasis to the collarbone and maybe elsewhere.

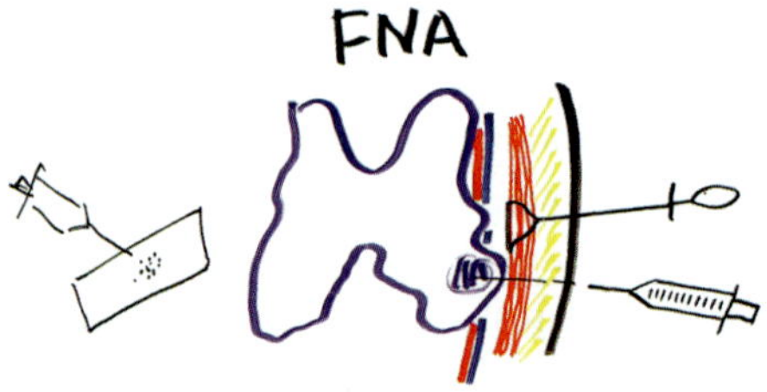

VIDEO 18.8. Fine-Needle Aspiration.

Transcript: Fine-needle aspiration is crucial to identifying thyroid nodules and whether they're benign or malignant. Here's a nice little drawing of a thyroid gland with a nodule in the left lobe. In the operating room, we might make an incision that goes through the skin, the fat, and the muscle, and then we would see this nodule and operate and take it out. But fine-needle aspiration means you're going to take a syringe and a fine needle—that's usually an 18 gauge, a 21 gauge, 25, 27—and stick that needle through the skin, through the fat, through the muscle, and into that nodule. And then that syringe is placed on a vacuum and little cells will slide up into the needle, and when you take that out, you'll take that syringe and spray that material on a slide, and the little bit of fluid and juice will put some cells there. A histopathologist can then tell by looking at those cells, this is a benign thyroid nodule or it's papillary thyroid cancer or medullary thyroid cancer. It's a very inexpensive, cheap test. The key thing is you've got to get the needle in the nodule without hurting the carotid or the jugular. It's a straightforward test, and it can be repeated multiple times. It's incredibly beneficial because most nodules are benign, and we'd like to not operate on benign nodules. This has revolutionized the way people practice thyroid surgery.

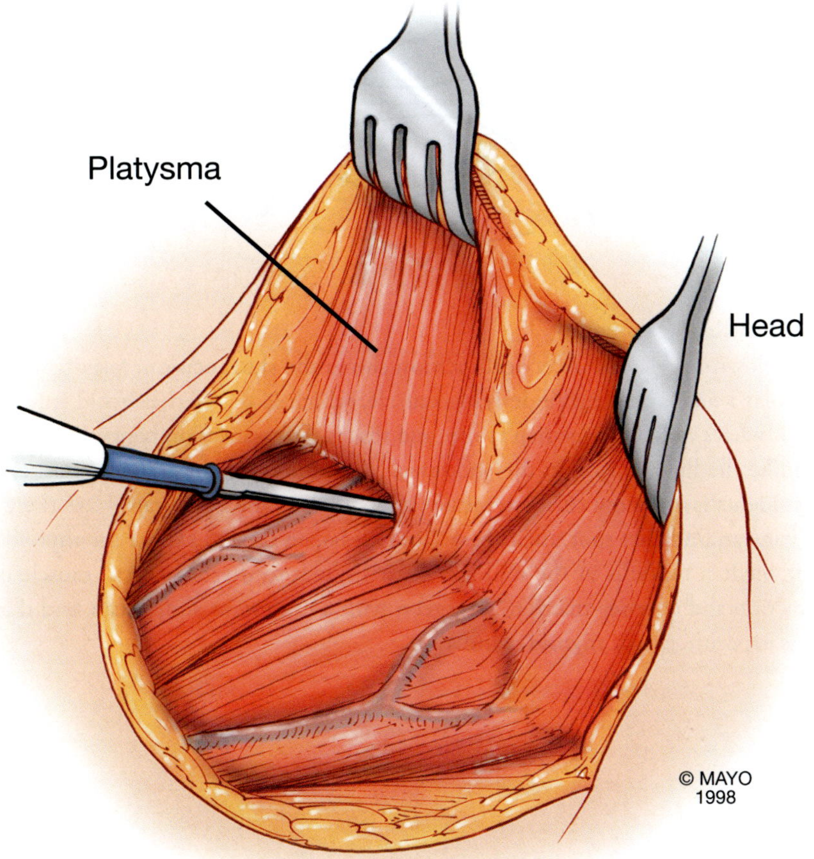

FIGURE 18.4. Transection and Elevation of the Platysma.

Thyroid Challenge Questions

18.1. Is there a middle thyroid artery?
18.2. What is the thyrocervical trunk?
18.3. What is the second most common thyroid cancer?
18.4. Does MEN involve thyroid cancer?
18.5. What is the tubercle of Zuckerkandl?
18.6. What is Plummer disease?
18.7. Is Graves disease treated surgically?
18.8. What does MACIS stand for?
18.9. Who was Emil T. Kocher?
18.10. What histologic characteristics does papillary thyroid carcinoma have?

(Answers appear on page 260)

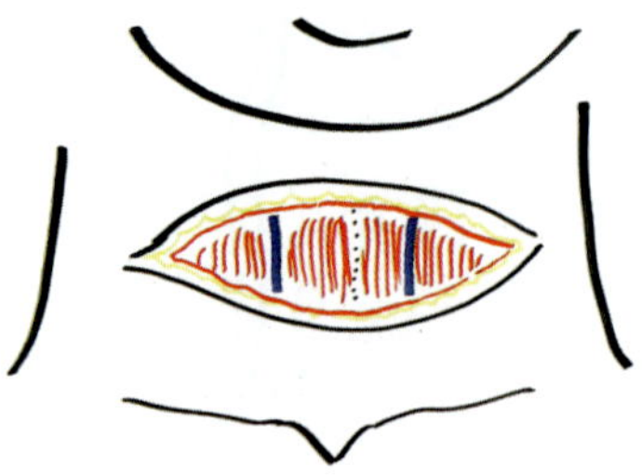

VIDEO 18.9. Median Raphe.

Transcript: This blown-up view of a cervical incision shows the skin incision, fatty tissue, the platysma, the anterior jugular veins, and then underlying muscle, which is the sternal hyoid muscle. In between here someplace is what's called the median raphe, and that is the connection between these muscles in the midline, much like the linea alba is in the abdomen. The important thing for thyroid and parathyroid surgeons and students is to know this is typically a bloodless plane. Very rarely are there blood vessels crossing. So if you can find that spot, then these 2 muscles open up and expose the thyroid gland. So the key thing is the median raphe is in the midline, sternal notch to thyroid notch, muscle on either side. With a little traction and counter-traction, a surgeon with a cautery or scalpel can find that space and it gives a bloodless exposure to our thyroid gland.

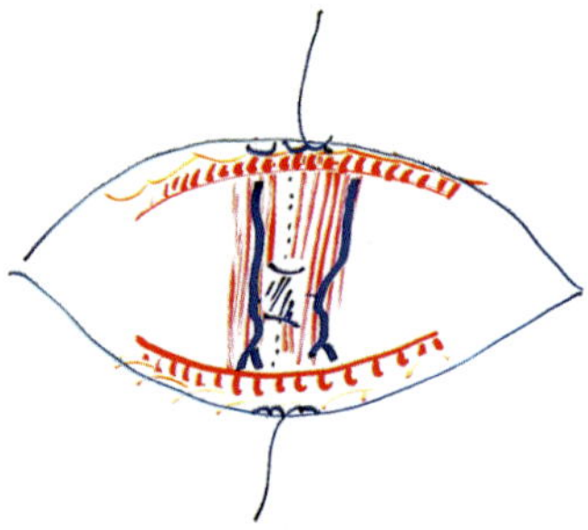

VIDEO 18.10. Exposure of Platysma.

Transcript: So the start of a thyroidectomy makes a typically curvilinear collar incision, and with retractors holding things back, we get exposure. Cutting through the fatty tissue, we see the platysma muscle, and we cut that carefully across; not too deep, because the anterior jugulars run anteriorly to the strap muscles, the so-called sternothyroid and sternohyoid muscles. This would be the sternohyoid muscle. We see those 2 blood vessels, and in-between someplace is what's called the median raphe, and for thyroid surgeons, this is an important landmark because it tends to be avascular. It's rare that a blood vessel crosses that, and to get exposure to the underlying thyroid gland, which is down underneath, the isthmus is right there, thyroid gland. You want to go through the median raphe and retract the sternohyoid muscles. Best access for a thyroidectomy, through the median raphe, being careful not to injure the anterior jugular veins.

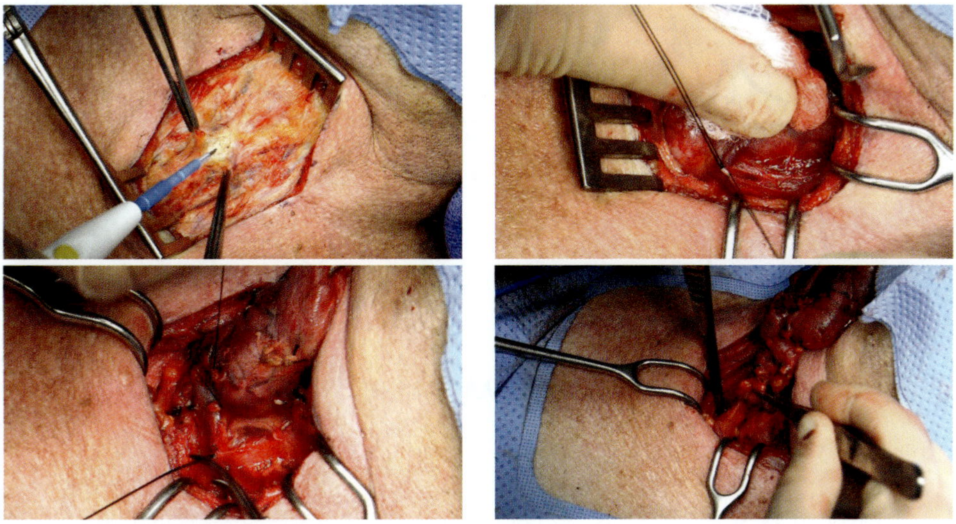

VIDEO 18.11. Thyroidectomy: Intraoperative.
Transcript: Thyroidectomy for somebody with multinodular disease. They've got a tennisball-size mass in their neck. Again, we need to go through the fatty tissue and platysma, raising some flaps up, and expose the median raphe. We've got anterior jugular veins going from the sternum to the left up toward the chin, and we're going to go through the median raphe with blood vessels on either side. A little right-angle clamp, trying to find that bloodless space between those anterior jugulars. We can see the strap muscle below, which would be the sternohyoid muscle. Sneaking up toward the notch of the thyroid gland, the chin is to the right.

We've gotten through the median raphe and now we're just taking a little bit of the cervical fascia, releasing things open so we have wide exposure to the thyroid isthmus. The question becomes, are we going to do a left thyroidectomy or right or both? We're going to start off with the patient's left side. We're looking over the shoulder here from the surgeon. That's the middle thyroid vein. We've ligated in continuity, we tie, tie, clip the bridge, and tie the sutures. And as we rotate further we might run into other blood vessels. Most times most people have a middle thyroid vein and multiple superior and inferior veins as well. So the superior pole is above us to the right, and we're trying to get control of the superior thyroid artery and the superior thyroid vein. We've got multiple Kocher clamps, and we're dividing the superior pole with a scissors, nice little cut. We've got a clamp above, and we'll tie that with 2-O silk suture, or others use clips or Harmonic scalpel. Trying to preserve a parathyroid gland. We've got our thumb pulling up on the tissue, the thyroid gland. Looks like there might be a little parathyroid, we might have to transplant if we devascularize it.

We're now looking for the nerve, and it's sitting right underneath it. It's a whitish little structure. Got to be careful of that whitish little structure; we don't want to divide that. It's a beautiful picture of the nerve. Teeny little vessel here. Nerve is in harm's way, be careful with that cautery, don't turn it on, keep your fingers away from the button if you use it as a dissector. As long as we know where the nerve is, we can be a little more bold and say all right, out it comes. If we have a parathyroid in that specimen, we should transplant it. This gland is being taken off the trachea. It's not a huge gland, but there might be a parathyroid there. That looks like fat, but if it's parathyroid, transplant it. Nice job with a left thyroid lobectomy.

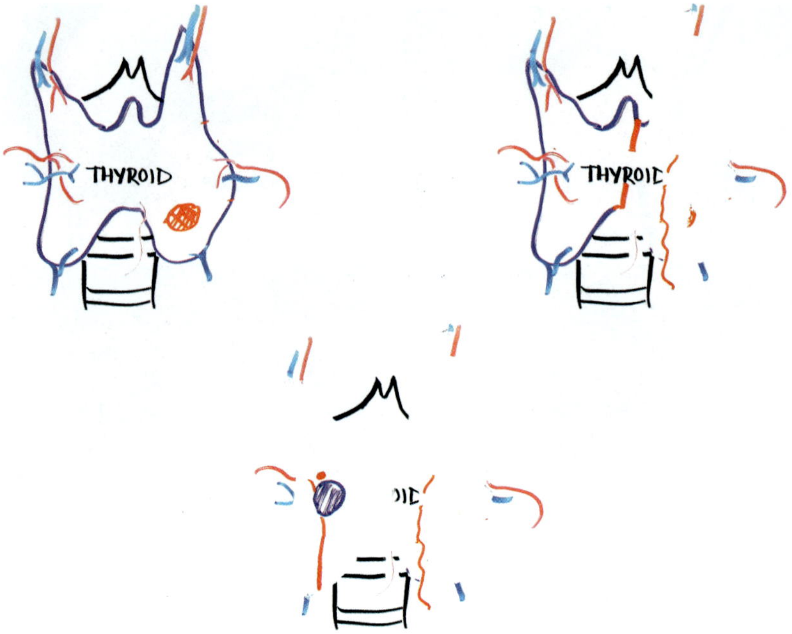

VIDEO 18.12. Lobectomy, Isthmectomy, Total, Near-Total.
Transcript: Perhaps we've got a lump in the thyroid gland, we biopsy, and it says papillary thyroid cancer or follicular thyroid cancer or we're really concerned about something. What's the treatment for that? Assuming the patient is fit for general anesthesia and is ready for surgery, most surgeons would agree that hemithyroidectomy, or so-called thyroid lobectomy, would be sort of the minimum treatment, so we want to take out at least half of the gland. So that means that you would divide the superior thyroid artery and vein, the middle thyroid vein, the inferior thyroid artery, and the inferior thyroid vein, being careful not to hurt the recurrent laryngeal nerve along the side. That's a thyroid lobectomy.

Most surgeons in the United States, if they had a cancer on 1 side, do a lobectomy plus an isthmectomy, and then take all or part of the right lobectomy. So a total thyroidectomy means exactly that; the entire thyroid gland is removed. A near-total thyroidectomy would be that operation that leaves a small remnant, perhaps, on my drawing scale, something like that, and it usually leaves a little bit of remnant to protect the recurrent laryngeal nerve that runs underneath it and perhaps a superior parathyroid gland. So, operations for thyroid cancer—lobectomy, plus isthmectomy, and then near-total (that's what this is), or total thyroidectomy. Those are the choices we have for surgery.

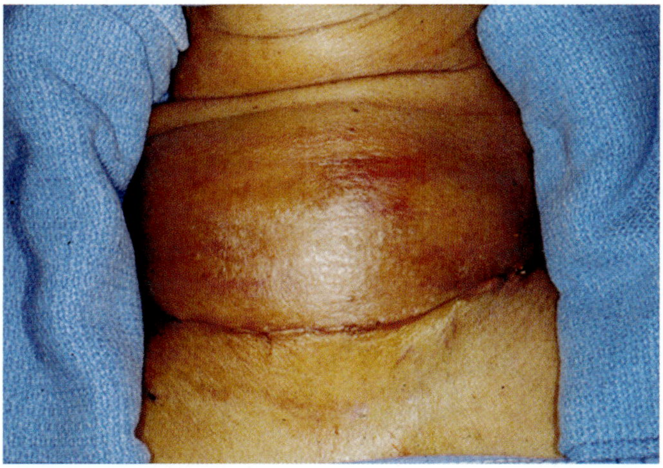

FIGURE 18.5. Postoperative Cervical Hematoma.

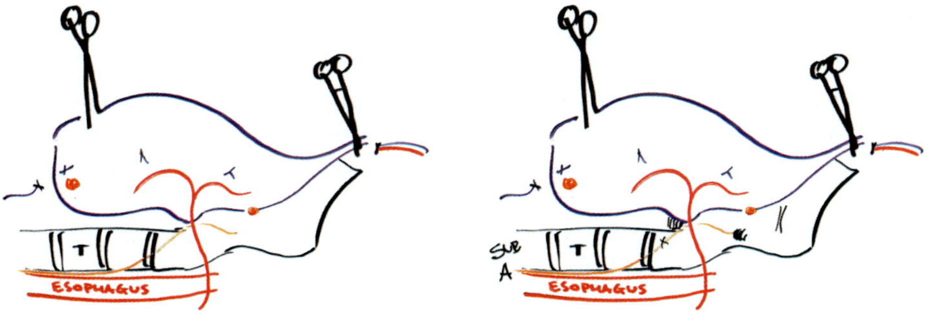

VIDEO 18.13. RLN.

Transcript: This is a side drawing. I'm thinking this is a drawing with the head here and the body here. This is the upper pole of the thyroid gland. The thyroid is being rotated off the esophagus and the trachea. The inferior thyroid artery sneaks up, supplies blood to both parathyroid glands. The trachea, underneath, just posterior. The so-called ligament of Berry and the tubercle of Zuckerkandl, the little bump where the genu of the recurrent laryngeal nerve, the little curve, occurs together. The recurrent laryngeal nerve lies within the tracheoesophageal groove. On the left side, it wraps around the aorta. On the right side, it's the subclavian artery. We don't want to hurt this nerve because it innervates all the intrinsic muscles except the cricothyroid muscle within the larynx. It's key to voice control. If you knock out 1 nerve on 1 side, you'll end up with a hoarse voice. If you knock out both nerves, on either side, you'll end up with obstruction or wide open for aspiration. We just can't afford that. So we want to preserve this.

We find it in the TE groove. It sneaks along the trachea, and it curves into the laryngeal musculature to innervate the vocal cords that lie underneath the thyroid cartilage. There's 1 on each side. One percent of people will have a nonrecurrent laryngeal nerve that's typically on the right side, where it doesn't wrap around the subclavian; it just goes straight into the larynx. About 1% to 2% of all thyroid operations end up in an injury somehow, either a permanent injury because of a thermal burn or cutting the nerve, or a transient injury, so-called neuropraxia. If we push on this thyroid hard enough and we stretch that

VIDEO 18.13. Continued

nerve, it may not work for several months, and this happens from time to time. So, take-home messages—recurrent laryngeal nerve lies within the TE groove, tracheoesophageal groove, it bumps up against the tubercle of Zuckerkandl and makes a curve, the genu of the nerve, and it innervates the vocal cords. The inferior thyroid artery typically lies anterior to it, but sometimes the artery can be posterior. Find the artery, find the tubercle of Zuckerkandl, the ligament of Berry, and that's where the recurrent laryngeal nerve will be.

Answers to Thyroid Challenge Questions

18.1. No.

18.2. The arterial branch off the subclavian artery that gives rise to the inferior thyroid artery.

18.3. Follicular cancer. Papillary cancer is most common. Metastatic thyroid cancer is third. Lymphoma and anaplastic cancers are rare.

18.4. Yes, MEN2.

18.5. It is an embryologic bud closely attached to the genu of the RLN.

18.6. Toxic multinodular goiter.

18.7. Sometimes; often, treatment is with medication or radioactive iodine.

18.8. MACIS is a scoring system used to predict survival for patients with papillary thyroid carcinoma. MACIS=metastasis, age, completeness of resection, invasion, size of cancer.

18.9. A Noble Prize–winning Swiss surgeon (1841-1917) who revolutionized thyroid surgery. He made it safe by meticulously ligating and dividing blood vessels.

18.10. Psammoma bodies.

19

Trauma Assessment and Surgery

Advanced Trauma Life Support Protocol

When the patient arrives in the emergency department, the primary survey should be for ABCDE: A, airway (Figure 19.1); B, breathing (Figure 19.2); C, circulation (Figure 19.3); D, disability (Figure 19.4); and E, exposure (Figure 19.5). Life-threatening issues are addressed as they are uncovered before advancing to the next step. A secondary survey is a head-to-toe physical examination and definitive care plan (Figure 19.6).

Clinical Presentations

Airway: When a patient is unable to speak, has a decreased level of consciousness, or has altered mental status, there is concern for a compromised airway. Breathing: Tension pneumothorax can be diagnosed clinically. Findings can include contralateral tracheal deviation, jugular venous distention, or absent breath sounds ipsilaterally; cardiac tamponade presents with tachycardia and the Beck triad (Video 19.1). Circulation: This is tested by palpation of pulses; other assessments include heart rate, BP, capillary refill, and skin. Disability: This is assessed from the mental status, pupils, and motor and sensory deficits (Glasgow Coma Scale [Video 19.2]). Exposure: The patient must be disrobed for complete inspection and digital rectal examination (secondary survey). Keep the patient warm to avoid hypothermia.

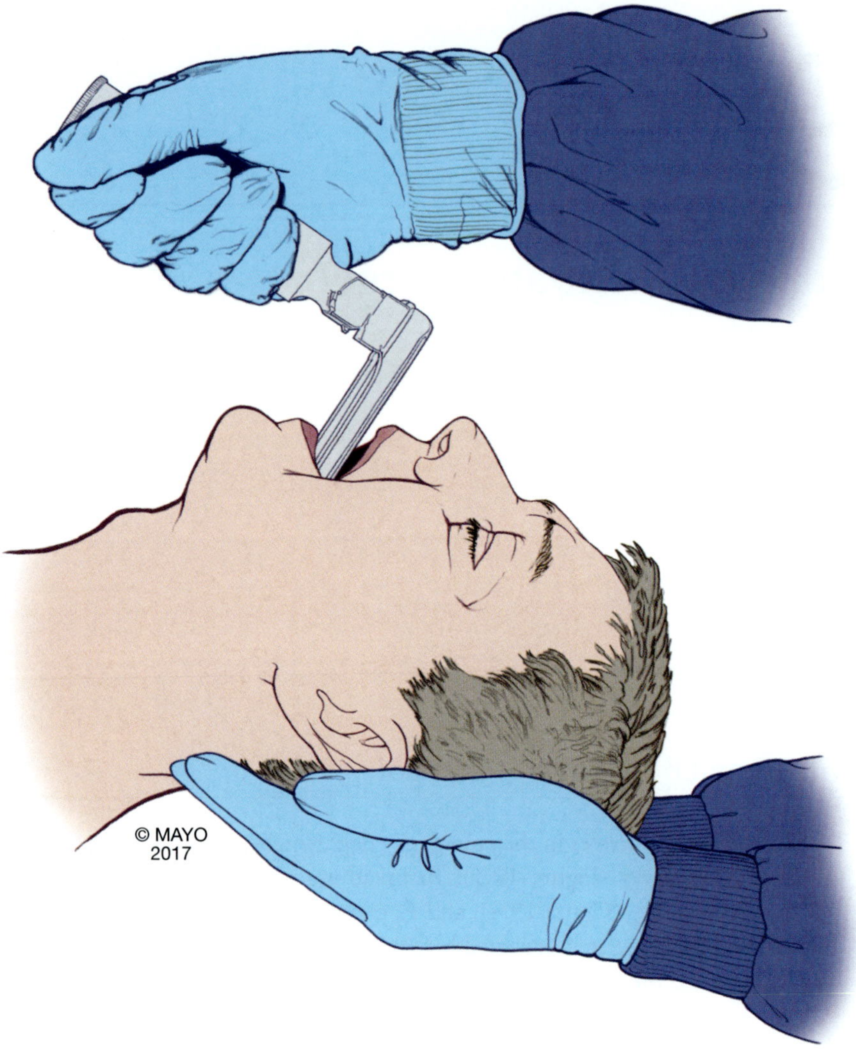

FIGURE 19.1. Establish Airway.

Imaging

CXR (Video 19.3) and pelvic radiographs may show evidence of fractures, bleeding, or perforation. FAST imaging looks for fluid or bleeding. Cardiac tamponade is diagnosed with US or echocardiography (Video 19.4). The best way to diagnose or rule out aortic injury is with CT angiography (Video 19.5).

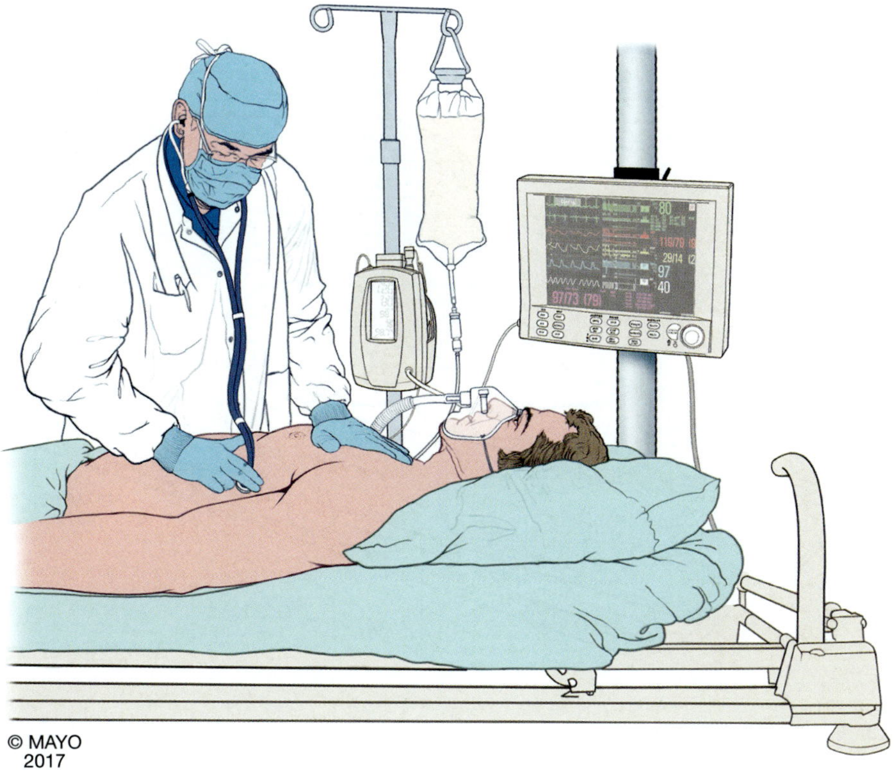
© MAYO
2017

FIGURE 19.2. Monitor Breathing.

Emergency Department Operations

If chin lift, jaw thrust, or endotracheal intubation are unsuccessful in establishing an airway, cricothyrotomy (Video 19.6) is indicated to provide an adequate airway. Needle thoracostomy, followed by tube thoracostomy, is the treatment for tension pneumothorax; cardiac tamponade is treated with a pericardial window (Video 19.7). Left thoracotomy is an intervention to allow access to cross-clamp the aorta (Video 19.8).

Wound care is also an important aspect of emergency department care. Once a patient is stabilized, attention can be given to meticulous wound care (Video 19.9).

Trauma Principles

- ABCs should be checked above all else.
- Make sure the patient has oxygen.
- Normothermia is ideal.
- Check vital signs often.
- Respond quickly with resuscitation (2 large-bore IV catheters and 2 L of IV fluids stat!).
- Stop the bleeding—sometimes the operating room is the safest place for a patient.

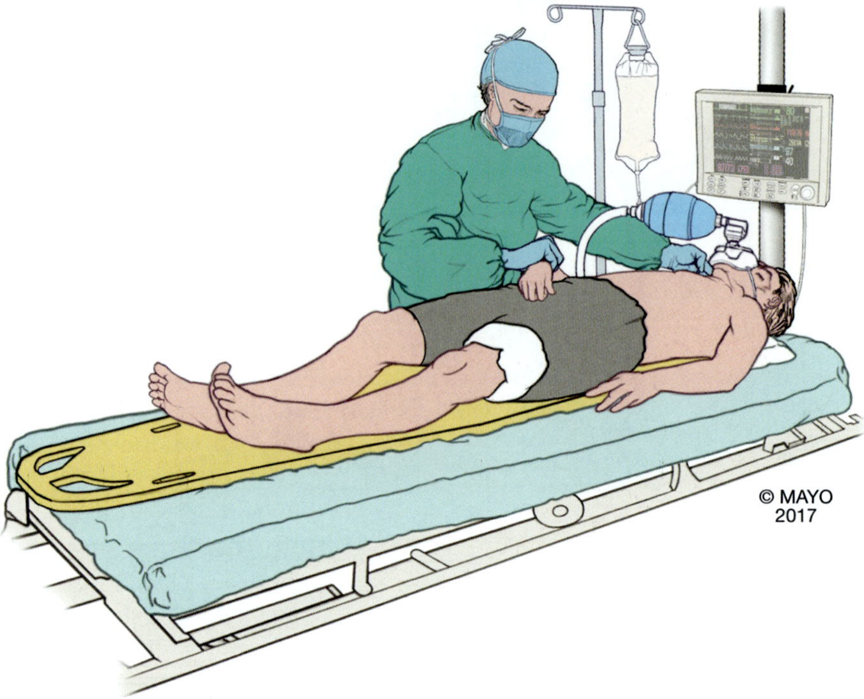

FIGURE 19.3. Check Circulation.

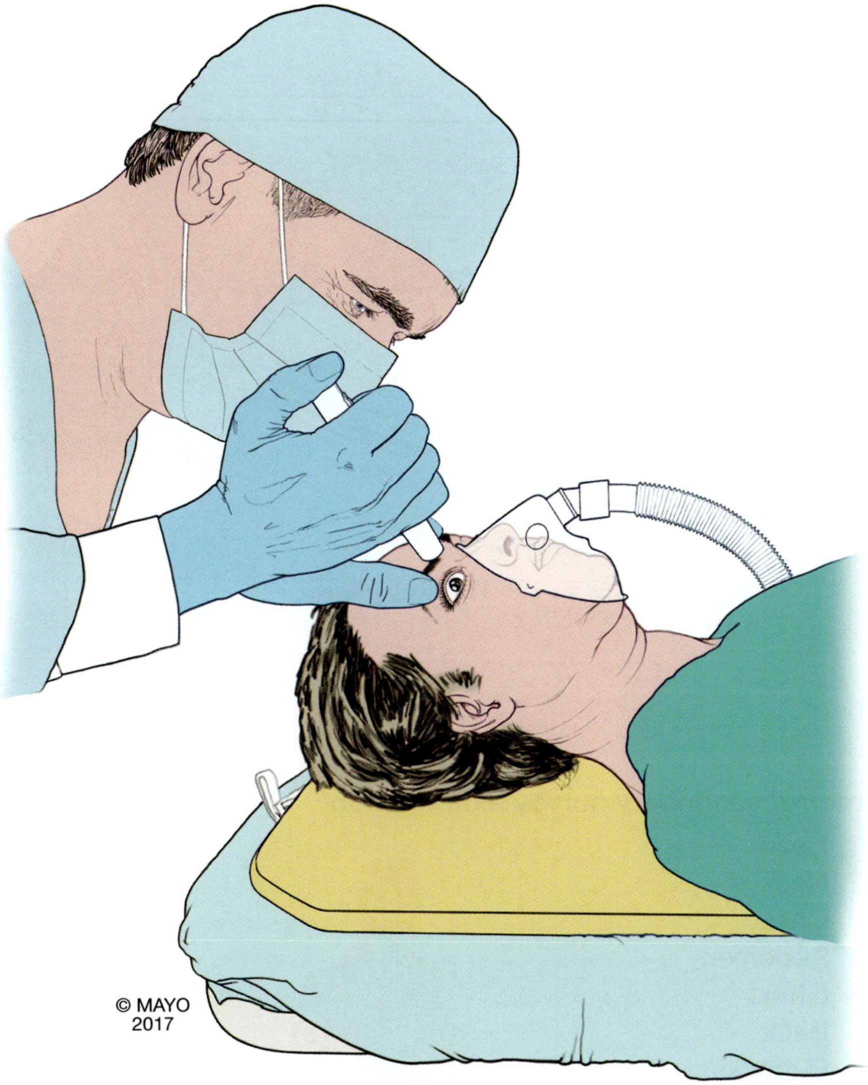

FIGURE 19.4. Assess Disability.

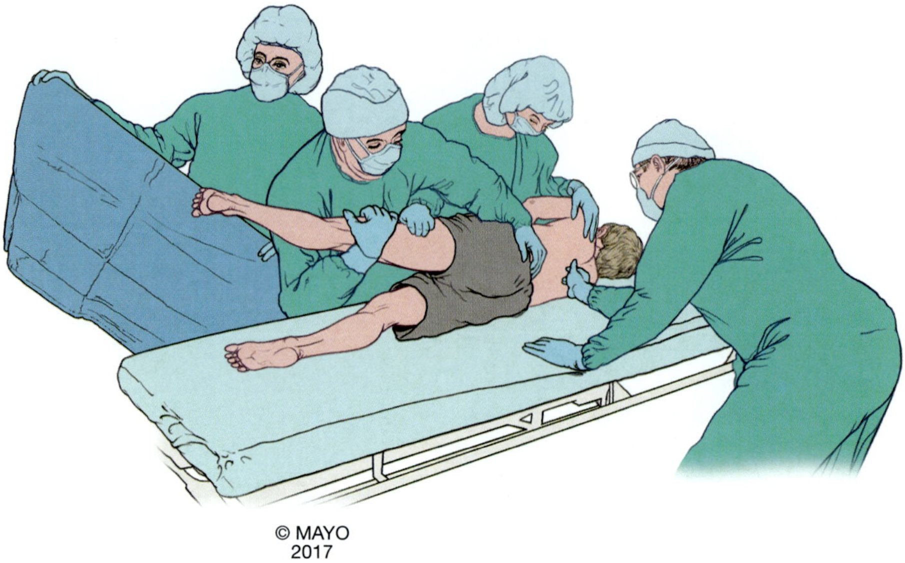

FIGURE 19.5. Expose Patient to Assess for Life-Threatening Issues.

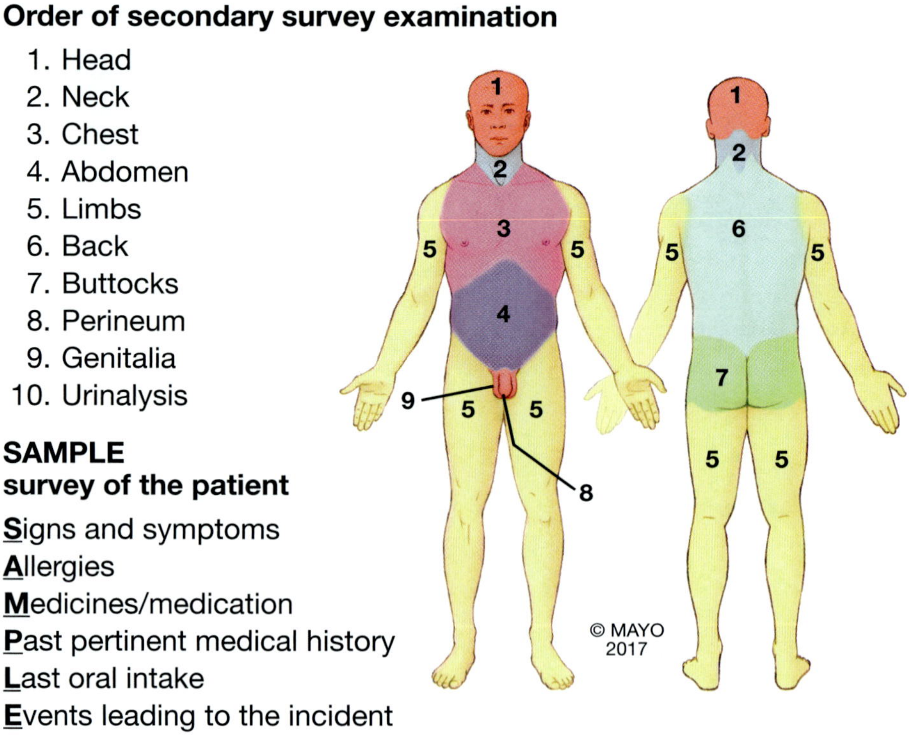

FIGURE 19.6. Perform a Physical Examination.

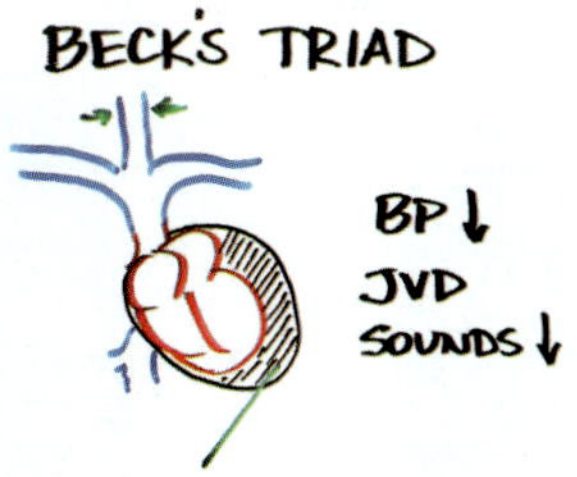

VIDEO 19.1. Beck Triad.
Transcript: Beck's triad is considered pathognomonic for acute cardiac tamponade. Dr Beck was a surgical trainee at Case Western when he noticed that some patients with low blood pressure, big veins in the neck—jugular venous distention. And when he listened to their heart, he couldn't hear it very well. And it turns out that you couldn't hear it very well because it was surrounded with fluid, either blood or water; a so-called pericardial effusion. And so in a trauma patient, this is not uncommon that people can get pericardial tamponade. And the treatment for that is pericardiocentesis, a needle in to drain that fluid out. If it continues to bleed then maybe surgery is warranted. But Beck's triad is hypotension, jugular venous distention, and muffled heart sounds.

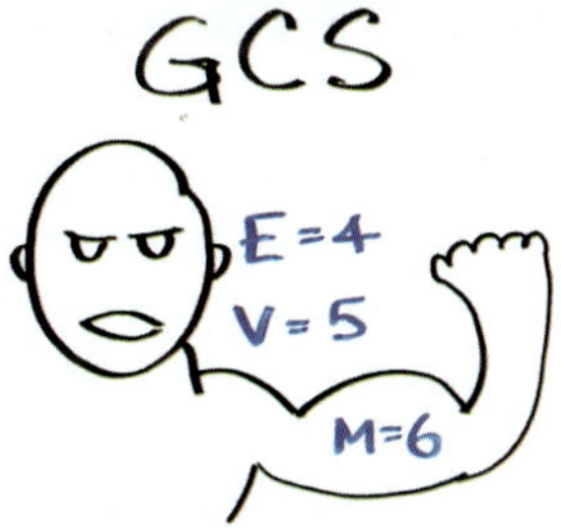

VIDEO 19.2. Glasgow Coma Scale.
Transcript: The Glasgow Coma Scale is a scoring system that basically looks at all trauma patients for 3 key things. It looks at their eyes; it looks at their verbal response; and their motor response. And it gives points for function with each one. For eyes you can get 4 points. For mouth or verbal you get 5, and for motor response you get 6. So a perfect score is 15. You and I have a GCS of 15 right now. The lowest score you can get is 1 point for each of those factors. If you had a score of 3 you would be in a deep coma. Patients with a score of 8 or less are in a coma.

Let me go over the Glasgow Coma Scale score with you just a bit. The eye opening response, if the eyelids open spontaneously that is a 4. If there is no response, that is a 1. And in-between they get 3 and 2 for speech and pain. Same thing with best verbal response; if they are oriented to time and place and they know what is going on they get a 5. If they are confused like somebody with a contusion or concussion, they will get a 4. If they have absolutely no response whatsoever to hollering and screaming at them, they will get a 1. And the motor response, there are 6 points available; obeys commands, moves to localized pain that is worth 5. But no response at all is a 1.

Glasgow Coma Scale score, 15 points; 8 or less is patient in a coma; meaning they need to be intubated. It is an important score and it is important to monitor it to see that it changes or doesn't change over time.

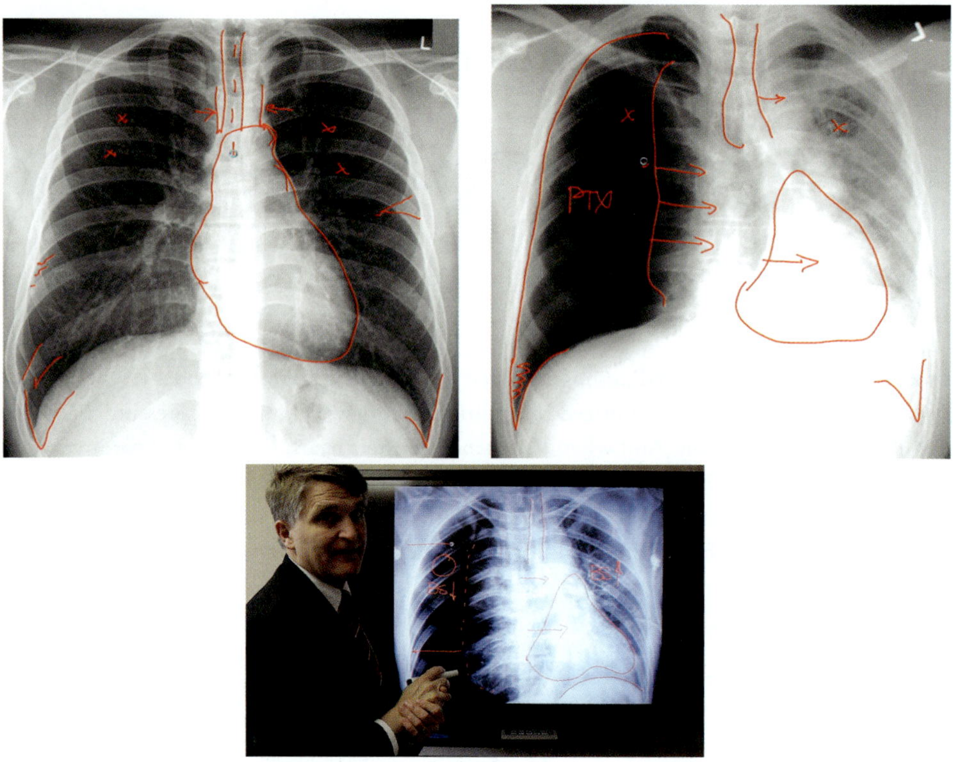

VIDEO 19.3. Trauma CXR.

Transcript: Chest x-ray for trauma evaluation is very important. Part of the secondary survey is sometimes something that we get very quickly. This is a beautiful chest x-ray of a trauma patient that probably sprained an ankle or broke a leg, because this is a stone-cold normal chest x-ray. We have got a small heart. No sign of an effusion. We can see the aortic knob. We can see the left atrium. We can see the right atrium. It is a small, thin mediastinum. We don't see any sort of rib fractures. We see a nice clear diaphragmatic sulcus. There is no fluid down here. And when we look specifically at the lung parenchyma, it looks the same on either side. We can see little markings all the way out to the edge. There is no evidence of pneumothorax. There is no fluid in the chest. There are no obvious rib fractures. The trachea, importantly, is midline—we can see that. And it is nice that it is a beautiful film here with spinal processes right behind it. We don't see any soft tissue damage. We don't see any clavicular injuries. This is a normal chest x-ray.

Let's take a peek at a couple of others. I hope you can look at this and say, "Wow" this is different, and something is going on. And honestly, something really bad has happened and we need to do something within 10 seconds or this patient is going to have a problem. So the good thing about looking down here in the diaphragm and the recesses, there is no fluid. That is good. On the other side, it is not there. So it likely means that there is either fluid or a lot more stuff on that side of the diaphragm. The trachea, where is the trachea? And it is kind of hard to see here, but it is drifted a little bit to the patient's left. The heart—where is the heart? The heart is stuck over here. It's been moved drastically to the patient's left. What about the lung parenchyma? We look at the density here, the opacity here versus the other side, they are not the same, and there is not symmetry involved. So something is drastically wrong, either on that side or this side, or potentially both. But I am going to suggest to you, the lung on the right side is

VIDEO 19.3. Continued

no longer touching the wall of the chest—the ribs and the musculature. This is what is called a pneumothorax. And importantly, it is not just a pneumothorax; it is what is called a tension pneumothorax. Because everything is moved, it's under pressure and there are so many bubbles of air leaking out from this injured lung that it is now displacing everything to the patient's left. What needs to happen immediately is a needle into the chest and let this air out and let the lung re-expand, let the heart drift back to normal, because this person potentially could be dead in 30 seconds or so. On this other side maybe there is some trauma and bruising, but right now what needs to happen is an alleviation of this tension pneumothorax.

Let's take a look at this chest x-ray. What do you see? Well, we don't see a diaphragm down at the bottom that usually means hyperinflation. We do see a diaphragm here. Alright—what else? Where is the trachea? It is tough to see it. It is tough to know exactly where it is. But it may be all the way over this way. It is pushed a little bit to the patient's left. Where is the heart? Again, it looks like it is further on the patient's left. And as before, we can see the lung on the patient's right side is decompressed and it is no longer up against the parietal peritoneum. We have got air in the right chest. And again, this is a pneumothorax, maybe not quite as graphic of a tension but it is moving things this way. Somebody needs to address this problem.

A key thing for a medical student, ideally you don't want to get this chest x-ray. When the patient comes in and they are short of breath and they are struggling, listen to this side. Breath sounds, probably not very evident. Breath sounds on this side, evident. Speak up with your residents and your staff, "Doctors, I don't hear any breath sounds on the right. I hear breath sounds on the left." And then we can sort of check and say, "Whoa, let's look at the neck. Maybe the veins are engorged. Maybe we have got a tension pneumothorax." In trauma resuscitation, if we are not sure and we don't hear sounds, a needle typically goes in and it goes, "puffffff" release. You have just saved somebody's life. Look for this, listen for this. Examine your patients carefully. Because you really don't want a chest x-ray—it's too late when you see this sign.

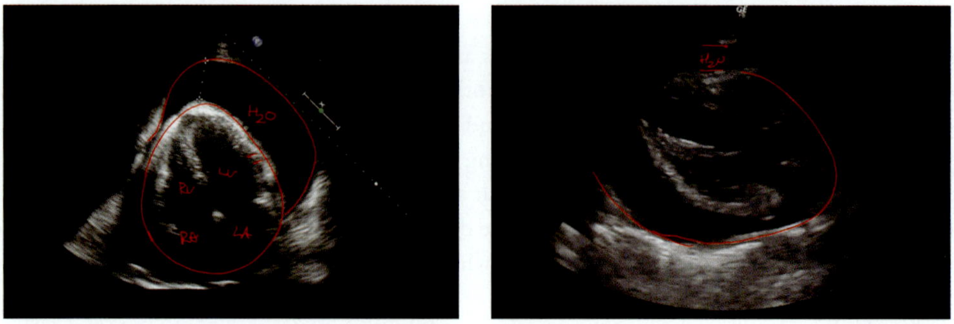

VIDEO 19.4. Echocardiogram for Cardiac Tamponade.

Transcript: It doesn't always happen in the emergency room, but sometimes people have bad problems of the heart. In a trauma scenario, it is either bleeding and a stab wound and those people go immediately to the operating room, or we find tamponade; fluid, a pericardial effusion. This is an echocardiogram, sort of the heart upside down. Everything is sort of backwards. The bottom here is the right atrium; the bottom here is the left atrium, left ventricle, right ventricle. This is a heart where the valves look like they are working pretty doggone normal.

Let me show you a couple of still photos that shows the fluid around the outside of the heart. So this echocardiogram, the still photo of it, is showing us the heart, sort of upside down here. And we have got our left ventricle, our left atrium, right atrium, and right ventricle. But important to note with ultrasound, is the echogenicity of what we are looking at. No echoes means anechoic. That is typically water. And you shouldn't have this big fluid cavity around the heart. That could be blood, but that is anechoic. As opposed to hyperechoic, that is musculature that is moving around there. So this is a picture of a pericardial effusion and if the patient is hypotensive with engorged neck veins and not good blood return, this is pericardial tamponade. And what this person needs is a needle or surgeon or somebody to get that fluid out of there. And this can be done easily with a needle if it is fluid. If it is blood, sometimes it doesn't want to come out very well and patients are taken emergently to the operating room.

Let's take a peek at another picture; tougher to look at here. But I am going to try to tell you that the pericardium is here on the outside and we look at this thing and we say, "We have got some fluid up here and maybe we have got some down here as well." But this is a less prominent picture of somebody that likely has pericardial effusion and if they are hypotensive and tachycardia that is pericardial tamponade, and for that, needs urgent treatment.

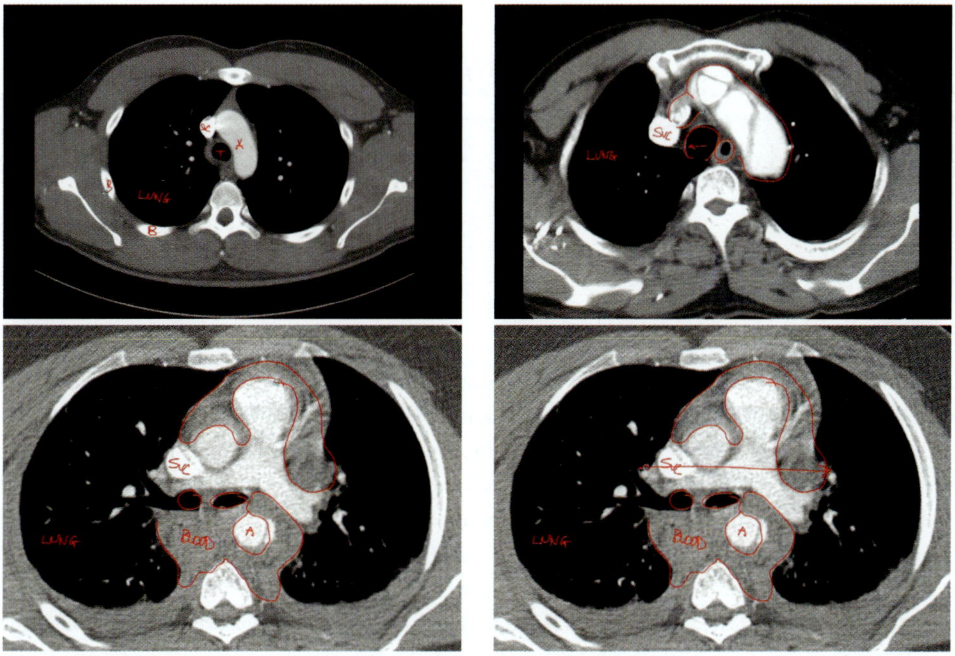

VIDEO 19.5. CT Angiography.

Transcript: Patients involved in critical motor vehicle accidents with deadly consequences or lots of injuries will oftentimes get a CT scan of the chest, abdomen, and pelvis. This is a CT scan that is a beautiful CT scan that shows contrast in the aorta and the superior vena cava, the trachea is midline and everything looks just fine. This person doesn't have any obvious problems in the chest. Remember black on a CT scan is lung or air. White is bone, these are ribs. We don't see any fractures. We see lots of muscles and a fit person.

Let's contrast that with this CT scan. Well, we can see lungs black, that looks just fine. We don't see any fluid in the chest. We see air in the esophagus and the trachea is maybe pushed a little bit to the patient's right. The muscles and everything on the outside seem not unreasonable. The SVC is sitting here, but it is this structure here that has got my attention. This is the aortic arch and it doesn't look normal. There is something decidedly wrong. There are flaps where the dye isn't inside the lumen. And this is what is called aortic dissection. This is a potentially lethal injury that needs emergent surgical intervention, endovascular repair, or careful treatment of this patient.

A different CT scan on a different patient. Again, lungs look pretty reasonable. Black, we have got contrast in the aorta, in the SVC, but we have also got something else that is going on here. We have got a trachea and bronchi might be right here, but we have all of this extra stuff, and it is blood. This is all blood, and it's all the way around here. It's within the mediastinum. This is what is called a hemomediastinum. That blood didn't just magically get there. We needed to fracture sternums, break blood vessels, and contuse lungs, but there is way too much blood in here. This person has a wide mediastinum. We sometimes can see that on a chest x-ray and then we would get this picture. This is somebody we need to be very careful about and think about a CT angiogram and find out is there aortic dissection, is there a transection, or is there obviously something else going on? But this is a markedly abnormal CT scan showing what is called a hemomediastinum.

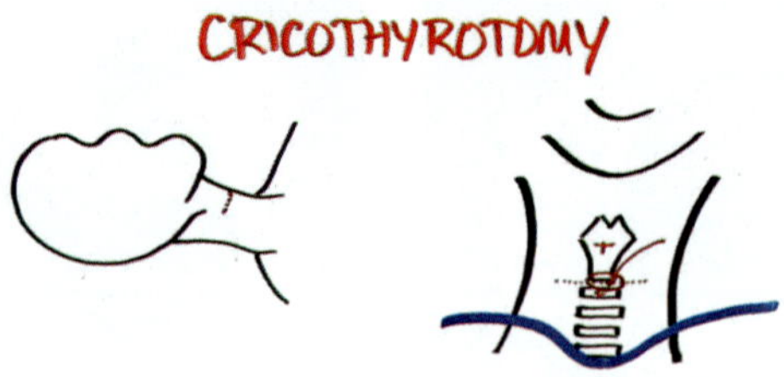

VIDEO 19.6. Cricothyrotomy.
Transcript: A cricothyrotomy is simplistically an incision that makes a hole between the thyroid cartilage and the cricoid cartilage. This is what is called a surgical airway. Tracheostomy is a surgical airway as well but that takes more time. A cricothyrotomy is a surgical emergency. Typically, an incision is placed on the neck with the patient out, passed out, unconscious, not being able to breathe. An incision is created between the thyroid cartilage and the cricoid cartilage. I usually make a transverse incision through the fatty tissue, through the platysma, and then what we want to do is go vertical through the median raphe spreading and then we will feel that space between the thyroid cartilage and the cricoid and we pop it with a Kelly clamp or a scalpel and we make a hole in this area right here. Then we need to slide in an endotracheal tube emergently—immediately giving oxygen and breaths. This can be a life-saving maneuver. I have done this 3 times and saved a life each time. But it is important to know when to do it. Patients are not breathing and don't have an airway or trying to breathe and don't have an airway. If you can't get an endotracheal tube in orally, or nasally, then cut to the chase and an incision on the neck, spread down to the cricoid membrane, pop the membrane, spread widely, and place the tube in and ventilate the patient. You will save somebody's life.

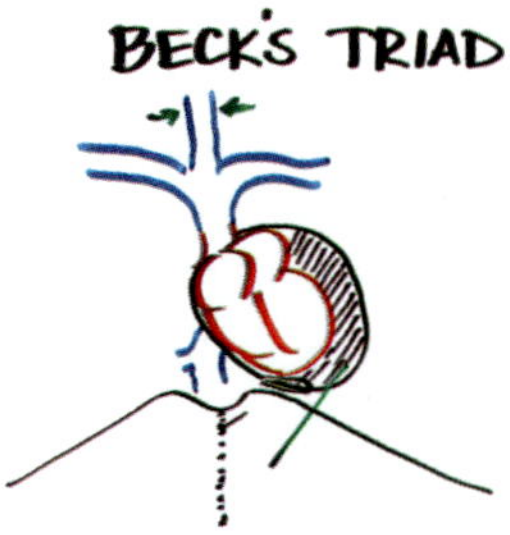

VIDEO 19.7. Pericardial Window.
Transcript: A pericardial window is useful especially when people have what is called "Beck's triad." Jugular venous distention, low blood pressure, and muffled heart sound. I previously told you about pericardiocentesis to get the fluid out, but if somebody is in harm's way and we have a rib cage and a xiphoid process, instead of sticking a needle in there, sometimes what has to be done is an operation through the midline, identify the diaphragm, split the diaphragm and look in and actually make a little hole in the pericardium, drain that fluid out. This is a temporizing feature. A needle sometimes is very good but sometimes blood doesn't come out through the needle. So, what is needed is called a pericardial window. Usually a midline incision down through the linea alba, up above the liver. Find the diaphragm and put a hole in the diaphragm, the pericardium will be right there, and with this fluid it will be butt up against it and we make a little incision in the pericardium with either scissors or electrocautery and remove that fluid. Then the question becomes, do we need an emergent sternotomy to repair bleeding from the inside, or can a little drainage tube solve the problem?

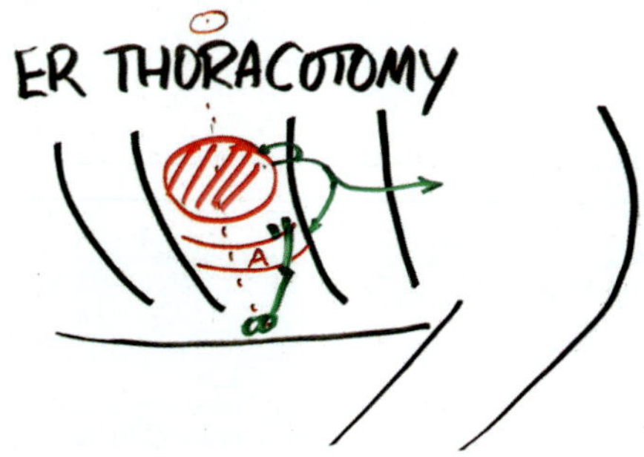

VIDEO 19.8. Thoracotomy. ER, emergency room.

Transcript: An ER thoracotomy is a rare procedure done by advanced surgeons and surgical trainees. The key to this is at the fourth or fifth intercostal space where the nipple areola complex is, we slide down and make a huge incision between the ribs, spread the ribs open, and hopefully we will find a beating heart on the inside, and posteriorly along the vertebral bodies, we will find an aorta. There are 2 major reasons for doing an ER thoracotomy: 1) to get to the heart, and 2) to get to the aorta. If there is bleeding from the heart, this is 1 access to it. More commonly people are doing ER thoracotomy for trying to get a clamp across the aorta, because now the aorta doesn't allow blood flow down to the rest of the body, but lets the blood flow to the head and keep the brain perfused, and back to the heart, and buys us some time. It is rarely done. It is better done if somebody is stabbed and immediately has hypotension and drops versus blunt trauma that happens very close to the hospital.

So in summary, an ER thoracotomy is rarely performed, but it is good in patients that have had penetrating injury, that have become unresponsive, become tachycardic, hypotensive, and then maybe no pulse whatsoever, swiftly getting into the chest. For blunt trauma patients it is less common, but if it is quickly after the accident. Again, lateral thoracotomy, expose the heart, expose the aorta, put the clamp across the aorta, and allow the blood to go back to the heart and into the head. This buys some time. It can be useful in some rare patients.

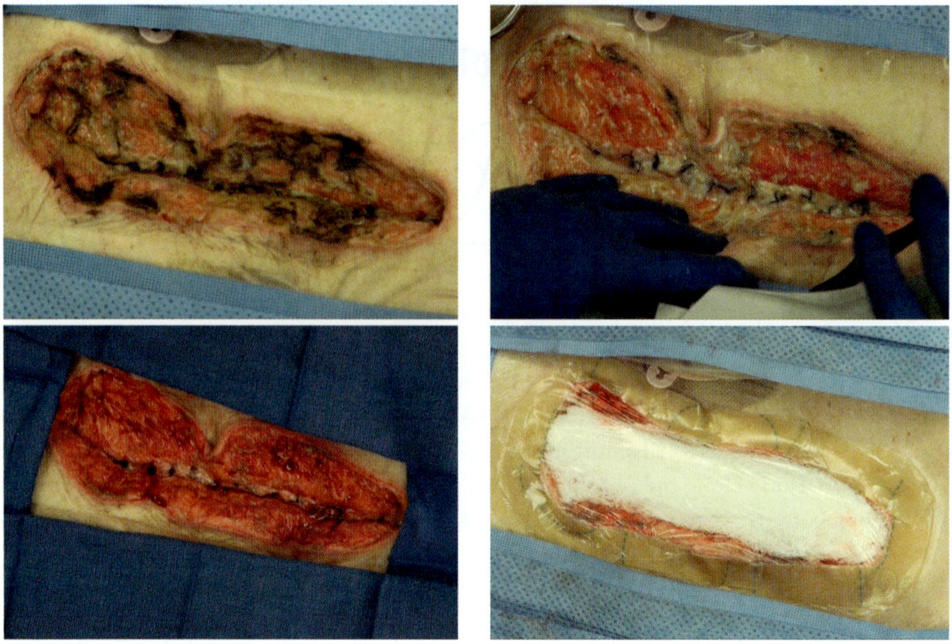

VIDEO 19.9. Open Wound Care.

Transcript: Most trauma surgery doesn't get videotaped because it is done so quickly with a gunshot wound or a bleeding spleen. But this is the reality of trauma surgery and hospital-based surgery. Somebody had a laparotomy and perhaps there was an injury, a traumatic injury, a gunshot wound to the colon or perforated diverticulitis.

This is a wound with the pubis to the left and xiphoid to the right. Somebody that had a bad intra-abdominal problem and now we have got a wound that has opened up and has a bit of dead tissue on it. And although this isn't the glamorous part of trauma surgery or general surgery, this is a critical portion for people taking care of patients with really bad problems. So this is a wound infection, wound breakdown, but the fascia is intact. I think you can see the bluish sutures interrupted where the fascia is intact and now we are going to try to get rid of all the dead tissue, the blackish tissue, and make it look pink and red and get it back down to bleeding tissue. We want to pick at it and get that dead stuff out of there, but not lose the sutures and not cause a dehiscence to the abdomen. And I think that you can sense that the team has done a nice job, they are back to bleeding tissue.

Try to stop the bleeding a little bit. This is a person with an ileostomy and protecting perhaps the left side of an anastomosis—we don't want this wound to break down. So they will take 20, 30, 40, or 50 minutes or more to clean this wound up and make it spotless. Where once there was dead tissue and a huge bacterial load, now we have got bleeding tissue that will granulate. And what we need to do now is to take super good care of this wound. And there are a lot of different ways to do that. One way is to put a wound vac in and an old fashioned way for the wound like this that is not quite ready yet to be closed up or do something exciting, is to put a simple piece of gauze in. And slide it in there and make the gauze stick to the sidewall if you can. You don't have to stuff a lot of it in; the idea is to just get it so that it touches the wall. This dressing will come off every day, couple times a day, and each time that the dressing is pulled out, it will pull with it some detritus and dead tissue and keep making that wound healthier and healthier.

The surgical team here is going to great lengths to put some protective things along the side of the skin so the skin edges themselves don't get beaten up and worn down and cause further infection. They are basically, lightly putting the gauze in. If anything, you don't need to pack it in. The idea is to make sure

VIDEO 19.9. Continued

the gauze touches the sidewalls which they have done here. It is done under sterile technique but pretty quickly. Bacteria on the skin or in that wound and that is why the dressing needs to be changed. Applying a little sticky material on the side in hopes of putting some protective plastic, rubber to avoid trauma to the skin, if you will.

Surgeons are meticulous about blood vessels, liver surgery, and a variety of things, but when push comes to shove, you need to be meticulous about wound care management and protect that wound and make it easier for the nurses to care in the ICU for this patient. Well done!

Trauma Assessment and Surgery Challenge Questions

19.1. What is the Beck triad?
19.2. What is the 1:1:1 rule?
19.3. What is the lethal triad in trauma?
19.4. What is the mortality rate associated with emergency department thoracotomy?
19.5. What is the halo sign?
19.6. Is bleeding from pelvic fractures most likely arterial or venous?
19.7. What is the treatment for skin injuries caused by human bites?
19.8. What is the most commonly injured abdominal organ in blunt trauma?
19.9. What is the treatment for a gunshot wound to the abdomen?
19.10. What is the diagnostic test of choice for an unstable patient with blunt trauma to the abdomen?

Answers to Trauma Assessment and Surgery Challenge Questions

19.1. Hypotension, muffled heart sounds, and jugular venous distention suggest cardiac tamponade.
19.2. For patients in hypovolemic shock: 1 unit packed red blood cells: 1 unit fresh frozen plasma: 1 unit platelets.
19.3. Acidosis, coagulopathy, and hypothermia.
19.4. Mortality is 95%.
19.5. Cerebrospinal fluid leaking from the nose or ear forms a "halo" around blood.
19.6. Venous, approximately 85% of the time.
19.7. Irrigate, do not close the wound, and antibiotics.
19.8. The liver.
19.9. Exploratory laparotomy (see Video 19.9).
19.10. FAST scan.

20

Vascular Surgery

Embryology

Blood vessels are formed from mesoderm-derived endothelial cells (Figure 20.1). Vasculogenesis is stimulated by vascular endothelial growth factor and placental growth factor. Formation of vessels from preexisting vessels is termed *angiogenesis* and occurs in both fetal and childhood development and sometimes in adulthood.

Anatomy

Arteries, arterioles, and capillaries carry blood from the heart to tissues; venules and veins return blood to the heart. Arteries have thick, muscular walls to help propel blood throughout the body; arterioles control the amount of resistance. Veins have thin walls and lower BP. Their lumens are larger in diameter than arteries and have valves that prevent backflow. Approximately two-thirds of blood volume is contained in veins. Blood vessels receive blood supply from the vasa vasorum (Figure 20.1).

Physiology

The force exerted by blood on the blood vessel wall is BP and is expressed in mm Hg. The relationship of blood circulation is as follows: flow = $\Delta P/R$ (difference in pressure/resistance). Radius (r) and length (L) of a blood vessel are factors that change the resistance: $R = L/r^4$.

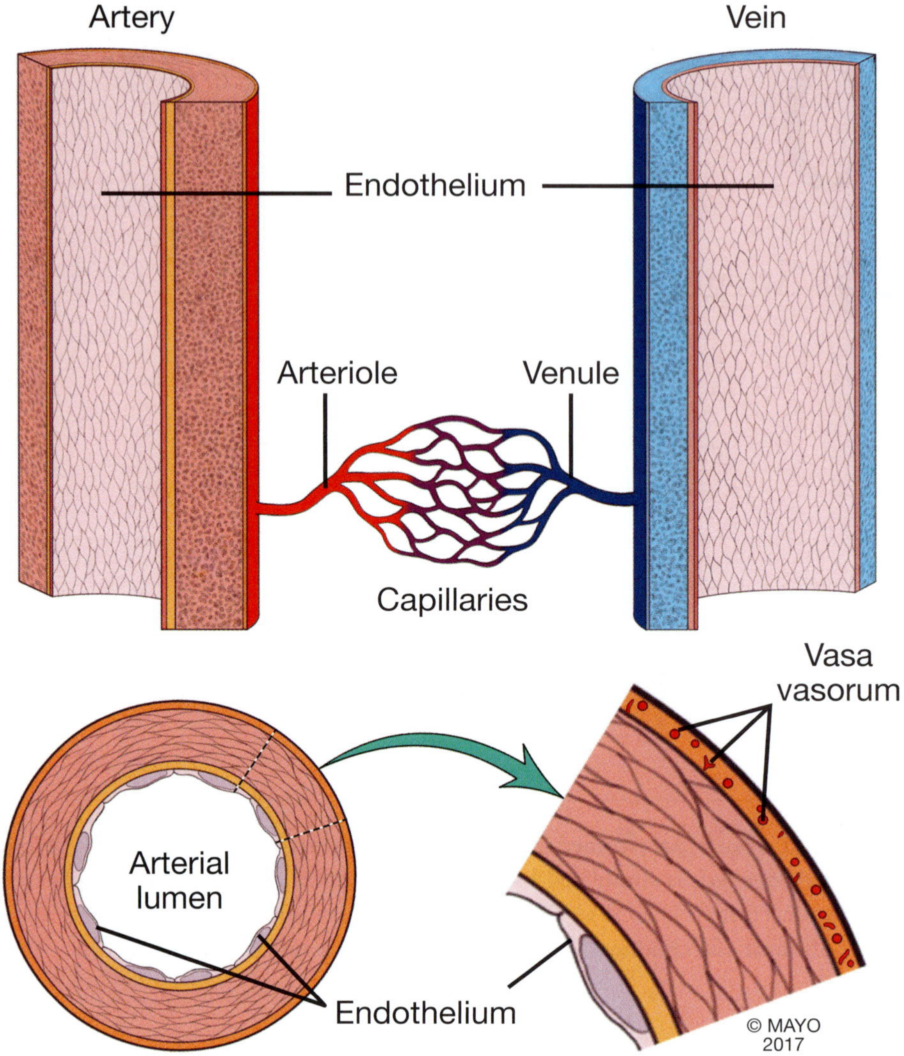

FIGURE 20.1. Anatomy of Arteries and Veins.

Clinical Presentation

Vascular diseases (atherosclerosis [Video 20.1], peripheral vascular disease [Video 20.2], renal artery stenosis [Video 20.3], disseminated intravascular coagulation [Video 20.4], aneurysms [Video 20.5], and cerebrovascular disease [Video 20.6]) present in various forms, such as bleeding, clotting, stroke, headache, and heart attack.

Imaging

Arteriography (Video 20.7) was the standard for evaluating arterial disease, but CT angiography (Video 20.8) and MRI (Video 20.9) are useful and ever improving.

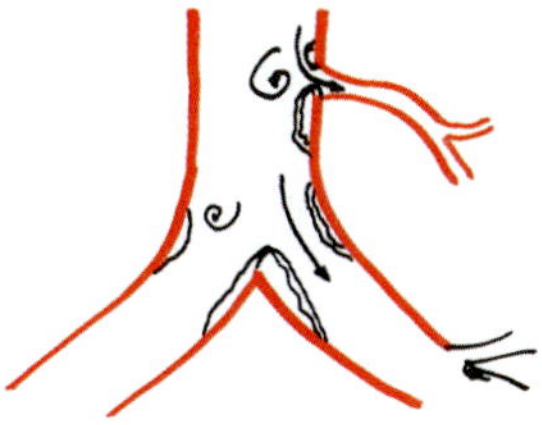

VIDEO 20.1. Atherosclerosis.

Transcript: Atherosclerosis happens to all of us in the United States. The risk factors for plaque buildup along the edge of the artery is very real. The older we get, the more the risk. The higher the blood pressure, the more the risk. The higher your cholesterol, glucose levels, the more fatty tissue you have; smoking and family history all contribute to this layering of the plaque over time. And at some point in time, that may narrow down the flow of blood. And if it does, that can lead to stroke or ischemia. You will most commonly find atherosclerosis at places where there is eddies, meaning where the blood flow isn't perfectly laminar. And that is usually where blood vessels take off here, the aorta, the iliacs, the IMA. I am trying to suggest that when it takes a turn like that, there is a current and it will make plaque build up on the sides next to it. So when you look at an arteriogram or CT scan, look at the blood vessels as they branch off and where they branch, look for the plaque. Atherosclerosis, it is a dangerous problem for all of us as we age.

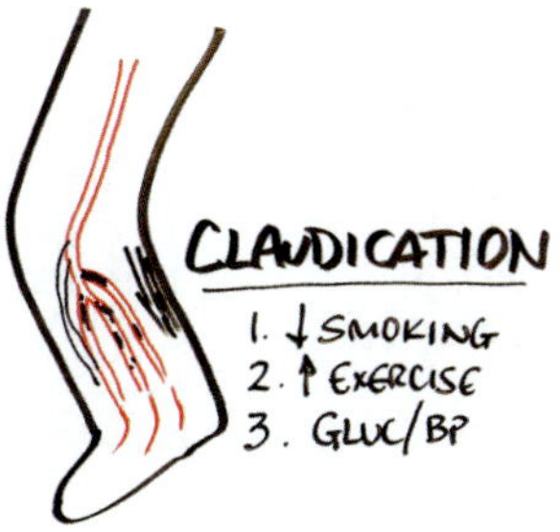

VIDEO 20.2. Peripheral Vascular Disease.

Transcript: Peripheral vascular disease is really nothing more than atherosclerosis of an extremity. Here I have tried to draw on the leg of a man perhaps that is a smoker and glucose is too high, and maybe his blood pressure is not good. Again, the blood slides down the superficial femoral into the popliteal and into 3 different branches down into the ankle and foot. If atherosclerosis develops and 1 of those arteries is knocked out, there is less blood flow. Fortunately, there is collateral flow, but if you get enough spots of blockage points, peripheral vascular disease will cause problems. And for a man like this we will think about what is called claudication. Claudication is pain with exertion. So an elderly gentleman may be walking his dog and doing just fine but he starts to notice that he can only go 3 or 4 blocks. Then 2 blocks, and then 1 block, and he gets terrible pain in his muscles, and that is because he is not getting blood flow and that is ischemia. So when you see somebody with claudication, pain in the muscles as they exert themselves: 1) stop the smoking, they cannot smoke, that will improve things greatly; 2) increase exercise, this will recruit and give us more collateral flow here; and 3) everything else health-wise; glucose, blood pressure, that sort of business. You usually don't need an operation to correct claudication. First things first, stop smoking, increase exercise, and medically manage things properly. But if at some point in time these vessels are blocked off, then some sort of a bypass or a stent will be useful to these people with peripheral vascular disease.

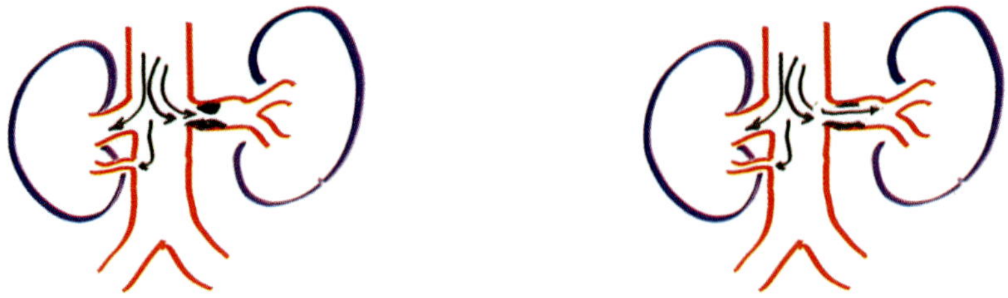

VIDEO 20.3. Renal Artery Stenosis.

Transcript: Renal artery stenosis is exactly that, a narrowing of the renal artery usually due to atherosclerosis, plaque, or the eddy set up, and it is tough for blood flow to get into that vessel. If that is the case and blood flow doesn't get into that kidney it is not going to work as well. The body will sense that and in fact try to send more fluid into the kidneys, raising the blood pressure. So somebody with a stenotic renal artery can have high blood pressure and can have serious problems, and can develop kidney failure. So the treatment for this is placing a stent or putting people on anticoagulation and allowing the blood to sneak through easier or surgical intervention, taking out the plaque, or putting a bypass. And it is important that when we look at people with high blood pressure, really high blood pressure, with kidney dysfunction, we need to think about renal artery stenosis. It is a life-threatening problem.

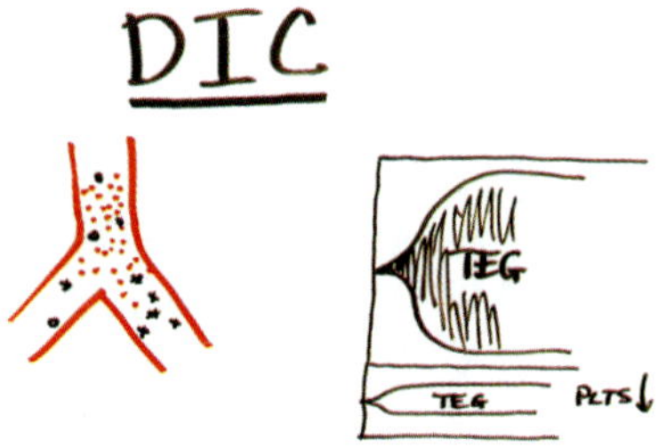

VIDEO 20.4. Disseminated Intravascular Coagulopathy. FFP indicates fresh frozen plasma.

Transcript: DIC is called disseminated intravascular coagulopathy. It basically means that beautiful harmonic system that works together with red blood cells, white blood cells, platelets, fibrin-split products, fibrinogen that washes through our bodies millions of times, over and over again, becomes abnormal. The platelets clot too much or they don't clot enough. As surgeons we see this sometimes with a variety of disorders: obstetrical problems, sepsis, malignancy, and traumatic brain injuries. And 1 of the things I would like you to know as a medical student about DIC is, think about obtaining a thromboelastogram, that is, TEG. They take a little blood, put it in a cup and that blood from that patient, they march it out over time and watch it spin and it creates a certain pattern. A normal pattern looks something like this. A skinny pattern, clotting pattern, may say too little platelets or too many fibrin-split products. This thromboelastogram allows intensivists, trauma surgeons, and others to give the right material to the patient. Some people need blood. Some people need plasma. Some people need FFP. And the TEG will allow us to help that. But first and foremost, the best way of curing DIC is eradicating the underlying problem. So if you have someone with sepsis, then draining the abscess would be good. If you have somebody with a cancer, removing the cancer. Somebody with a traumatic injury, well you can't take that back, but you have got to care for them. But think about the TEG. It might give you the chance to save somebody's life.

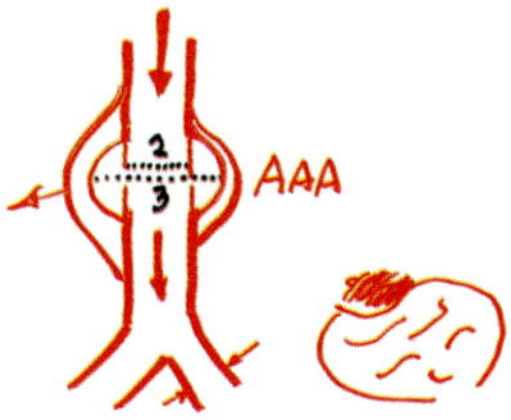

VIDEO 20.5. Aneurysms.

Transcript: Aneurysms are by definition a blood vessel, typically an artery, flowing through that should keep the same width, diameter, radius of a vessel until it gives off branches and then it will get smaller and smaller. But an aneurysm is when it gets 50% bigger than it should be. So here I am suggesting a normal abdominal aortic vessel is 2 cm across, this distance right here. If it was 3 cm across, and then became back to 2, this would be an abdominal aortic aneurysm.

So a blood vessel in the brain may be tiny, 3 mm, 2 mm, but if it swells out more than 50% it too is an aneurysm. And the problem with aneurysms is that vessel, that wall gets bigger and bigger over time, more and more pressure builds on that and this wants to burst out. And an aneurysm that bursts out in the abdomen, patients will bleed to death. A small little aneurysm in the brain that bursts out, they won't bleed to death, but there will be enough blood flow that it will create a hematoma and pressure on the rest of somebody's brain. And then that person will meet their maker.

So the key thing for an aneurysm is diagnosing it and then deciding what to do about it. If it is gigantic, if a 2-cm abdominal aortic vessel becomes 10 cm, that needs to be treated right away. If it is just 2.4, that is not big enough to call it an aneurysm. Let's sit tight and watch. Sometimes blood pressure and medication can do the thing to correct and not need any treatment for aneurysm. But when it gets above 50%, then that is something that probably every year that people should begin having an examine and assessing as it's getting bigger; because the more quickly it gets big, the more dangerous it is.

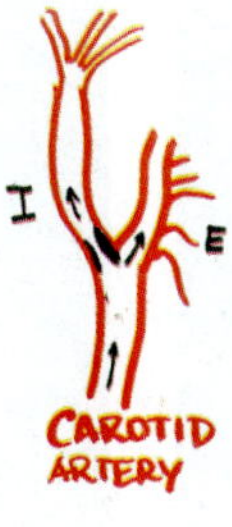

VIDEO 20.6. Cerebrovascular Disease.

Transcript: Cerebrovascular disease is a group of diseases basically most commonly affected by atherosclerosis of the blood vessels that supply the brain. So if this is our common carotid artery, it branches into an external and an internal. The internal goes up into the brain. The external goes to the neck and the face and the musculature of the face. The carotid artery, the common carotid, most importantly gives blood to the brain, and that is where we think about cerebrovascular disease, usually at the bifurcation of the external and internal carotid vessels. And either removing that plaque, or if there is a clot, an embolus, or

VIDEO 20.6. Continued

a narrowing or scarring, will allow that patient normal survival. What we know is over time is if plaque develops and we get plaque at 50% of the lumen, patients still do just fine. But as we get to 60%, 70%, and 80% stenosis, meaning only 10% or 20% is open, people can have symptomatic problems. They can get a stroke. Some of these folks will completely shut off the carotid artery. It is an amazing thing that you can have collateral flow and that patient can still be just fine. But most people will become symptomatic when they have a little wisp running through there. And they either need medicine or surgical intervention. And if it is surgical, it is with a stent or a carotid atherosclerosis plaque removal. Those are big operations with high risk, but they are done very safely in the United States, less than 1% of people have a really bad outcome.

So cerebrovascular disease causes a variety of problems. You can have a stroke, you can have confusion, and you can have dementia, a variety of problems when you don't get enough blood flow. Things for you to think about as a medical student: think about the internal carotid artery and atherosclerosis. How are you going to remediate that problem?

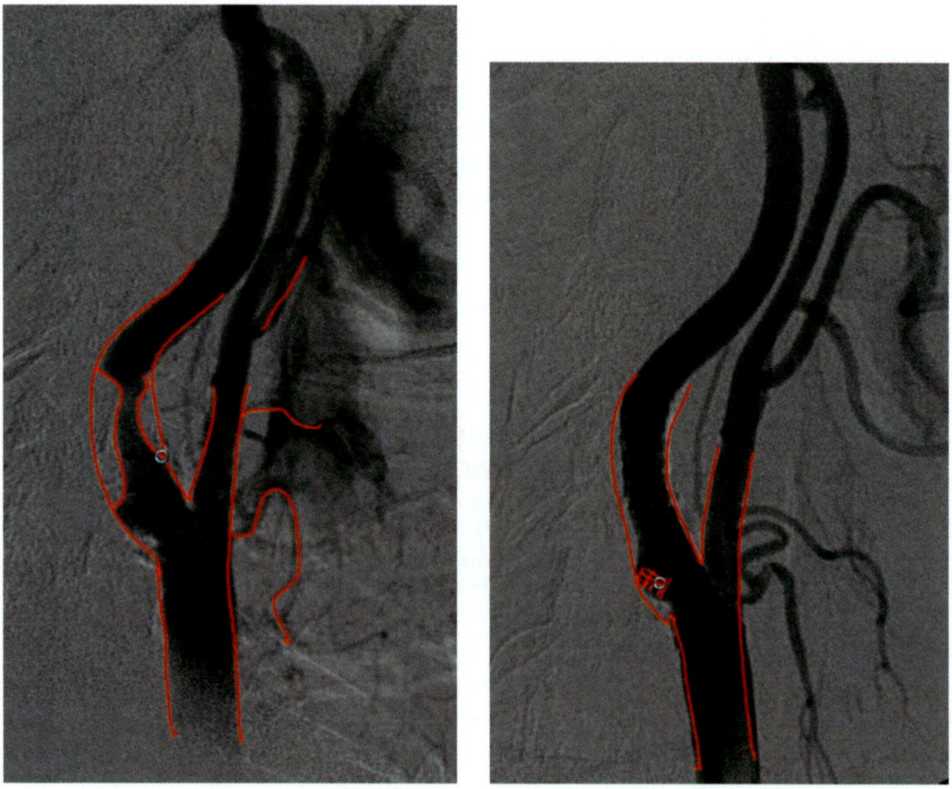

VIDEO 20.7. Arteriography.

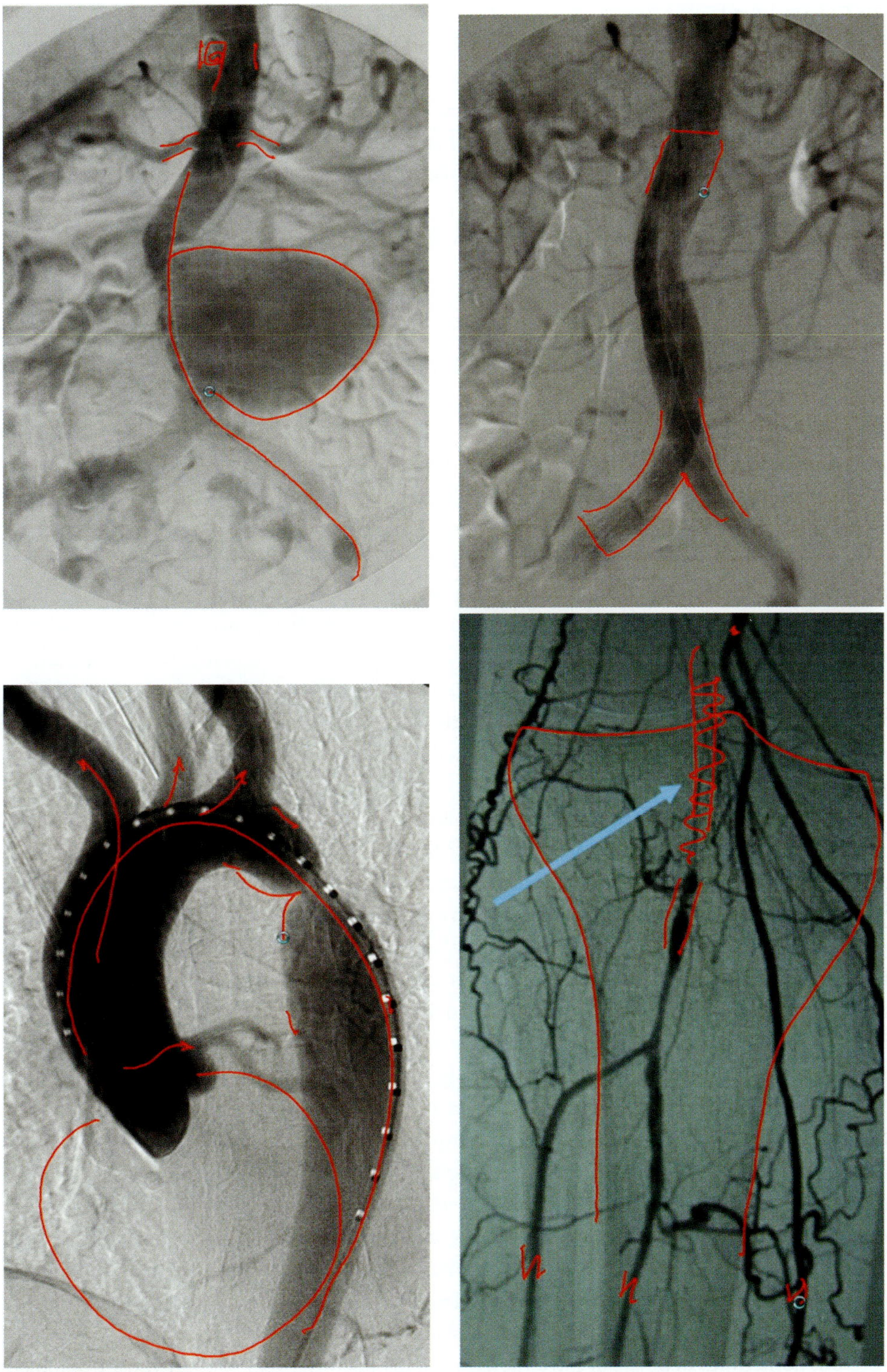

VIDEO 20.7. Continued

Transcript: Arteriography was described a century ago and it has been utilized for surgeons and medical doctors alike to care for patients like this. What is this? This is an arteriogram with dye in the common

VIDEO 20.7. Continued

carotid artery that branches off into the external carotid artery. The superior thyroid artery is the first branch and then there are other branches that come off of it. But this is the part we want to look at that the arteriogram is so helpful for. This is the internal carotid artery and you can see that there is plaque here. It is kind of like a cancer of the colon only this is blood vessels or dye shooting through and it is narrowed here. This is somebody with atherosclerosis. And they are going to have a stroke if we don't do something positive to help them.

Surgeons historically would make an incision and cut that plaque out. But there are other ways of doing that nowadays.

This is the same patient, maybe a few minutes or an hour after a procedure. And I don't know if you can tell but, common carotid, external, and now the internal looks nice and smooth here. And maybe you get a sense that there is some different sort of gradient there. There is a stent, it's a metallic stent, and it is basically from there to here, and it's inside the blood vessel now. And so now the blood can go through that stent and come up and the person has less risk of having a stroke. It is an amazing sort of technology and the arteriogram allows us to see it and then to repair it.

This is an arteriogram as well; specifically it is called an aortogram because we are looking at the aorta. Can you see the catheter coming through the patient's left groin? Sneaking all the way up into a relatively normal aorta here with a catheter, and they shoot some dye and the dye, the contrast is placed into the aorta. And we see kidneys. We see vessels. And then we can see something that is far bigger than it should be. This is an aneurysm. An aneurysm by definition is something that is more than 50% bigger than the artery above and below. So if this is a normal aorta here, and a normal down here, 50% would be something about yeah big. This is a dangerous aneurysm. If this thing bursts, this patient is going to perish. So the same sort of thing we shot the arteriogram, the dye lets us know. The iliac vessels may be okay, but we have got an aneurysm of the aorta. And we are either going to fix it with surgical technique or some sort of stenting technique.

This is another picture, a different picture of an aneurysm. It's important when you are looking at an arteriogram, where are the blood vessels coming off? So if these are the kidneys, the left renal or the right renal, we have got to say, "Alright, this is above that or below that and what are we going to occlude?" Or we look at it carefully and say, "Hey, those aren't the renals, this is the splenic artery. And this is the common hepatic artery." This is a thoracoabdominal aneurysm; much more difficult to repair. A difficult procedure, but it is crucial that we understand the anatomy of the arteriogram.

This is a wonderful picture after somebody had their aneurysm fixed. We can see the stent, here, sneaking up, stent on the other side and both iliacs and it extends all the way up underneath here. This is repaired. This is somebody that used to have a huge aneurysm here. Now the blood sneaks through the stent and doesn't put any pressure on that aneurysm and it doesn't burst. This is a life-saving procedure.

This is another type of aortogram. Now we are up at the top of the arch of the aorta. So if the heart was visualized, it would be right here. But we have got this catheter coming in from below and they have left it right above the aortic valve and dye starts in and maybe it starts into the coronary vessels and the dye sneaks up through the innominate, the carotids, and then the subclavians in the carotid. What is interesting about this is there is an abnormality. I think you can see it. Look carefully at that aorta. It's this big here, it's this big here, but right here it is tiny. This is what is called a coarctation of the aorta. And it typically happens congenitally. It is somebody who was born with this. But this patient was found to have this at age 66. Sometimes people can have these problems for other reasons, but the aorta looks so nice that I am thinking that this young man was born as a child with a small little stenosis there. And over the course of time, we have to figure out how to fix those things.

VIDEO 20.7. Continued

This is a different picture in a different patient. Twisted and turned and I am confused looking at it. But the catheter is in there. Dye is set up and likely 3 big vessels coming off the arch here. Then what the question is is there something abnormal? And sometimes it is as simple as a funny little squiggly line that says could be a dissection. The flap of the endothelium maybe tearing away.

Another look, another different picture. Again, this is an aortogram, this arteriogram. We see 3 normal looking vessels, the vessels themselves look healthy. Now the question becomes, is this normal aorta? It looks like it. Is this normal aorta? It does. This looks bigger. The aorta shouldn't get bigger as it goes down and usually what that means is after a narrowing, things get a little bit smaller and the blood flow has to be much quicker and it pushes things out. So there may be a narrowing here in this arch of the aortogram.

Lastly, let me show you some pictures of arteriograms in the leg. If you can see behind it here the tibia, the bone is sitting like this, that is the tibia. And sliding down from above should be a popliteal vessel, but there really isn't any until about right here. We can see it. We have given dye up in the groin. The superficial femoral artery is still intact up here, but there is clotting in this region—atherosclerosis. The blood vessels downstream and the tibial vessels look good. But we are going to need to repair that. The blue arrow shows us a narrowing. And I will be danged, look at that! A stent placed in that section of the popliteal vessel. The stent goes from here to maybe here. And now there is no problem at all and it looks like the blood flows beautifully through there. This is somebody that had ischemia of the foot, they would get claudication and pain in the foot and now because of the arteriogram, we see there is a problem and it also allows us to fix it either surgically or with stent—so-called endovascular procedures.

Operation

Preoperatively, patients must understand that nonoperative treatments such as smoking cessation, increasing physical activity, lowering blood pressure, lowering the cholesterol value, and lowering the blood glucose value will improve peripheral vascular disease. The tenets of vascular surgery (Video 20.10) involve excellent exposure, proximal and distal control of vessels, tension-free anastomoses, adequate runoff and inflow, and maximizing perfusion.

Complications

Postoperative concerns include bleeding, clotting, ischemia, stroke, and myocardial infarction.

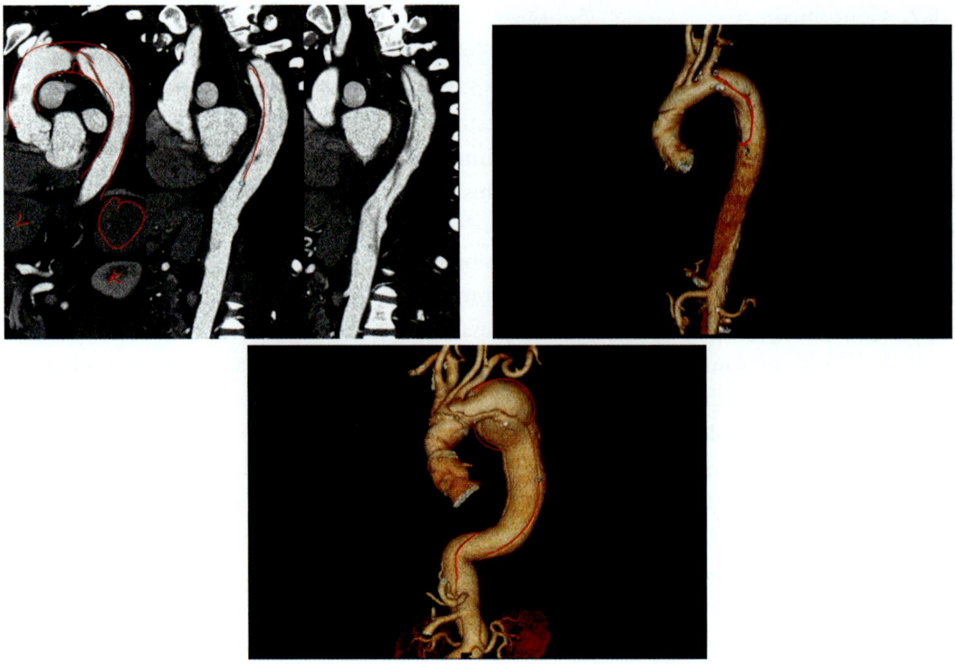

VIDEO 20.8. CT Angiography.

Transcript: So there is classic, sort of old fashioned arteriography where somebody puts a needle in an artery and injects the dye. This is a CT angiography where somebody is putting some dye into the vein and letting the dye swirl around. Here are 3 cuts of the same patient. Importantly, what I need you to know is, this is the arch of the aorta sneaking around down into the abdomen with a spleen down here, and the liver here, and a kidney here. If we put dye in and wait long enough, we can take a look and see what is happening. It is less invasive; you don't have to poke a hole into somebody's artery. But these are 3 cuts may be a little bit delayed and little different sections of them. We can see there is something abnormal from the aorta. Can you see it? A couple of different things: this little narrowing makes me ponder, "Alright, does this person have a coarctation?" But most importantly what is abnormal is this funny little line, this black little line. That shouldn't be in the middle of a blood vessel. That's a dissection. That's a flap of endothelium. A flap, the intima of the artery has been cut, the pressure was high, and it tore. And now you have got a waving bedsheet, if you will, in the middle of this tube, and that is a real problem because those things can dissect and they can cause weakness. They can occlude blood vessels. So this is a wonderful cut with a CT scan using intravenous dye showing us an aortic dissection.

Here is one cut, an axial cut, that was a longitudinal cut; this is an axial cut where we can see the trachea, we can see the vertebral bodies, and then we see the arch of the aorta. And this is the arch here, nicely depicted, it looks pretty reasonable except again this is the same patient. This is this flap of intima and it shouldn't be there. It is holding on and it's going to be in the way and it is going to allow clotting and all sorts of different problems. Whether surgery or medicine or endovascular treatment, but that needs to be fixed.

CT is a wonderful tool because now we can take those CT pictures and reconstruct them and just give the surgeon and the cardiologist or the radiologist the things they are looking for. So this is a reconstructed sort of a 3-D image of the CT scan. It's the same patient. And we can see what? We can see this intimal dissection, this flap, and that is not how it should be. We can turn it and rotate it and surgeons can decide, "We need to approach from the left or the right or when we cut in here we want to make an incision here

VIDEO 20.8. Continued
or we want to make an incision here." Or, the interventionalist might say, "Yes, we can pass a catheter up and put a stent in and block that off." The key thing is to know where is that flap emanating from. Lots of different pictures to look at this.

Here is another CT reconstructed picture. This is somebody that looks like they have an aneurysm of the arch. They also have these funny little lines down here. Is this somebody with an intimal flap as well? I am not an expert and we need a radiologist and a cardiologist and a cardiac surgeon and a vascular surgeon to figure this out. But it is a wonderful opportunity when minute details where less than a millimeter of effectiveness take a look at these things.

Another reconstruction showing you plaque—this whitish material in the aorta. And then we can say, "Alright, we have got an aneurysm here." And the key thing now is so many of these operations are done percutaneously. The key thing that the person needs to know is the vascular or cardiac or interventional cardiologist is can they get safely in, "There is a lot of plaque there, maybe it is safer on this side. Can you get the catheter in? Or is there too much tortuosity? We might not be able to do that because eventually we are going to put a stent up." So this is a wonderful opportunity to look and see where the plaque is, where the kinks are, and then is there enough space between the big blood vessels up above for this stent to sit in there? It is called seating it.

Another picture of a reconstructed CT angiography. What do you see? Hopefully you see what I see. Simplistically it is actually a pretty nice looking aorta. Very little plaque. It looks very nice. A beautiful take off of the main 3 vessels off the arch. But what doesn't look so good here is a tight stenosis, a so-called coarctation of the aorta. And either needs an operation to open this up or a stent placed in between it. And nowadays the stent works pretty doggone well.

And this is what it looks like after the repair. A stent has been placed in there to correct that. It is not perfect like the rest of the aorta, but instead of having a narrowing that was down to less than 50% of the flow through there, this person's blood pressure will drop, they will feel better, they will have more fitness, and they will be able to live a more normal life.

Vascular Surgery Challenge Questions

20.1. What is the Mayo vein?
20.2. What is blue toe syndrome?
20.3. What are the 6 Ps of acute arterial occlusion?
20.4. What is the most common cause of embolus from the heart?
20.5. What is the most common cause of abdominal aortic aneurysm?
20.6. What is the normal abdominal aorta diameter?
20.7. If the IMA is sacrificed in abdominal aortic aneurysm surgery, what is a postoperative concern?
20.8. What are the most common bacteria in aortic graft infections?
20.9. Which vein crosses the abdominal aorta?
20.10. What are risk factors for splenic aneurysm rupture?
(Answers appear on page 290)

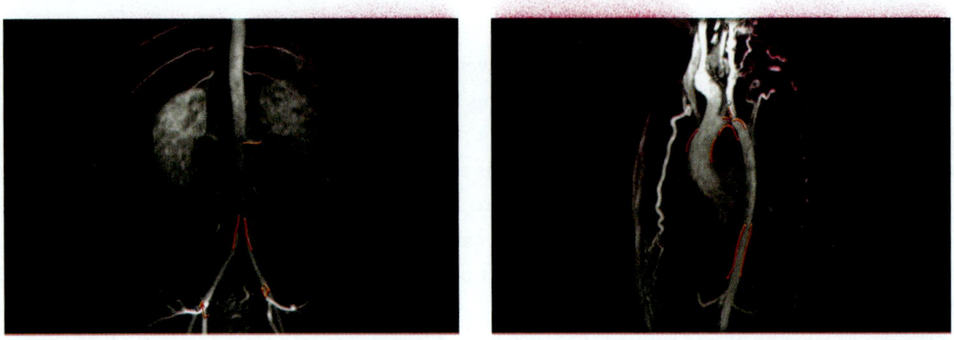

VIDEO 20.9. MRI.

Transcript: Another way to look at blood vessels is using MRI, magnetic resonance imaging. The neat thing about MRI is it doesn't have radiation so it's not dangerous to the patient. The bad thing is that it is kind of claustrophobic right now, but that test is getting better. So if we have an MRI of the aorta, we can get pretty nice pictures. We can see 2 kidneys on either side; the aorta looks good, no obvious abnormalities. This looks pretty doggone normal. Intercostal vessels, aorta, right renal, left renal, we have got the bifurcation of the iliacs, coming down the internal and external iliac artery. It is a beautiful picture and it shows us that this is a normal person. They don't have any problems.

Contrary, this is an abnormal picture of a MRI scan. And again, when we look at this, most of the blood vessels look pretty normal. I don't see much atherosclerosis. Nice arch. But again I think you can see a subtlety here. As we sneak up here, this person has a coarctation of the aorta. And the interesting thing is it takes off where the left common carotid is, it may be a dangerous problem and they may be having a stroke, or light-headedness, or they are having all sorts of other issues. But this is an MRI scan, no radiation. The downside is you can't treat right now using an MRI; whereas, arteriography and fluoroscopy, you can actually do something. Here with MRI it is less useful that way. But the idea of not using radiation is very effective and the MRI scans are becoming more and more granular. We are seeing things less than a millimeter and that makes it very effective for interventionalists, radiologists, surgeons, and the like to take care of our patients.

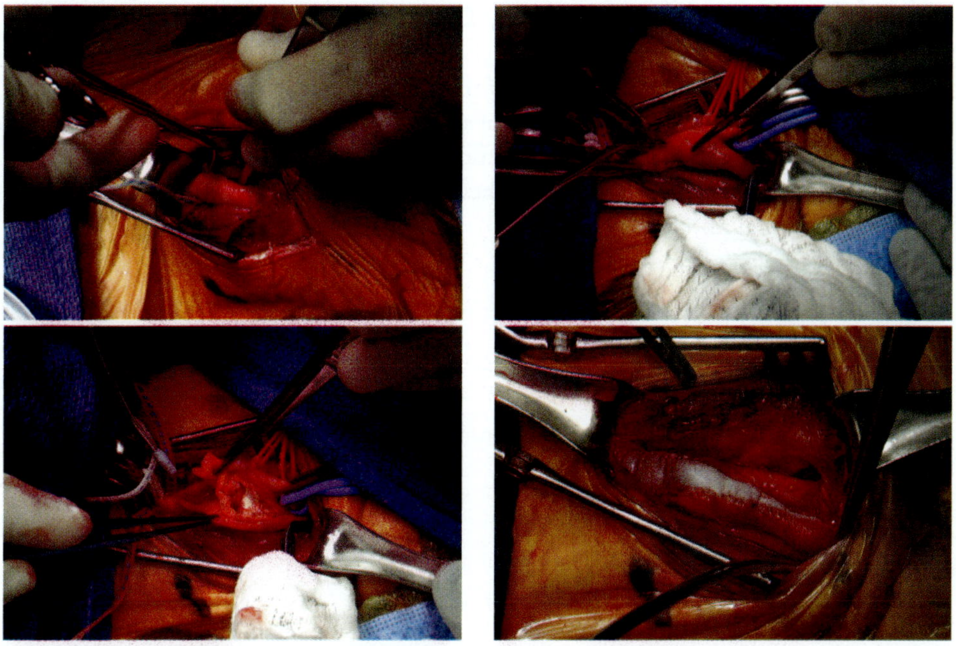

VIDEO 20.10. Carotid Endarterectomy: Intraoperative.

Transcript: Carotid endarterectomy—the chin is up, we are on the patient's left side making an incision along the sternocleidomastoid. We can see it there and we are going to sneak down in, looking for the jugular vein, and the carotid artery. A little cervical fascia opening up, sharp dissection, going to sneak around the carotid artery. Common carotid coming out of the chest below us to the left, it is going to divide. We have got a little Rummel tourniquet–type instrument. In case we run into bleeding, we can kink that off. Beautiful picture of artery and vein. Careful dissection, not hurting the vagus nerve. We have got little vascular threads that we can kink off blood vessels if we run into trouble. We have got branches of the external above us, likely the superior thyroid artery. We have got the internal carotid below us. We have got these vessel loops, blue and red, color coded to know what they are around. If a surgeon would get in trouble or would have to use a shunt it is nice to have that control.

So now what we do is we occlude inflow and outflow. We open up this carotid vessel. This is somebody that has had a stroke in the past or had difficulties. We have got vascular clamps on so there shouldn't be much bleeding if at all. An 11-blade scalpel with a scissors, Potts scissors, allows us to open up and we see crud in the wall—atherosclerosis. Made a nice arteriotomy. Opening things up. And we are going to dissect that plaque off. You see how it comes nicely off the intima there. Beautiful! We want to get every last little piece of plaque that we can. And now rather than just sewing that arteriotomy closed we are going to put a patch on it. It is too easy to close it and stricture it down and narrow the vessel. This little patch made up of a variety of different materials allows us to make a little bit bigger opening, better lumen and less problems postoperatively. Got to be careful to let go of the clamps in an opportune time, we don't want to wash atherosclerotic plaque into the brain. Nicely done!

Answers to Vascular Surgery Challenge Questions

20.1. Vein overlying the pylorus of the stomach: vena prepylorica.
20.2. Microemboli from a proximal arterial plaque causing intermittent painful toes (or fingers) with bluish discoloration.
20.3. Pain, paralysis, pallor, paresthesia, poikilothermia, and pulselessness.
20.4. Atrial fibrillation.
20.5. Atherosclerosis (95%).
20.6. Normal diameter is 2 cm.
20.7. Colonic ischemia.
20.8. *Staphylococcus aureus*, *Staphylococcus epidermidis*.
20.9. The left renal vein.
20.10. Pregnancy, hypertension, trauma, and size of the aneurysm.

Index

Figures and videos are indicated by *f* and *V* following the page number